Transforming Healthcare Infrastructure

In recent years, unprecedented demographic aging has placed considerable strain on outdated healthcare systems, exacerbating existing challenges and creating new ones. Geriatric care, in particular, necessitates a multidisciplinary approach involving architects and engineers alongside healthcare professionals. Emerging technologies such as artificial intelligence (AI), digital healthcare, adaptive systems, inclusive policies, and biodegradable materials offer promising avenues for systematic improvements in healthcare delivery. *Transforming Healthcare Infrastructure* addresses the issues of demographic aging and embracing digital transformations such as AI and offers timely insights into the evolving landscape of healthcare. It also emphasizes the necessity for all stakeholders to embrace these changes for the betterment of healthcare delivery and outcomes. This book serves as a definitive resource for healthcare professionals at all levels, from frontline workers to administrators, as well as researchers and students across various disciplines. Engineers, policymakers, architects, and environmentalists within the healthcare sector will also find it indispensable.

Key Features:

- Offers timely insights into the evolving landscape of healthcare.
- Explores emerging technologies such as AI, Internet of Things (IoT), adaptive systems, and biodegradable materials used for healthcare solutions.
- Emphasizes the necessity for all stakeholders to embrace these changes for the betterment of healthcare delivery and outcomes.

Transforming Healthcare Infrastructure

Edited by
David S-K. Ting and Jacqueline A. Stagner

CRC Press
Taylor & Francis Group
Boca Raton London New York

CRC Press is an imprint of the
Taylor & Francis Group, an **informa** business

Designed cover image: Shutterstock

First edition published 2026
by CRC Press
2385 NW Executive Center Drive, Suite 320, Boca Raton FL 33431

and by CRC Press
4 Park Square, Milton Park, Abingdon, Oxon, OX14 4RN

CRC Press is an imprint of Taylor & Francis Group, LLC

ISBN: 978-1-032-84559-3 (hbk)
ISBN: 978-1-032-84560-9 (pbk)
ISBN: 978-1-003-51383-4 (ebk)

DOI: 10.1201/9781003513834

Typeset in Times
by codeMantra

Contents

Preface

Albert Einstein proclaimed, "In the midst of every crisis lies great opportunity." Crisis may be too strong a word to describe the present healthcare situation. To say the least, there are more than a few pressing challenges. This volume aims at complementing existing efforts in mending and improving our healthcare. Experts from diverse fields are brought together to disseminate a multidisciplinary approach to addressing the challenges of aging, technology, and sustainable design.

In Chapter 1, "In the Trenches: Current Challenges in Healthcare Delivery," **Zulfkar Qadrie**, **Mudasir Maqbool**, and **Mohd Altaf Dar** present some of the grave challenges with the way we deliver care. The COVID-19 pandemic and the threat of climate change are wake-up calls. Existing hurdles include inequitable access, workforce shortages, financial limits, and outmoded technologies. These challenges are worse for middle- and low-income countries, which also tend to lose their already-scarce medical staff to developed nations. Financial sustainability and technological breakthroughs are essential to solving the problem. To effectuate the solutions, an integrated approach that includes key agents such as clinicians, administrators, policymakers, and technologists is proposed by **Tasnia Nabil** and **Julia Aman**. They view healthcare as a complex adaptive system in Chapter 2, "Health Innovation as a Complex Adaptive System." It is found that adaptive, patient-centric solutions can scale across diverse settings. To overcome barriers to innovation, it is time to remove perceived field boundaries between engineering, behavioral science, and socio-political governance. "The transformation of healthcare infrastructure lies in the recognition that complexity is not a barrier but a strength." This is principally echoed by **Mohit Goswami** in Chapter 3, "Service Innovation in Healthcare: Perspective from Organizational, Societal, and Technological Dimensions." Demographic changes, regulatory policies, and advancements in technologies are key drivers, while resistance to change, resource limitations, data security concerns, and interoperability challenges are obstacles to overcome. Integrating regulatory incentives, technological advancements, and patient engagement is needed to sustain innovation in healthcare services. The current situation in India is the topic of Chapter 4, "Recent Initiatives in Revamping Healthcare Policies and Programs in India: A Review of Progress and Challenges." **Bhaskar Behera, Jiban Kumar Behera**, and **Manojit Bhattacharya** draw our attention to the vital role of healthcare in income generation and employment growth in India. To continue these forward strides that have taken place in India, rural-urban disparities, and workforce and financial sustainability must be enforced to safeguard continual success. Inclusive transportation must be provided for the aging population to access healthcare. India's national urban transport policy (NUTP) is scrutinized by **Shashikant Nishant Sharma** and **Kavita Dehalwar** in Chapter 5, "Examining the Inclusivity of India's National Urban Transport Policy for Senior Citizens." It is heartwarming to learn that NUTP promotes the integration of public transport, non-motorized transport, and paratransit services to furnish seamless connectivity and reduce travel time for older adults. They recommend (i) Improved Physical Accessibility, (ii) Audio-Visual

Announcement Systems, (iii) Subsidized Travel and Optimized Scheduling, (iv) Training Programs for Transport Staff, (v) Integration of Smart Technology, (vi) Strengthening Public Participation and Feedback Mechanisms, and (vii) Last-Mile Connectivity and Safe Transit Environments.

Are there prevailing diseases and illnesses that demand special attention? In Chapter 6, "Increasing Burden of Non-Communicable Diseases on Health Systems in Aging Populations and Possible Approaches to Lessen the Burden," **Berrak Itır Aylı** reveals the rising prevalence of non-communicable diseases. Of these, cardiovascular diseases, cancer, chronic respiratory diseases, and diabetes are at the forefront, seriously burdening health systems globally. Transitioning from traditional models designed to treat acute and infectious diseases toward integrated models is required. Patient-centered care, proactive prevention strategies, and policies aimed at lowering behavioral risk factors and socioeconomic disparities are needed. A serious health issue, depression, continues its increasing trend post-COVID-19. Intestinal microbiota for treating this and other convoluted etiopathogenesis of neuropsychiatric disorders is still in its infancy. This is the topic of Chapter 7, "A New Option for the Treatment of Neuropsychiatric Diseases: Fecal Microbiota Transplantation?" **Alper Evrensel** enlightens us with the history, new findings, and obstacles of this potentially efficacious treatment. The earliest record of the application of fecal microbiota transplantation (via mouth, i.e., ingestion) appears as early as the third century, during the Dong-jin dynasty according to Reference 111 of Evrensel's chapter. A key obstacle concerns the ethics of moving the experimental trials of fecal microbiota transplantation from animals to humans. Concerning mental well-being, the environment we live in plays a significant role. **Kheir M. Al-Kodmany** integrates health, sustainability, and urban vitality in tall building design in Chapter 8, "Elevating Wellness: Integrating Health, Sustainability, and Urban Vitality in Tall Building Design." With urbanization, tall buildings are becoming vital contributors to occupant wellness, environmental sustainability, and urban health. The path forward is to catalyze healthier, more sustainable, and resilient urban features. This requires a collaborative, interdisciplinary approach that unites architects, urban planners, engineers, policymakers, and communities.

On the topic of the health of the environment, replacing the widespread use of harmful plastics with biodegradable alternatives in the healthcare environment can lead the way. **Velur Ved Vikash Reddy**, **Prasanthi Chidipudi**, **Sujatha Alla**, and **Nagesh Bheesetty** scrutinize the transformative potential of biodegradable alternatives to traditional plastics in Chapter 9, "Replacing Harmful Plastics with Biodegradable Alternatives: Innovations and Applications in Healthcare." They convey numerous healthcare settings that have proven the replacement of plastics with eco-friendly biodegradable materials to be cost-effective. What about healthcare electronic products, where the technologies are advancing at an ever-increasing rate? A circular economy is the answer to this problem. **Fatemeh Abedi, Ulla A. Saari, Maria Smolander, Liisa Hakola, Tilak Lakshmana, and Thomas M. Kraft** expound on this in Chapter 10, "Circular Sustainable Electronics from Design and Manufacturing to Business Models." They highlight the importance of designing products with easily separable, reusable, or recyclable electronic parts. Doing so not only reduces their environmental impact but also extends product life cycles. It is time to adopt circular economic principles in healthcare.

How are current healthcare systems doing? The volume concludes with such an analysis of European Union healthcare by **Fazıl Gökgöz** and **Engin Yalçın**, "Analyzing the Healthcare Performances of EU countries via Decision Method." As a fundamental structure, the performance of healthcare speaks to the well-being of the nation. Using a multicriteria decision-making framework, they evaluated EU countries based on healthcare expenditure, hospital bed complement, health personnel, and life expectancy at birth and found Germany and France to be the champions. More importantly, their exhaustive approach, which considers trade-offs between key indicators, reveals the strengths and weaknesses of the systems. These details lead the way in sustaining the strengths while mitigating the weaknesses.

Acknowledgments

It would have been impossible for the two concerned editors to engineer such a timely volume that encompasses far beyond their profession without the 26 experts from diverse backgrounds who brought their respective expertise and formed this edition. The amazing publishing team led by Joseph Clements is commended for their trust in us and their guidance throughout the journey. Providence transforms this impossible into the possible.

David S-K. Ting and Jacqueline A. Stagner
Turbulence & Energy Laboratory
University of Windsor

Editors

Dr. David S-K. Ting is the founder of the Turbulence & Energy Laboratory. He supervises research students mostly on flow turbulence and renewable energy in the Department of Mechanical, Automotive, and Materials Engineering at the University of Windsor. He has co/supervised 90 plus (post)graduate students, co-authored over 190 journal papers, authored 5 textbooks, and co-edited over 30 volumes.

Dr. Jacqueline A. Stagner is the Undergraduate Programs Coordinator in the Faculty of Engineering at the University of Windsor. She is also an adjunct Associate Professor in the Department of Mechanical, Automotive, and Materials Engineering. Her current research focuses on bettering the next generations through sustainable engineering and living. She has co-edited 16 volumes since she first embarked on this rewarding calling in 2020.

Contributors

Fatemeh Abedi
Industrial Engineering & Management
Faculty of Management & Business
Tampere University
Tampere, Finland

Kheir M. Al-Kodmany
College of Urban Planning and Public Affairs

Sujatha Alla
Engineering Management and Systems Engineering
Old Dominion University
Norfolk, Virginia

Julia Aman
Turbulence and Energy Laboratory
University of Windsor
Windsor, Canada

Berrak Itır Aylı
Institute of Public Health
Graduate School of Health Sciences
Hacettepe University
Ankara, Turkey

Bhaskar Behera
Department of Biosciences and Biotechnology
Fakir Mohan University
Balasore, Odisha, India

Jiban Kumar Behera
Department of Zoology
Fakir Mohan University
Balasore, Odisha, India

Manojit Bhattacharya
Department of Zoology
Fakir Mohan University
Balasore, Odisha, India

Nagesh Bheesetty
Engineering Management and Systems Engineering
Old Dominion University
Norfolk, Virginia

Prasanthi Chidipudi
Joint School of Public Health
Old Dominion University
Norfolk, Virginia

Mohd Altaf Dar
Department of Pharmacology
CT Institute of Pharmaceutical Sciences
PTU
Jalandhar, Punjab, India

Kavita Dehalwar
Department of Planning and Architecture
Maulana Azad National Institute of Technology
Bhopal, Madhya Pradesh, India

Alper Evrensel
Department of Psychiatry
Uskudar University
Istanbul, Turkey
and
NP Brain Hospital
Istanbul, Turkey

Fazıl Gökgöz
Faculty of Political Sciences
Ankara University
Ankara, Turkey

Mohit Goswami
Operations Management Group and Quantitative Techniques
Indian Institute of Management Raipur
Raipur, India

Liisa Hakola
Technical Research Centre of Finland Ltd (VTT)
Espoo, Finland

Thomas M. Kraft
Technical Research Centre of Finland Ltd (VTT)
Kaitoväylä, Oulu, Finland

Tilak Lakshmana
Sensors and Embedded Systems
IoT Hardware Center of Excellence
Essity Hygiene and Health AB
Gothenburg, Sweden

Mudasir Maqbool
Department of Pharmaceutical Sciences
University of Kashmir
Hazratbal, Jammu and Kashmir, India

Tasnia Nabil
School of Biomedical Engineering
Marnix E Heersink School of Biomedical Innovation
McMaster University
Hamilton, Canada

Zulfkar Qadrie
Department of Pharmacology
Government Medical College Baramulla
Jammu and Kashmir, India

Velur V. V. Reddy
Department of Social Work
Norfolk State University
Norfolk, Virginia

Ulla A. Saari
Industrial Engineering & Management
Faculty of Management & Business
Tampere University
Tampere, Finland

Shashikant Nishant Sharma
Department of Planning and Architecture
Maulana Azad National Institute of Technology
Bhopal, India

Maria Smolander
Technical Research Centre of Finland Ltd (VTT)
Espoo, Finland

Engin Yalçın
Faculty of Economics and Administrative Sciences
Fırat University
Elazığ, Turkey

1 In the Trenches
Current Challenges in Healthcare Delivery

Zulfkar Qadrie, Mudasir Maqbool, and Mohd Altaf Dar

1.1 INTRODUCTION

Healthcare delivery encompasses the systems, techniques, and processes by which healthcare services are administered to individuals and communities. It includes a wide array of services, ranging from preventive care and primary health interventions to intricate hospital treatments and specialist medical procedures. Healthcare delivery is fundamental to public health, offering vital services that promote the well-being and lifespan of populations. Efficient healthcare provision can markedly improve quality of life by preventing illnesses, controlling chronic ailments, and enhancing overall health results (Kamel Boulos, Wilson, & Clauson, 2018).

The provision of healthcare is critically significant, especially in the contemporary age where global health is increasingly linked to political, economic, and social elements. Healthcare is a paramount problem in all countries, ranging from high-income nations to low-resource situations. It affects a society's economic productivity, social stability, and equitable access to services. An effective healthcare delivery system can enhance community health, alleviate disease load, and enable individuals to lead productive lives (Hayoun & Gannot, 2025).

Conversely, inefficiencies, injustices, and systemic failures may exacerbate health disparities, diminish treatment quality, and escalate healthcare expenditures. The healthcare delivery system consists of multiple components, including healthcare professionals (HCPs; physicians, nurses, specialists, and technicians), healthcare organizations (hospitals, clinics, private practices), health insurance institutions, governmental bodies, pharmaceutical corporations, and technological innovators (Merner et al., 2023). All of these institutions must collaborate to guarantee that care is accessible, inexpensive, and of superior quality. Efficient collaboration among these entities is crucial for establishing a system capable of addressing both standard medical requirements and intricate health emergencies (Gola, Brambilla, Barach, Signorelli, & Capolongo, 2020).

Contemporary healthcare systems are progressively transitioning from treating individual patients to managing populations, a notion commonly known as "population health management." This methodology considers the overarching socioeconomic determinants of health, including income, education, housing, and

DOI: 10.1201/9781003513834-1

environment, which significantly influence health outcomes (Ostini et al., 2021). Furthermore, technological breakthroughs, such as electronic health records (EHRs), artificial intelligence (AI), and telemedicine, are revolutionizing healthcare delivery, enhancing its efficiency, accessibility, and personalization. Nonetheless, these advances present both opportunities and problems, rendering healthcare delivery a perpetually developing domain (O'Sullivan, McGrail, & Russell, 2017).

1.1.1 Context of Current Challenges

Healthcare systems globally are facing various challenges due to rapid advancements in medical technology, evolving demographics, and transforming social and economic landscapes. The persistent challenges of healthcare delivery are intensified by public health crises, political instability, economic disparities, and environmental changes. The COVID-19 pandemic underscored the vulnerability of global healthcare systems and revealed numerous long-standing, overlooked vulnerabilities. The epidemic exerted significant pressure on healthcare systems worldwide (Almalki, Fitzgerald, & Clark, 2011; Gautam, Thakrar, Akinyemi, & Mahr, 2020). Hospitals, already functioning at full capacity in numerous nations, were inundated with patients afflicted by the virus, driving many systems to the verge of failure. Numerous places had shortages of essential medical supplies, HCPs, and intensive care units (ICUs), hindering health workers' ability to deliver sufficient care. The crisis exposed disparities in healthcare access and delivery, disproportionately impacting marginalized and vulnerable people throughout the pandemic and highlighting their lack of access to timely, quality care (Voumard et al., 2018).

The health inequities shown by COVID-19 are long-standing issues, having persisted for decades; yet, the pandemic underscored the fundamental deficiencies inherent in global healthcare systems. In addition to the pandemic, healthcare systems are contending with the ongoing challenge of escalating healthcare expenses. Developed and emerging nations encounter difficulties in reconciling the growing demand for healthcare services with constrained resources (Forriol & Vaquero, 2012). The aging population significantly contributes to escalating prices, since elderly persons often possess more intricate and persistent health ailments necessitating continuous care. The increasing incidence of chronic diseases, including diabetes, cardiovascular conditions, and mental health issues, exacerbates the burden on healthcare resources and necessitates innovative care strategies. The worldwide healthcare workforce is concurrently confronting a crisis (Somberg, 2009).

Deficiencies in healthcare personnel, especially in rural and neglected regions, are resulting in service supply shortages. The psychological and physical strain on HCPs, intensified by extended hours, elevated stress levels, and burnout, is a significant factor contributing to the difficulties encountered by healthcare systems. Moreover, workforce diversity continues to pose an issue, as specific communities are underrepresented in healthcare professions, exacerbating health inequities. A further difficulty pertains to the increasing demand for digital transformation in healthcare (Adebayo et al., 2020).

Despite the considerable promise of innovations such as telemedicine, AI, and big data to enhance care delivery, numerous healthcare systems are encountering difficulties in their efficient implementation. Data privacy, cybersecurity, and the digital divide present challenges, resulting in certain groups lacking access to essential digital tools required to leverage these breakthroughs. Moreover, healthcare providers and institutions frequently encounter opposition to the use of new technologies, attributable to expenses, training demands, and apprehension regarding the disruption of existing procedures (Zehravi, Maqbool, & Ara, 2021b).

Climate change presents a burgeoning challenge for healthcare systems. With the escalation of extreme weather events, environmental pollution, and emerging disease patterns linked to climate change, healthcare systems will face heightened demands for response (Wang, Rao, Wu, & Liu, 2013). Healthcare institutions must exhibit resilience to natural disasters, while public health systems must adjust to evolving disease epidemiology and increasing health hazards linked to environmental conditions. These difficulties are interrelated, necessitating a coordinated, systemic strategy for resolution. Healthcare systems must evolve to be more adaptive, inclusive, and sustainable in order to address present demands and future uncertainty (Kelly, 1985).

We aim to examine the contemporary challenges in healthcare delivery, elucidate the complexities confronting modern healthcare systems, and provide viable solutions to these problems. The primary obstacles encountered by healthcare providers, organizations, governments, and patients, focusing on how these issues contribute to inefficiencies, disparities, and escalating prices, will be identified and analyzed. A comprehensive analysis of the linked difficulties in healthcare delivery and the critical necessity for systemic reform will be provided.

In this chapter we will identify issues and examine potential remedies to rectify shortcomings in healthcare delivery systems. These solutions will concentrate on technical improvements while also analyzing legislative interventions, workforce initiatives, and financial reforms that may facilitate the development of more effective and equitable healthcare systems.

We will examine the significance of patient-centered care, highlighting the necessity of transitioning to a more personalized and inclusive methodology that prioritizes individual needs and preferences. Real-world examples and case studies to address these problems will be presented, emphasizing both effective interventions and instances of systemic failure. These examples will furnish tangible evidence of effective and ineffective practices, imparting significant insights for future healthcare policy and implementation. At the conclusion of the chapter, readers will possess an enhanced comprehension of the contemporary healthcare delivery landscape, the problems confronting healthcare systems, and the diverse solutions required to address these issues. We will enhance the discourse on developing more resilient, accessible, and efficient healthcare systems that address the changing requirements of global populations (Zehravi, Maqbool, & Ara, 2021a).

Figure 1.1 highlights the key challenges in healthcare value delivery, including a broken ecosystem, misaligned goals, and the transition from volume-based to value-based care. It also emphasizes issues such as data management, financial pressure, regulatory complexities, and the need for innovation. Addressing these obstacles is crucial for achieving more efficient, equitable, and patient-centered healthcare systems (Bowling & Bond, 2001).

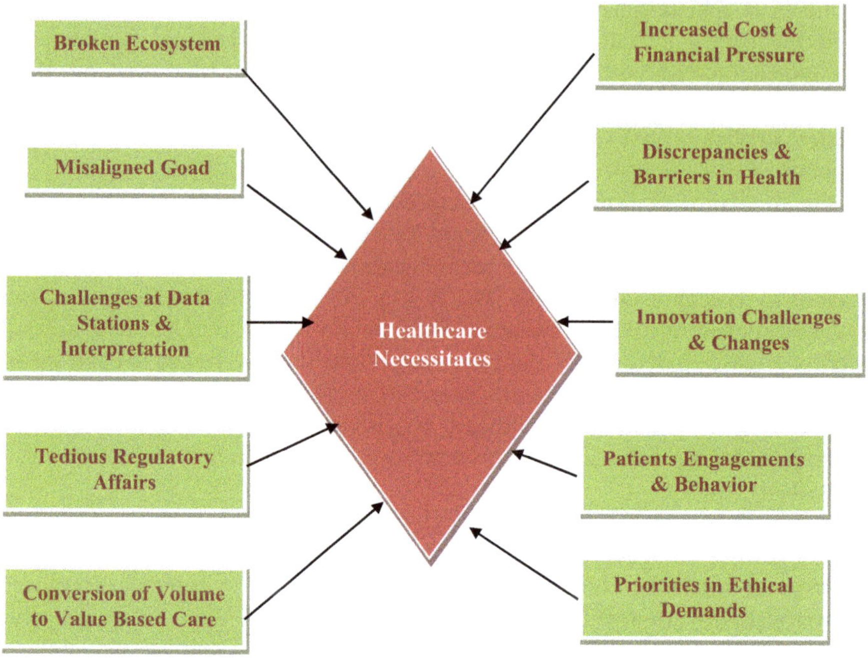

FIGURE 1.1 Healthcare value delivery and its necessities.

1.1.2 The Healthcare System Landscape

Healthcare infrastructure denotes the physical and organizational frameworks that facilitate the provision of healthcare services. The infrastructure includes hospitals, clinics, primary care centers, mental health institutions, and public health initiatives. It encompasses not just physical structures but also the labor, technology, policies, and financial mechanisms that guarantee the availability of healthcare services to the population. An effective healthcare infrastructure is essential for enhancing the health and well-being of individuals and populations (Choi, 2023; Guttman et al., 2021).

1.1.2.1 Hospitals and Specialized Care

Hospitals constitute the foundation of healthcare delivery systems in numerous nations. They offer intricate medical services, encompassing operations, emergency care, acute care, and specialty therapies. Large metropolitan hospitals in the United States, such as the Mayo Clinic in Rochester, Minnesota, and Massachusetts General Hospital in Boston, provide advanced medical care and draw patients from national and international locations. These hospitals deliver superior care, frequently providing novel therapies unavailable in other facilities (Dennett et al., 2021; Peters, Kooij, Lenferink, van Harten, & Doggen, 2021). Nevertheless, hospitals sometimes incur high expenses related to both building and operations costs, and they may be less accessible in rural and neglected regions. In numerous low- and middle-income countries (LMICs), hospitals are predominantly situated in urban areas, resulting in rural communities lacking access to emergency services or specialized medical treatment (White, Kosar, Rahman, & Mor, 2020).

In sub-Saharan Africa, hospitals are predominantly situated in capital cities, necessitating long-distance travel for rural populations to access medical care. The problem is worsened by insufficient infrastructure, which further restricts access. Conversely, primary care services are the cornerstone of healthcare systems in numerous nations, especially those emphasizing preventive treatment (Gruen, Weeramanthri, Knight, & Bailie, 2004). Primary care centers serve as the initial point of contact for persons pursuing healthcare, overseeing basic health issues, preventive services, and referrals to specialists when required. Countries with a strong primary care system, such as Sweden and the Netherlands, have superior health results at reduced costs. In the Netherlands, primary care physicians serve as gatekeepers, orchestrating patient care to avert superfluous hospital visits and successfully manage chronic conditions (Bowling & Bond, 2001; Zehravi, Maqbool, & Ara, 2023a).

Figure 1.2 outlines the complications stemming from India's fragmented healthcare system, including inconsistent access to healthcare facilities, cost variations in treatment, and inefficient use of resources. It also highlights critical issues such as a shortage of HCPs and limited healthcare insurance coverage. These challenges undermine the effectiveness and equity of healthcare delivery in the country (Bogler, Liu, Cadesky, & Bell, 2021).

1.1.2.2 Mental Health Services

Mental health services constitute an essential, but frequently neglected, component of healthcare infrastructure. Mental health is an escalating global concern; nonetheless, services are often insufficient or underfunded. In affluent nations such as the

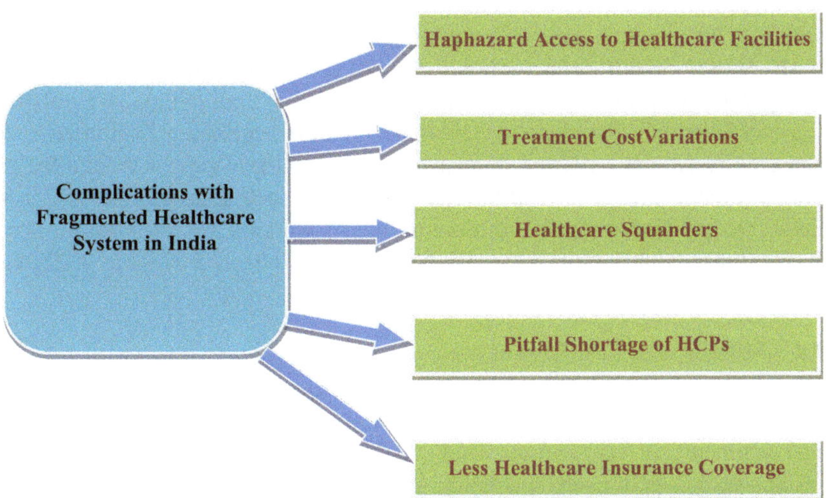

FIGURE 1.2 Complications with fragmented healthcare system in India.

United States, mental health services are frequently disjointed, characterized by protracted waiting periods and restricted access to care for those in need of psychiatric intervention (Shinfuku, 1998).

In numerous LMICs, the circumstances are exacerbated by a significant deficiency of mental health experts and the pervasive stigma surrounding mental health issues. In India, there are about 0.3 psychiatrists per 100,000 individuals, significantly lower than the global average. Countries such as Australia have advanced mental healthcare by implementing government-funded programs designed to enhance access to services (Zhao, Liu, Hu, Chen, & Sun, 2017). The Headspace initiative provides mental health services for youth, including counseling, early intervention, and crisis care. Likewise, the National Health Service (NHS) of the United Kingdom has implemented mental health services in conjunction with physical health treatments, fostering a more cohesive healthcare model. Notwithstanding these endeavors, mental health services continue to be inadequate in numerous regions globally, underscoring the necessity for investment in mental health infrastructure (Whiteford, 2017).

1.1.2.3 Health Access Disparities

Healthcare access and quality disparities are prevalent, especially between high-income and low-income nations. In industrialized countries, healthcare access is more comprehensive yet frequently inequitable, with factors such as geographic location, insurance coverage, and care affordability restricting access for some populations. In the United States, those lacking insurance or possessing insufficient coverage encounter substantial obstacles to obtaining appropriate care (Beroukhim, Mahabamunuge, & Pal, 2022). The Affordable Care Act (ACA) has broadened healthcare access for millions; nonetheless, gaps remain, especially in rural regions where healthcare facilities and professionals are limited. Conversely, numerous developing nations encounter even greater difficulties. The deficiency of infrastructure and resources in rural regions, coupled with insufficient funding for public health initiatives, results in many individuals not obtaining the necessary care (Tepper et al., 2022).

In Kenya, there are around 2.2 healthcare workers per 1,000 individuals, well below the World Health Organization's (WHO) recommendation of 4.5 healthcare workers per 1,000 individuals. Consequently, numerous individuals in rural Kenya must go considerable distances to access the nearest healthcare institution, which can be excessively costly or time-intensive. Rectifying these gaps is crucial for guaranteeing equitable access to healthcare. Approaches such as mobile health clinics, telemedicine, and investment in community health workers are essential for accessing disadvantaged communities (McKinney, Kelm, Windsor, & Keyser, 2024; Talati et al., 2018; Zehravi, Maqbool, & Ara, 2023b).

1.1.2.4 Stakeholders in Healthcare

Healthcare delivery encompasses various stakeholders, each significantly influencing the system's functionality, efficiency, and accessibility. The stakeholders comprise governments, private entities, HCPs, patients, insurers, and policymakers. The actions and decisions of each stakeholder influence the overall efficacy of healthcare delivery, and their collaboration is vital for establishing a coherent system (Pastorino et al., 2019).

1.1.2.5 Governments

Governments are key entities in healthcare provision, tasked with regulation, financing, and policy formulation. In several nations, especially those with universal health coverage (UHC), the government serves as the principal financier and supervisor of healthcare services. In the United Kingdom, the government finances the NHS, which offers healthcare services to all citizens at no cost at the time of delivery (Mubin et al., 2021).

In Canada, the government offers UHC, guaranteeing that all Canadians can receive essential medical treatments without financial obstacles. In nations such as Germany and France, healthcare systems are organized around social health insurance, wherein both employers and employees contribute to a compulsory insurance fund. The government supervises the management of these funds, guaranteeing fair access to healthcare services (Jones et al., 2012).

Governments play a pivotal role in formulating healthcare policy, guaranteeing that healthcare delivery corresponds with public health interests. During the COVID-19 pandemic, governments globally were tasked with overseeing public health precautions, such as lockdowns, healthcare facility readiness, and vaccine delivery (Henneker & Reed, 2012).

1.1.2.6 Private Organizations and Insurers

Private entities, such as insurance firms, pharmaceutical corporations, and private healthcare providers, exert considerable influence on healthcare delivery. Private insurers offer coverage for healthcare expenses, especially in nations lacking national health systems. In the United States, private insurance is pivotal in healthcare access, with private insurers covering a substantial segment of the population, especially via employer-sponsored policies. Private healthcare providers augment the public healthcare system by delivering specialist services and elective procedures (Terkola, Antoñanzas, & Postma, 2019).

The Mayo Clinic and Cleveland Clinic in the United States exemplify private healthcare providers delivering exceptional medical services. Nevertheless, dependence on private providers might intensify healthcare disparities, as individuals with lower incomes or insufficient insurance coverage may be unable to pay such services. Pharmaceutical companies are essential to healthcare provision as they produce drugs and vaccines, fostering therapeutic innovation (Malik, Prescott, Khalid, Hashmi, & Kiani, 2021). Nonetheless, elevated pharmaceutical costs in both affluent and impoverished nations constitute a substantial obstacle to access, particularly for chronic ailments. The exorbitant expense of hepatitis C therapies has been a significant concern, with several life-saving medications priced at tens of thousands of dollars annually (Ng, Kim, & Suri, 2022).

1.1.2.7 Healthcare Workers

HCPs, encompassing physicians, nurses, specialists, and allied health practitioners, provide the foundation of healthcare provision. They deliver direct patient care and are crucial in the prevention, diagnosis, and treatment of disorders. HCPs globally have substantial obstacles, such as burnout, extended working hours, and inadequate compensation. The COVID-19 pandemic intensified these issues, subjecting HCPs to significant stress, fatigue, and emotional burdens due to the increase in cases (AlJohani, Karuppiah, Al Mutairi, & Al Mutair, 2021).

A national survey in the United States revealed that approximately 60% of HCPs reported having burnout. The training, recruiting, and retention of healthcare workers continue to pose substantial obstacles, especially in rural and underserved regions. India experiences a significant deficit of healthcare experts, having merely 9.2 doctors per 10,000 individuals, in contrast to 26 doctors per 10,000 individuals in the United States. This mismatch results in inequitable access to healthcare and inferior health outcomes, especially in rural regions (Carbone et al., 2022).

1.1.2.8 Patients

Patients are the primary beneficiaries of healthcare services, and their wants and preferences are fundamental to care delivery. Recently, there has been a transition toward patient-centered care, which underscores the significance of including patients as active partners in their healthcare. In the United States, the Patient Protection and Affordable Care Act promotes patient-centered care approaches aimed at enhancing patient satisfaction, involvement, and health outcomes (Chung, McKenna, & Cooper, 2020).

Patients are increasingly becoming knowledgeable and engaged in their healthcare, especially due to the proliferation of digital health technologies. Telemedicine, mobile health applications, and patient portals enable individuals to monitor their health, obtain medical counsel, and manage chronic disorders at a distance. Nonetheless, obstacles persist regarding equity, as many people lack access to the internet or digital resources (Sun et al., 2023).

1.1.2.9 Recent Trends in Healthcare Delivery

Recent trends are transforming healthcare delivery, propelled by technological innovations, demographic shifts, and evolving patient expectations. Telemedicine, the provision of healthcare services through digital platforms, has expanded considerably in recent years. It gained particular prominence during the COVID-19 epidemic, when healthcare systems were compelled to transition to remote consultations to minimize in-person interactions. Telemedicine enables patients to engage with healthcare practitioners from their residences, enhancing accessibility to healthcare, especially in rural or underserved regions (Sloan et al., 2014). In Canada, telemedicine has been extensively utilized in distant provinces to link patients with specialists in major hubs. Nonetheless, obstacles such as legal constraints, payment complications, and the digital divide hinder the extensive implementation of telemedicine (K. B. Johnson et al., 2021).

Conversely, personalized medicine, which customizes therapies according to an individual's genetic composition, lifestyle, and environment, is another trend influencing healthcare delivery. Progress in genomes and biotechnology is allowing healthcare practitioners to deliver more accurate and efficacious therapies. Targeted therapies in oncology have transformed cancer treatment by utilizing medications that specifically target mutations in cancer cells, leading to improved outcomes. Nonetheless, the substantial expense of genetic testing and individualized therapies continues to impede wider use (Dar, Maqbool, & Ara, 2023; Mefford et al., 2021).

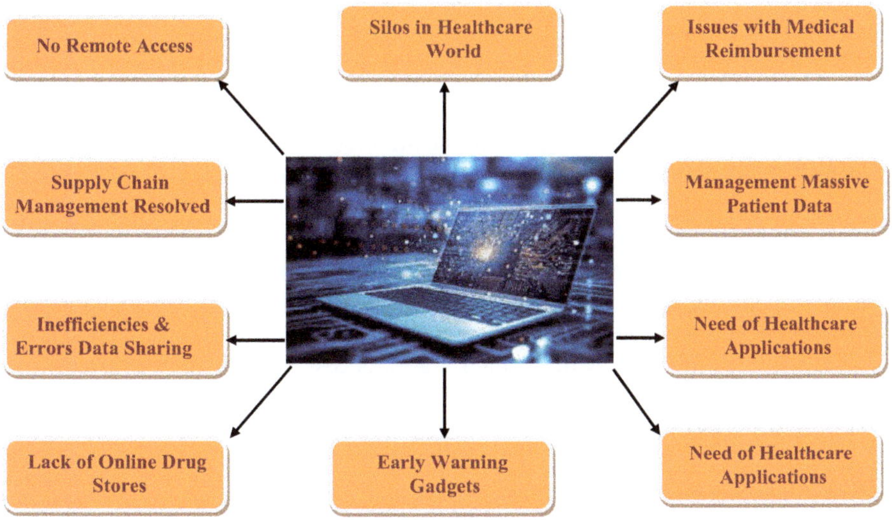

FIGURE 1.3 Current technology that can solve top ten issues in healthcare.

Figure 1.3 highlights how current technologies can address critical issues in healthcare, including lack of remote access, healthcare silos, and difficulties with medical reimbursement. It emphasizes the role of technology in managing large patient data, improving supply chain management, and providing early warning gadgets (Mefford et al., 2021).

Additionally, the need for healthcare applications and better data sharing is crucial for enhancing efficiency and reducing errors in the healthcare system. Digital health technology, including wearable gadgets, mobile health applications, and EHRs, is revolutionizing healthcare delivery (Ban et al., 2024). Wearable gadgets such as Fitbit and Apple Watch enable patients to monitor their physical activity, heart rate, and manage chronic illnesses such as diabetes. These devices furnish real-time info to healthcare providers, facilitating better individualized care (Mefford et al., 2020).

Digital health applications assist patients in managing illnesses such as asthma, diabetes, and hypertension by delivering reminders, monitoring progress, and giving health education. The incorporation of these technologies into healthcare delivery promotes efficiency, improves patient engagement, and provides novel methods for managing chronic conditions. Nonetheless, issues about data privacy, security, and equity must be resolved to fully leverage the potential of digital health (Tran et al., 2012).

1.1.3 Key Challenges in Healthcare Delivery

The healthcare delivery system encounters numerous obstacles that impede its capacity to offer effective and equitable care to all patients. The challenges encompass access and equity concerns, manpower shortages, budgetary limitations, technology integration, and policy restraints. Confronting these difficulties necessitates a comprehensive and multifaceted strategy for transforming healthcare systems worldwide (Brown, 2020; Fennell & Flood, 1998). This section will examine critical concerns in healthcare delivery, including accessibility, workforce challenges, financial pressures, the incorporation of new technologies, patient-centered treatment, regulatory obstacles, and the effects of public health crises, accompanied by real-world examples when applicable (M. Maqbool et al., 2021; Waterson, 2021).

1.1.3.1 Accessibility and Equity

Access to healthcare services is a significant challenge for healthcare delivery systems worldwide. Access to healthcare is frequently inequitable, with notable gaps evident across economic, geographical, social, and cultural dimensions. In numerous high-income nations, such as the United States, access to healthcare is affected by economic variables, such as insurance coverage. Despite insurance, high-deductible plans and out-of-pocket expenses can render healthcare costly for low-income persons (Northridge, Kumar, & Kaur, 2020; Purkey & MacKenzie, 2019). A survey revealed that over 40% of insured Americans had postponed or forwent treatment due to financial apprehensions. Geographical obstacles constitute a significant factor. In rural regions, healthcare access is sometimes constrained by a shortage of doctors, especially specialists, and the considerable distance patients must traverse to access medical facilities (Levesque, Harris, & Russell, 2013).

In nations such as India, Brazil, and South Africa, healthcare services are frequently centralized in urban areas, resulting in rural populations facing considerable obstacles to access, including extensive travel distances, insufficient infrastructure, and a scarcity of well-educated medical personnel. In India, merely 2% of physicians operate in rural regions, despite a significant share of the population living in those areas. Consequently, rural inhabitants encounter significant health hazards, particularly concerning chronic ailments such as diabetes and hypertension, which necessitate consistent maintenance (Gwyther et al., 2019; Kurpas et al., 2018).

1.1.3.2 Cultural and Social Barriers

Cultural and socioeconomic issues significantly restrict access to healthcare. Language challenges, cultural perceptions of healthcare, and skepticism about medical institutions might hinder underprivileged people from accessing care. Immigrant communities and racial minorities, especially in nations such as the United States, encounter discrimination in healthcare environments, resulting in diminished participation with the system. Research indicates that Black Americans are more susceptible to medical abuse and are less likely to obtain sufficient pain management than their white counterparts (Sangaleti, Schveitzer, Peduzzi, Zoboli, & Soares, 2017).

The pandemic has intensified this issue, as communities of color faced elevated rates of infection, hospitalization, and mortality from COVID-19, primarily because of existing inequities in healthcare access and outcomes. The WHO asserts that mitigating these disparities necessitates a holistic strategy, encompassing the enhancement of healthcare coverage for marginalized communities, the advancement of cultural competence in healthcare provision, and the allocation of resources toward outreach initiatives to involve at-risk populations (Rubel & Garro, 1992; Sohal, Sohal, King-Shier, & Khan, 2015).

1.1.3.3 Workforce Issues

A major obstacle in global healthcare delivery is the scarcity of HCPs, especially in low-income and rural regions. The shortfall arises from multiple sources, such as an aging workforce, heightened demand for healthcare services, and prolonged training durations necessary to cultivate qualified experts. Sub-Saharan Africa has only 2.3 healthcare workers per 1,000 individuals, significantly lower than the global average of 7.7 per 1,000 individuals (Franco, Lima, & Giovanella, 2021; Garnelo et al., 2020).

The deficiency of healthcare personnel results in extended wait times, diminished access to care, and overburdened medical staff, ultimately undermining the quality of healthcare services. The deficiency of HCPs in India, especially in rural regions, has resulted in dependence on a limited cadre of overburdened doctors and nurses, hindering the provision of sufficient care. Many developing countries face analogous challenges in recruiting and retaining medical personnel within their healthcare systems (M. Maqbool, Bekele, & Fekadu, 2022; Mitton, Dionne, Masucci, Wong, & Law, 2011).

Burnout constitutes a significant concern within the healthcare sector, especially as the demands placed on HCPs persistently escalate. Prolonged shifts, emotional strain, and physical fatigue contribute to burnout, resulting in care errors, elevated turnover rates, and diminished quality of care. The COVID-19 pandemic has markedly intensified this issue, as healthcare staff was inundated by the volume of patients and the intricacy of treatment necessitated by the virus. A research in the United States indicated that about 50% of HCPs had signs of burnout, such as emotional tiredness and depersonalization (Norcross & Wampold, 2011).

Alongside workforce shortages, there exist deficiencies in the training of healthcare personnel. Numerous healthcare systems, particularly in resource-limited nations, exhibit inadequate investment in educational and training initiatives. This is especially apparent in specialist domains such as mental healthcare, cancer, and geriatric medicine, where there is an increasing need for qualified practitioners but restricted training options. In Nigeria, there exists a critical deficit of mental health experts, with only 0.3 psychiatrists per 100,000 individuals, in contrast to 12 psychiatrists per 100,000 individuals in affluent nations such as the United Kingdom (da Silva et al., 2023; Prince, 2023).

The migration of competent HCPs from LMICs to higher-income nations in pursuit of superior remuneration, improved working conditions, and enhanced career prospects is another factor exacerbating labor difficulties. This "brain drain" intensifies the deficiency of trained HCPs in nations that require them the most. The emigration of HCPs from nations such as the Philippines, India, and Zimbabwe to countries such as the United States, the United Kingdom, and Australia results in a deficit of healthcare workers to adequately serve their people (Leightley & Murphy, 2023; St Clair et al., 2017).

1.1.3.4 Financial Strain

The escalating expenses of healthcare services constitute one of the foremost difficulties confronting healthcare systems globally. The escalation in healthcare expenditures is propelled by multiple variables, such as the aging demographic, technology innovations, the growing incidence of chronic illnesses, and elevated administrative expenses. In the United States, healthcare expenses have more than doubled in the past 20 years, with national health expenditures currently surpassing 18% of GDP (Abrams et al., 2021; Smith et al., 2022). This escalation has been especially onerous for people and families that incur a substantial share of the expenses via elevated premiums, deductibles, and co-pays (Wang et al., 2013).

In Europe, although healthcare expenses are typically lower than in the United States, several nations are experiencing financial pressure due to an aging demographic and the rising incidence of chronic illnesses. In Italy, healthcare expenditures are anticipated to rise by 2.5% each year owing to the aging demographic, exerting considerable strain on the healthcare budget (Kadakia et al., 2022; R. Maqbool, Maqbool, Zehravi, & Ara, 2021a).

Healthcare systems in numerous LMICs encounter considerable financial limitations. In these areas, healthcare expenditure is frequently constrained, resulting in inadequate infrastructure, insufficient personnel, and substandard services. In sub-Saharan Africa, health expenditure per capita is under $100, significantly lower than the WHO's recommended $1,000 per capita to guarantee access to fundamental healthcare (Blinder, 2022). Consequently, numerous countries in this region are unable of delivering essential healthcare services to their populations, resulting in adverse health outcomes and avoidable fatalities (Wu & Moss, 2023).

A further financial obstacle is the framework of healthcare insurance. In nations such as the United States, where private insurance is predominant, healthcare expenses are frequently elevated, and coverage is disjointed. The ACA has increased insurance accessibility for numerous Americans; nonetheless, substantial coverage gaps persist, resulting in millions remaining uninsured. Conversely, nations with universal healthcare systems, such as the United Kingdom and Canada, offer healthcare services to all residents, mostly financed through taxation. Although universal systems typically exhibit greater cost efficiency, they may suffer from underfunding, resulting in prolonged wait times and diminished quality of treatment in specific areas. Optimal resource allocation is a significant issue in global healthcare systems (Ehsan et al., 2023; Smith, Mendoza, Lowenstein, & Shih, 2021).

Healthcare delivery frequently experiences waste due to resource misallocation, overutilization of medical services, and administrative inefficiencies. A survey by the Institute of Medicine estimates that as much as 30% of healthcare expenditure in the United States is superfluous, stemming from unneeded tests, treatments, and procedures. The objective is to distribute resources efficiently to guarantee that healthcare systems deliver high-quality services while minimizing financial waste due to inefficiencies (Longo et al., 2020; R. Maqbool, Maqbool, Zehravi, & Ara, 2021b).

1.1.3.5 Technology Integration and Data Management

The incorporation of emerging technologies, including EHRs, AI, and telemedicine, has the capacity to revolutionize healthcare delivery. EHR systems enable healthcare practitioners to preserve a digital record of patient history, facilitating information sharing, minimizing medical errors, and enhancing patient outcomes. In the United States, the utilization of EHRs has become prevalent, with more than 80%

of physicians employing them. Likewise, AI is progressively employed to examine medical data, identify ailments, and create individualized treatment strategies (Zeng, Li, Pan, Chen, & Pan, 2021).

Although emerging technologies provide substantial advantages, they simultaneously provoke apprehensions over data privacy and cybersecurity. The heightened utilization of digital health tools presents risks of patient data breaches, potentially undermining confidentiality and diminishing trust in healthcare systems. A 2020 poll revealed that 70% of healthcare businesses encountered a data breach in the preceding year, emphasizing the necessity for enhanced data security protocols (Reddy, 2024).

Conversely, numerous healthcare systems, especially in LMICs, persist in utilizing antiquated technologies, which may impede efficiency and the quality of care. In India, numerous hospitals continue to depend on paper-based records, hindering the prompt and precise sharing of patient information. Resistance to the adoption of new technology, whether stemming from financial constraints, insufficient training, or apprehension regarding disruption, constitutes an additional impediment to advancement. This aversion to innovation may result in inefficiency and inadequate patient care (von Gerich et al., 2022; Xie et al., 2021).

1.1.3.6 Patient-Centered Care

A significant transformation in contemporary healthcare is the transition to patient-centered care, which prioritizes patient engagement in their healthcare decisions. This transition encounters multiple obstacles, such as communication disparities between patients and clinicians, insufficient tailored treatment alternatives, and cultural impediments to effective care. Effective communication is crucial for patient involvement. Nonetheless, in numerous healthcare systems, communication between patients and physicians frequently proves inadequate (Barry & Edgman-Levitan, 2012; Khan et al., 2025).

Figure 1.4 emphasizes the principles of patient-oriented healthcare, focusing on aligning goals with patient care and ensuring collaborative, coordinated, and accessible healthcare services. It underscores the importance of including families in healthcare decisions, respecting their viewpoints, and prioritizing both physical and emotional well-being. Transparency and ease of delivery are also key elements in enhancing the overall patient experience (Barry & Edgman-Levitan, 2012).

Research indicates that healthcare personnel often inadequately communicate diagnoses, treatment alternatives, or possible adverse effects to patients, resulting in uncertainty and discontent. Moreover, patients from minority backgrounds may encounter linguistic obstacles, hence exacerbating communication difficulties. Cultural competence is an additional obstacle in delivering patient-centered care. Healthcare practitioners must comprehend and honor patients' cultural origins to deliver suitable care. Nevertheless, HCPs frequently lack the requisite expertise to meet the cultural demands of varied communities. In the United States, Hispanic and Black patients may encounter difficulties in obtaining culturally responsive care, resulting in inferior health outcomes (Altaf Dar, Maqbool, Ara, & Zehravi, 2023; Lamb & Wang, 2020).

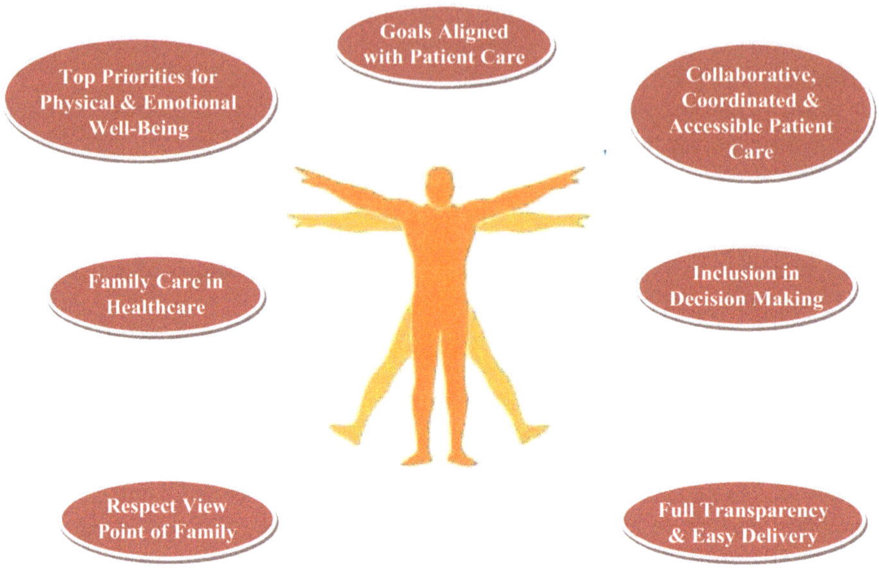
Goals Aligned with Patient Care
Top Priorities for Physical & Emotional Well-Being
Collaborative, Coordinated & Accessible Patient Care
Family Care in Healthcare
Inclusion in Decision Making
Respect View Point of Family
Full Transparency & Easy Delivery

FIGURE 1.4 Patient-oriented healthcare.

1.1.3.7 Policy and Regulatory Hurdles

Healthcare rules and policies are essential in influencing healthcare delivery. Government policies concerning healthcare financing, insurance coverage, and reimbursement rates can either enhance or obstruct access to care. In the United States, the fragmented healthcare system, dependent on private insurance, presents considerable obstacles to access, especially for persons with lower incomes. In Canada, despite the existence of universal healthcare coverage, financial limitations and prolonged wait times for non-emergency services have emerged as significant concerns (Ayati et al., 2021; T, Kumar, & R, 2024).

1.1.3.8 Public Health Crises and Pandemics

The resilience and efficacy of the healthcare system are perpetually challenged during public health emergencies and pandemics, which can strain resources, reveal systemic weaknesses, and intensify existing health disparities. Healthcare systems must be equipped to confront both urgent health threats and the enduring consequences for public health and safety, stemming from the worldwide proliferation of infectious illnesses and the difficulties posed by climate change (Burkle, Bradt, & Ryan, 2021).

The COVID-19 pandemic exemplifies a significant and recent disruption to healthcare delivery caused by a global health disaster. Global healthcare systems, particularly in low- and middle-income nations, were ill-equipped for the significant increase in demand for medical services. Hospitals in Italy, Spain, and the United States were inundated, with ICUs at maximum capacity, and HCPs saw unparalleled levels of stress, exhaustion, and virus exposure (Burkle, Bradt, Green, & Ryan, 2021).

The pandemic revealed substantial deficiencies in healthcare system readiness, including insufficient personal protective equipment (PPE), ventilators, and testing infrastructure. Furthermore, the epidemic underscored concerns regarding healthcare accessibility and equity. Marginalized groups, such as racial minorities, the elderly, and individuals with pre-existing diseases, saw a disproportionate impact from the virus, affecting both infection rates and the quality of care provided (Sugand, Park, Aframian, Gupte, & Sarraf, 2024). The differences were particularly pronounced in the United States, where Black and Hispanic populations faced elevated rates of hospitalization and mortality from COVID-19 as a result of systemic inequities in healthcare access (Sweet et al., 2020).

Pandemics such as COVID-19 not only overwhelm physical healthcare resources but also exert pressure on mental health infrastructure. The social isolation, fear, and uncertainty induced by the epidemic led to heightened incidences of anxiety, sadness, and post-traumatic stress disorder (PTSD), exacerbating the strain on already overextended mental health facilities. Healthcare systems, particularly in industrialized countries, rapidly adjusted by expediting the use of telemedicine, AI-driven diagnostics, and remote care platforms. In the United Kingdom, the NHS swiftly augmented its telehealth services, facilitating virtual consultations to alleviate the strain on traditional healthcare facilities (Myhre et al., 2022).

These developments may be crucial for alleviating the effects of future pandemics, allowing healthcare systems to maintain operations during crises. The epidemic exposed deficiencies in the global response, notwithstanding the considerable problems encountered by numerous countries. Global cooperation was essential for disseminating crucial information, guaranteeing fair access to resources, and expediting vaccine development (Johnson, Cahill, Choate, Roelfs, & Walsh, 2021). Initiatives such as COVAX, spearheaded by the WHO, GAVI, and many international entities, aimed to guarantee that low- and middle-income nations received COVID-19 vaccines, underscoring the significance of equitable access in alleviating the effects of global health emergencies (Blinder, 2022).

Although pandemics such as COVID-19 have prominently influenced the global health agenda in recent years, climate change is emerging as a comparably important long-term danger to healthcare systems and patient safety (Imperato, LaRosa, Kavaler, Benker, & Schechter, 2011). Increasing global temperatures, severe weather phenomena, air contamination, and alterations in disease patterns attributable to climate change present distinct and cumulative threats to public health and healthcare systems. Severe weather phenomena, such as hurricanes, floods, and wildfires, inflict catastrophic consequences on healthcare infrastructure, displacing communities and damaging hospitals, clinics, and other medical facilities. The 2020 COVID-19 pandemic coincided with catastrophic wildfires in Australia, which impaired healthcare services during a period when the system was already contending with the epidemic (Cai et al., 2022). Hospitals in California and other regions of the United States were compelled to adapt to the dual challenges of a pandemic and wildfires, which not only stretched resources but also inflicted environmental harm that impacted the health of both patients and healthcare personnel (Myhre et al., 2022).

Moreover, increasing temperatures and modified weather patterns introduce additional health hazards by broadening the geographical distribution of diseases such as malaria, dengue, and Zika virus (Oza et al., 2023). Warmer climates facilitate the multiplication of mosquitoes that transmit these diseases, resulting in heightened prevalence in formerly untouched regions. For instance, East Africa has experienced an increase in malaria incidence attributed to altered rainfall patterns, but Zika virus epidemics have been associated with meteorological changes generated by El Niño. Healthcare systems in sub-Saharan Africa and Southeast Asia are more susceptible to vector-borne diseases, necessitating prompt public health interventions, including extensive pesticide application and robust surveillance systems (Smith et al., 2022).

The psychological effects of climate change must not be overlooked (Eisman, Kim, Salloum, Shuman, & Glasgow, 2022). Severe weather phenomena, displacement caused by natural calamities, and the unpredictability of climate change add to stress, anxiety, and depression among impacted communities. Individuals who have lost their homes and livelihoods due to storms, floods, or droughts frequently experience post-traumatic stress, resulting in enduring mental health issues. Mental health treatments should be incorporated into disaster response methods; yet, numerous healthcare systems in poor nations lack the necessary resources to adequately meet these demands (Van Nguyen et al., 2022).

The safety of patients is directly influenced by these environmental elements. Severe weather phenomena, atmospheric contamination, and increasing temperatures can aggravate pre-existing diseases such as asthma, cardiovascular ailments, and heatstroke, hence elevating the danger for susceptible populations. Older folks and individuals with pre-existing health issues are especially vulnerable to heatwaves. The WHO reports that heatwaves cause thousands of fatalities annually, especially in areas such as Southern Europe, North America, and Asia. An innovative solution to this challenge has been the creation of climate-resilient healthcare infrastructure (Correia & Willis, 2022). This encompasses the design of healthcare facilities capable of withstanding severe weather occurrences and the implementation of sustainable methods to mitigate the environmental impact of healthcare delivery (Mitton et al., 2011).

In Bangladesh, healthcare facilities are being constructed with flood-resistant infrastructure to alleviate the effects of rising sea levels and flooding. In a similar vein, solar-powered health clinics in Africa are enhancing healthcare delivery in areas with restricted energy access, illustrating how environmentally aware planning may bolster the resilience of healthcare systems (James et al., 2023). Governments must pursue policy measures to mitigate the health effects of climate change. Integrating climate change adaptation and mitigation strategies into national health systems is essential for enduring health resilience. The WHO's Climate and Health Program offers technical support to nations on adapting health systems to climate change, emphasizing vulnerable populations, disease surveillance, and disaster preparedness (Watson, Staton, Grella, Scott, & Dennis, 2022).

1.1.4 Case Studies and Real-World Examples

Case studies offer significant insights into the practical difficulties and solutions in healthcare delivery. They emphasize how many areas and nations have confronted various healthcare challenges, ranging from rectifying systemic failures to effectively executing creative solutions. This section will analyze two notable examples: one in which a healthcare system encountered substantial difficulties, and another in which a successful intervention markedly enhanced healthcare delivery (Ham, 2020b). Example 1: The NHS Struggles During COVID-19: The NHS in the United Kingdom is one of the largest publicly funded healthcare systems globally, recognized for delivering universal healthcare to all inhabitants. However, when the COVID-19 pandemic emerged in early 2020, the NHS, similar to several healthcare systems worldwide, experienced significant pressure (Ham, 2020a).

1.1.4.1 Challenges Faced by the NHS

As the epidemic proliferated throughout the United Kingdom, the NHS encountered numerous significant obstacles that tested the health system's capacities. The principal concern was the overwhelming number of patients necessitating acute care, particularly during the initial phases of the pandemic. Hospitals were swiftly inundated, with ICU beds at full capacity, resulting in minimal availability for non-COVID patients. The situation was aggravated by the absence of PPE and ventilators, resulting in considerable logistical challenges. The United Kingdom's NHS Test and Trace system, intended to monitor and mitigate the infection, encountered criticism for its sluggish response and poor efficacy in curbing the virus's spread (Nandhra & Benson, 2022).

This situation was exacerbated by staffing shortages as healthcare personnel contracted COVID-19 or encountered quarantine protocols, hence diminishing the number of frontline workers available for patient care. Furthermore, non-COVID care was postponed as hospitals prioritized COVID patients, resulting in a backlog of critical treatments for those with chronic diseases such as cancer, heart disease, and diabetes. Reports indicate that as many as 50,000 individuals in the United Kingdom succumbed due to delays in routine and emergency care during the initial wave of the epidemic (Benedetto, Goodwin, Kendall, Uppal, & Akowuah, 2020).

1.1.4.2 Response and Adaptation

In reaction to these unparalleled problems, the NHS instituted various emergency measures to address the influx of cases and maintain the functionality of healthcare services. The Nightingale Hospitals initiative established temporary field hospitals in large convention centers and exposition halls nationwide to enhance critical care capacity. These provisional facilities offered assistance to hospitals inundated with COVID-19 cases; nonetheless, many remained underutilized due to staffing challenges and logistical limitations. Furthermore, the NHS increased its telemedicine services to enable patients to consult with physicians remotely (Mouawad et al., 2021). This was a critical action, as it allowed patients to obtain care without burdening hospitals and jeopardizing further exposure to the infection. Telemedicine services were swiftly incorporated into the NHS, providing virtual consultations for many concerns, including mental health assistance and chronic disease management. This transition was especially advantageous in delivering uninterrupted care to patients who may have struggled to access services during lockdowns (Beswick et al., 2004; Jalal, Bardhan, Sanders, & Illing, 2019).

Notwithstanding these endeavors, the NHS's response underscored critical deficiencies within the UK healthcare system, encompassing inadequate budget, workforce shortages, and insufficient pandemic preparedness. The crisis demonstrated the NHS's resilience and capacity to react, successfully vaccinating millions in a brief timeframe via extensive immunization initiatives. Despite the challenges faced by the NHS during the pandemic, its capacity for swift mobilization and resource expansion, exemplified by the rapid establishment of new hospital facilities and the adoption of telemedicine, imparted significant insights for future healthcare readiness (Jalal, Schirwani, & Bardhan, 2021). Although numerous healthcare systems globally faced challenges in service delivery during the COVID-19 epidemic, certain regions devised unique strategies to surmount their constraints. India, with a population over 1.3 billion, encountered significant obstacles in delivering healthcare to its rural populace (Example 2). More than 60% of India's population resides in rural regions, where healthcare access is constrained by distance, inadequate infrastructure, and a deficiency of healthcare personnel (Maniruzzaman et al., 2022).

1.1.4.3 Telemedicine in Rural India

In response to these issues, the Indian government, in collaboration with commercial sector partners, instituted telemedicine programs to enhance healthcare accessibility in remote and underserved regions. Telemedicine has demonstrated significant efficacy in rural India, where access to urban healthcare services is sometimes arduous and costly. Telemedicine enables people in rural regions to consult healthcare specialists remotely, thus minimizing the necessity for extensive travel for medical services (Dash, Aarthy, & Mohan, 2021).

An exemplary telemedicine program in India is eSanjeevani, a platform established by the Ministry of Health and Family Welfare. The technology links patients in rural regions with physicians and specialists in urban centers, facilitating remote consultations through video calls. This method is crucial for mitigating healthcare disparities in remote regions where expert access is restricted (Ramasamy, Mishra, Kannan, Namperumalsamy, & Sen, 2021).

The eSanjeevani portal has been extensively utilized in multiple states, such as Uttar Pradesh, Tamil Nadu, and Himachal Pradesh, and has enabled over 15 million consultations since its launch. Alongside eSanjeevani, numerous more telemedicine programs have been established in partnership with the private sector. Apollo Telemedicine has established a network of telemedicine clinics that offer virtual consultations for patients in isolated regions. Through collaboration with local healthcare providers and pharmacists, these telemedicine programs have successfully broadened healthcare access to some of the most marginalized populations in India (Aneja & Arora, 2021; Peri, Bagchi, & Baveja, 2022).

Figure 1.5 outlines key challenges in India's National Health Policies, including inadequate awareness and health education, which hinder effective healthcare utilization. It also highlights issues such as reduced and unaffordable access to healthcare, financial barriers, uneven distribution of healthcare resources, and insufficient infrastructure and technology. These challenges must be addressed to improve the accessibility and effectiveness of healthcare across the country (Hersh et al., 2001).

1.1.4.4 Impact and Successes

The efficacy of telemedicine in India is shown in its beneficial influence on healthcare provision in rural regions. A research by the WHO indicates that telemedicine

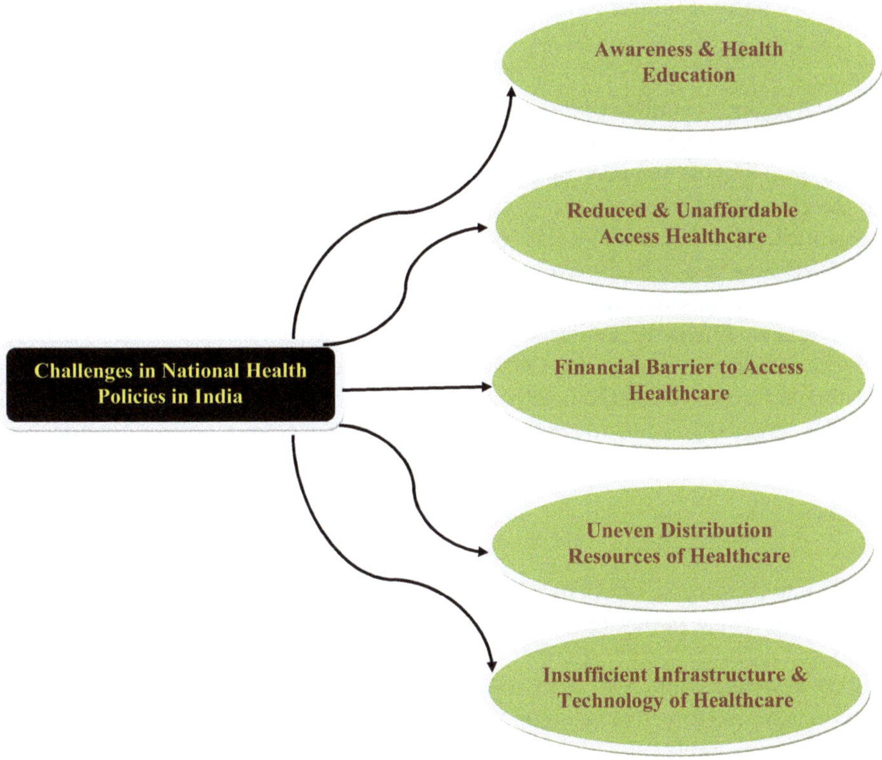

FIGURE 1.5 National health policy in India—challenges.

has alleviated the strain on local healthcare facilities, which frequently face resource limitations and excessive demands. It has enhanced patient outcomes by facilitating access to prompt and specialized care that might otherwise be inaccessible. Telemedicine has significantly enhanced mother and child health in rural India (Venkataraman, Fatma, Edirippulige, & Ramamohan, 2024). Pregnant women in isolated regions can now access prenatal care, consultations, and postnatal follow-up via telemedicine systems. This has resulted in a decrease in maternal and newborn mortality rates in certain places (R. Maqbool et al., 2021a).

Furthermore, telemedicine has been essential in mental healthcare. Mental health practitioners are limited in rural India, and telemedicine has facilitated remote access to counseling and therapy, which has been particularly crucial during the pandemic when mental health demands increased (Marques, Bartuska, Cohen, & Youn, 2020). Furthermore, telemedicine has facilitated the remote monitoring of chronic illnesses, including diabetes and hypertension, by healthcare specialists. This has proven especially beneficial for patients necessitating routine examinations and ongoing care, guaranteeing they do not overlook critical consultations. The Tamil Nadu Telemedicine Project enables diabetic patients in rural regions to remotely monitor their blood sugar levels and communicate the results to their physicians, who offer comments and modify treatment programs accordingly (Nath, Mishra, Padhy, & Ranjan, 2020).

1.1.4.5 Challenges and Future Prospects

Notwithstanding its achievements, numerous obstacles impede the extensive implementation of telemedicine in India. The principal concern is the digital divide; numerous rural regions continue to lack dependable internet connectivity and the requisite infrastructure for high-quality video consultations. Moreover, apprehensions over data privacy and the safeguarding of patient information must be resolved to guarantee the efficacy of telemedicine systems. Furthermore, the efficacy of telemedicine is significantly influenced by the training and competencies of healthcare practitioners (Dubey et al., 2020). To guarantee the efficacy of telemedicine, HCPs must receive comprehensive training in utilizing digital platforms and conducting virtual consultations. Telemedicine has significantly transformed rural healthcare delivery in India, especially during the COVID-19 pandemic. Telemedicine is an essential instrument for narrowing the healthcare gap between urban and rural populations in India by enhancing access to care, minimizing travel expenses, and facilitating more effective resource utilization (Ganapathy et al., 2020).

1.1.5 Strategies for Overcoming Challenges

Addressing the diverse issues in healthcare delivery necessitates a multifaceted strategy encompassing policy reform, technological advancements, financial solutions, workforce assistance, and international collaboration. Each of these measures can address systemic challenges, enhance efficiency, and guarantee fair access to care. We will examine effective solutions to tackle the existing issues in healthcare delivery, offering examples and ideas from various global contexts (Blinder, 2022).

1.1.5.1 Policy Reform

A crucial method to address healthcare delivery difficulties is through policy reform that guarantees expanded access to care. Universal healthcare, which ensures that all residents have access to basic services without experiencing financial distress, is a system implemented by nations such as Canada, France, and the United Kingdom. Enhancing healthcare accessibility via public insurance or nationalized healthcare systems guarantees that financial obstacles do not hinder persons from obtaining essential care. The ACA in the United States sought to enhance healthcare accessibility by broadening Medicaid coverage and establishing health insurance exchanges, so offering more Americans affordable health insurance (Zehravi et al., 2021b). Nonetheless, considerable disparities persist, particularly in states that declined Medicaid expansion. A prospective policy reform may involve extending Medicaid coverage to the remaining states, thus offering a more extensive safety net for low-income individuals (Mouawad et al., 2021).

A crucial element of policy reform is tackling the regional inequities in healthcare access. One approach to remedy this issue is by enhancing mobile health services and telemedicine in underprivileged rural regions. The eSanjeevani telemedicine platform in India enables patients in rural regions to consult with physicians in urban cities, thus mitigating geographical obstacles. Global expansion of such projects, particularly in places such as Africa with restricted healthcare access, can facilitate the provision of medical services to individuals in need (Hersh et al., 2001).

Workforce challenges, such as staffing deficiencies and employee burnout, constitute substantial obstacles to efficient healthcare provision. Policy improvements must tackle these concerns by enhancing working conditions, offering improved compensation, and rewarding employment in underserved regions (Sloan et al., 2014).

Countries such as Norway and Finland have successfully retained HCPs by offering competitive remuneration, facilitating work-life balance, and ensuring continuous professional growth. Moreover, student loan forgiveness initiatives for HCPs serving in underprivileged regions, similar to those implemented in the United States, might be broadened to encourage healthcare practitioners to operate in rural or economically disadvantaged areas. Government measures promoting the equitable allocation of the healthcare personnel can guarantee that marginalized people obtain timely and sufficient care (Oza et al., 2023; Sugand et al., 2024).

1.1.5.2 Technological Innovations

Technological advancements can effectively mitigate obstacles in healthcare delivery. AI is progressively utilized to enhance diagnostics, forecast illness progression, and formulate individualized treatment strategies. AI-driven tools are employed to aid radiologists in detecting abnormalities in medical imaging, such as malignancies or fractures, with enhanced precision and efficiency compared to human doctors alone. This could diminish diagnostic inaccuracies and enhance patient outcomes, particularly in environments with a deficit of qualified medical personnel (Reddy, 2024).

In oncology, AI is currently employed to evaluate extensive datasets from clinical trials, medical records, and genetic testing to offer individualized therapy alternatives depending on an individual's genetic composition. The advancement of tailored therapeutics in oncology, exemplified by treatments for breast and lung cancer, illustrates the transformative impact of AI and genetics on healthcare. These technologies can assist in determining the most efficacious treatments for individual patients, resulting in improved outcomes and reduced unwanted effects (Ayati et al., 2021).

Telemedicine is another technical advancement capable of surmounting obstacles in healthcare delivery. Telemedicine enables healthcare providers to remotely confer with patients, diminishing the necessity for in-person visits, especially for non-emergency matters. This is especially beneficial in rural and underserved regions, where access to healthcare services may be restricted (Gautam et al., 2020; Jones et al., 2012). Throughout the COVID-19 epidemic, telemedicine witnessed substantial expansion as healthcare systems transitioned to distant care to mitigate transmission risk. Teladoc Health, a prominent telemedicine service provider in the United States, reported a 300% surge in telehealth consultations during the epidemic (Brown, 2020).

Africa's mHealth Initiative seeks to deliver remote healthcare services to rural populations through mobile phones. These services encompass consultations, health education, and remote monitoring of chronic illnesses, such as hypertension and diabetes. Telemedicine provides an economical and scalable approach to enhance healthcare accessibility, particularly in areas with inadequate healthcare infrastructure. Governments could enhance telemedicine adoption by providing financial subsidies or incorporating telehealth services into national insurance programs (Venkataraman et al., 2024; Zehravi et al., 2021a).

1.1.5.3 Financial Solutions

Innovative financial solutions are essential to mitigate escalating healthcare costs and ensure sustainability. One strategy is the implementation of public-private partnerships (PPPs), which utilize public resources and private sector experience to enhance healthcare delivery. In nations such as Singapore, PPPs have effectively been employed to augment healthcare infrastructure, including the establishment of hospitals and clinics, and to improve service delivery (Benedetto et al., 2020). Singapore Health Services (SingHealth) partners with commercial enterprises to offer a variety of medical services, encompassing specialized care and testing. This partnership enables the government to concentrate on delivering essential healthcare services, while the private sector enhances the public system by providing superior treatment and advancing medical technologies (Forriol & Vaquero, 2012).

Healthcare systems must investigate novel insurance arrangements to enhance the affordability and accessibility of healthcare. Universal health insurance programs, exemplified by those in Germany and Canada, have demonstrated efficacy in lowering healthcare expenditures while guaranteeing access to essential treatments for all individuals. Nevertheless, numerous countries continue to depend significantly on private insurance systems, thereby depriving poor populations of access to cheap healthcare. A possible answer is the implementation of sliding scale insurance plans, wherein individuals pay rates according to their income. This concept is implemented in nations such as Mexico, where the government's Seguro Popular program offers health insurance to low-income citizens at a subsidized rate. Such solutions can alleviate the financial strain on individuals while maintaining the fiscal sustainability of the healthcare system (McKinney et al., 2024).

1.1.5.4 Workforce Training and Support

An essential technique for addressing workforce difficulties is the enhancement of training, mental health services, and retention initiatives for healthcare personnel. In numerous nations, HCPs encounter substantial mental health issues stemming from elevated stress and burnout levels. Resolving these difficulties is crucial to guarantee that healthcare personnel have adequate support in their roles and can deliver superior care. Countries such as Norway have effectively established mental health support initiatives for HCPs, offering counseling services, stress management training, and an emphasis on work-life balance (da Silva et al., 2023). Furthermore, providing continuing education opportunities and mentorship programs can enhance job satisfaction and diminish turnover rates (Venkataraman et al., 2024).

A vital component of workforce development is the enhancement of medical education and the provision of opportunities for HCPs to specialize in neglected regions. Scholarship programs, such as the U.S. National Health Service Corps, provide financial aid to medical students who commit to serving in underprivileged regions for a specified duration. This concept could be enhanced to incentivize additional HCPs to serve in rural and economically disadvantaged areas (Zehravi et al., 2023a).

1.1.5.5 International Cooperation

Challenges in healthcare delivery transcend borders; international collaboration is crucial for tackling concerns such as pandemics, health disparities, and resource deficiencies. International institutions, such as the WHO, United Nations (UN), and Global Fund, are essential in orchestrating global health programs and offering technical assistance to nations in need. The Global Fund to Fight AIDS, Tuberculosis, and Malaria has effectively mobilized resources to address infectious diseases in low-income nations (Marques et al., 2020). This partnership among governments, NGOs, and private sector entities has preserved millions of lives by facilitating access to essential pharmaceuticals and healthcare services in resource-limited environments (Norcross & Wampold, 2011).

Cross-border collaboration is crucial during health crises, such as the COVID-19 epidemic, where prompt access to information, resources, and expertise is essential. The COVAX effort is a global collaboration designed to guarantee fair access to COVID-19 vaccinations. COVAX has facilitated the delivery of vaccinations to LMICs by consolidating resources and knowledge from governments, pharmaceutical corporations, and international organizations, thereby overcoming limitations in vaccine access (Smith et al., 2021). An additional instance is the European Union's reaction to the refugee crisis, wherein member nations cooperated to deliver healthcare services to displaced individuals. This encompassed the creation of provisional healthcare facilities, mobile clinics, and telemedicine services to assist refugees and migrants (Zehravi et al., 2021b).

Global healthcare standards, such as those established by the WHO, facilitate uniform adherence to fundamental quality benchmarks in healthcare provision across nations (Myhre et al., 2022). These standards can serve as a criterion for enhancing healthcare systems, especially in resource-limited environments. Establishing global standards for vital health services enables countries to collaborate in enhancing the quality and accessibility of healthcare globally (Kadakia et al., 2022).

Figure 1.6 outlines the key factors for a stable healthcare system, including broad strategic perspectives, preventive measures for health promotion, and quality assurance. It also highlights the importance of accountability at both institutional and personal levels, along with addressing environmental concerns. These elements are essential for creating a sustainable and effective healthcare system (Fennell & Flood, 1998).

1.1.6 The Future of Healthcare Delivery

The future of healthcare delivery will be influenced by technological advancements, sustainability issues, and the urgent requirement for global equity as healthcare systems worldwide progress. Advancements in AI, precision medicine, and sophisticated diagnostics will transform healthcare delivery, enhancing personalization, efficiency, and accessibility. Nonetheless, as these technologies progress, the enduring viability of healthcare systems and initiatives to tackle global healthcare inequities will be pivotal in determining the future of healthcare delivery. This section will examine developing trends, evaluate the sustainability of healthcare systems, and consider global initiatives designed to mitigate gaps and foster fair healthcare worldwide (Zehravi et al., 2023b).

The future of healthcare delivery will be profoundly shaped by technological breakthroughs, especially in AI, precision medicine, and sophisticated diagnostics.

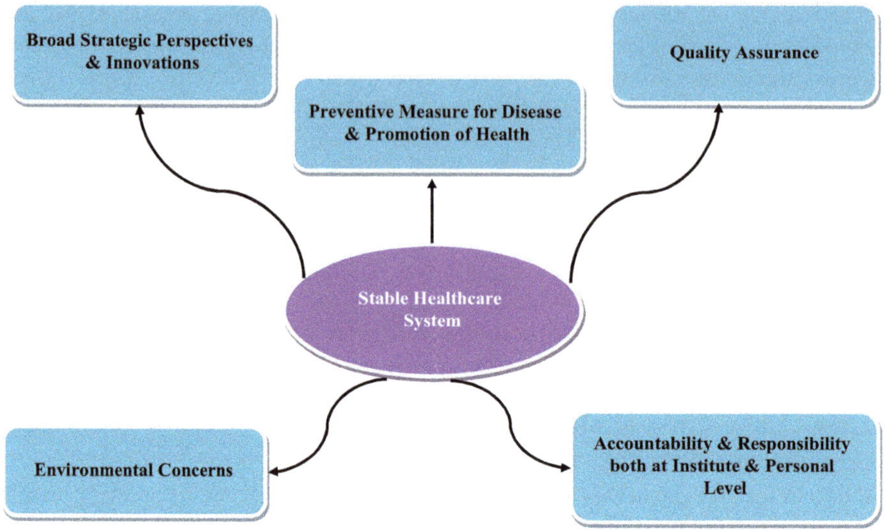

FIGURE 1.6 Sustainable healthcare system.

These advances are currently revolutionizing healthcare procedures and will persist in broadening their scope and influence in the forthcoming decades. AI and machine learning are leading the transformation of healthcare. AI can now analyze extensive datasets to identify patterns that may elude human observation, facilitating swifter and more precise diagnoses (Nath et al., 2020).

AI algorithms are currently employed to evaluate medical pictures, including X-rays and magnetic resonance images, with accuracy levels that are comparable to or above those of radiologists. A prominent instance is the AI system created by Google Health, which can identify breast cancer in mammography with accuracy comparable to that of seasoned radiologists (Wu & Moss, 2023). This technique has the potential to markedly decrease the time and expenses related to identifying intricate diseases, resulting in earlier identification and improved outcomes. In addition to diagnostics, AI is set to improve patient care by forecasting health complications before their occurrence. Through predictive analytics, AI models may evaluate patient data and provide early indicators of prospective illnesses, such as heart disease or diabetes, facilitating proactive treatment and alleviating pressure on healthcare systems (Aneja & Arora, 2021).

AI-driven platforms such as Babylon Health provide consumers virtual health consultations informed by their symptoms and medical history, facilitating prompt guidance without the necessity of an in-person doctor visit. A burgeoning trend is precision medicine, which customizes treatment protocols based on an individual's genetic composition, lifestyle, and environmental influences (O'Sullivan et al., 2017). This tailored strategy seeks to enhance treatment effectiveness and minimize adverse effects by delivering customized treatments informed by patients' genetic profiles. Genetic profiling is currently employed in cancer treatment, allowing medications to be customized according to the unique mutations in a patient's tumor, resulting in more successful interventions. CAR-T cell therapy, an immunotherapeutic approach for specific cancers, exemplifies precision medicine, providing hope to patients with otherwise incurable malignancies (Zeng et al., 2021).

Alongside AI and precision medicine, the future of healthcare delivery will be shaped by sophisticated diagnostics. Wearable health devices and remote monitoring technology provide continuous health tracking for patients. Devices such as smartwatches and fitness trackers may measure vital signs, including heart rate, blood pressure, and blood oxygen levels, in real time. This ongoing surveillance facilitates the prompt identification of possible health concerns, resulting in expedited actions (Dubey et al., 2020). The Apple Watch features an ECG capability, enabling users to monitor their cardiac rhythms and identify indications of atrial fibrillation, a condition that may result in strokes if not addressed. The incorporation of these technologies into everyday life will enhance healthcare accessibility and personalization, enabling individuals to manage their health proactively and fostering a transition from reactive to preventive care. The problem lies in guaranteeing that these advances are accessible to everyone, especially marginalized communities lacking access to advanced technologies (Whiteford, 2017).

1.1.6.1 Sustainability

Although technological improvements provide significant potential for enhancing healthcare delivery, sustainability continues to be a paramount issue for healthcare systems globally. The future of healthcare will hinge on the development of systems that are economically sustainable, environmentally sound, and resilient to forthcoming problems. Financial sustainability represents a significant concern for healthcare systems, especially in LMICs. The escalating expenses of healthcare services, alongside an aging demographic and the rising incidence of chronic illnesses, is exerting considerable strain on healthcare resources. In the United States, healthcare expenditures constitute over 18% of GDP, with projections indicating a growth due to an aging population and rising healthcare demands (Ramasamy et al., 2021).

To achieve long-term financial sustainability, healthcare systems must investigate novel funding mechanisms, including PPPs, pay-for-performance frameworks, and value-based care models. These methodologies emphasize providing value to patients and enhancing health outcomes rather than merely compensating for services done. In Sweden, the government has instituted a pay-for-performance model that incentivizes healthcare providers to offer high-quality care and achieve patient satisfaction objectives. This paradigm promotes efficiency, minimizes waste, and enhances overall healthcare quality (Lamb & Wang, 2020).

Environmental sustainability is an increasingly significant issue in healthcare. The healthcare sector significantly contributes to global carbon emissions due to substantial energy use, waste generation, and reliance on disposable medical products. A research published in *The Lancet* indicates that the global healthcare sector contributes approximately 4.4% of net greenhouse gas emissions. To alleviate this impact, healthcare institutions must implement more sustainable practices, including the utilization of renewable energy sources, waste reduction, and the enhancement of digital record usage to minimize paper consumption (Levesque et al., 2013). The NHS in the United Kingdom has pledged to be the first national health system to attain net-zero carbon emissions by 2040, thereby serving as a model for healthcare systems worldwide to implement ecologically sustainable practices (Beswick et al., 2004).

The sustainability of healthcare systems will ultimately rely on their resistance to crises, including pandemics, natural catastrophes, and economic shocks. The COVID-19 pandemic has demonstrated the necessity for healthcare systems to be flexible and adaptable in response to unforeseen obstacles. Enhancing healthcare infrastructure, optimizing supply chain management, and investing in digital health technologies are critical measures for developing more resilient systems capable of enduring future crises (Gwyther et al., 2019).

1.1.6.2 Global Healthcare Equity

Global healthcare equity represents a critical challenge for the future of healthcare delivery. Healthcare gaps between high-income and low-income nations, as well as within nations, persist in restricting access to care and worsening health outcomes for at-risk groups. The WHO reports that about 50% of the global population still lacks access to vital health services, with sub-Saharan Africa seeing the most significant adverse health effects. International collaboration is a crucial step in attaining global healthcare parity (Ng et al., 2022).

Through the exchange of knowledge, resources, and best practices, nations may collaboratively tackle shared healthcare concerns. Global health efforts such as COVAX, which has played a crucial role in ensuring equitable access to COVID-19 vaccines, show the efficacy of international collaboration. COVAX, spearheaded by the WHO, GAVI, and the Coalition for Epidemic Preparedness Innovations (CEPI), has facilitated the distribution of vaccinations to LMICs, guaranteeing that no nation is excluded in the battle against the pandemic (Ehsan et al., 2023).

Alongside solving global health problems, international collaboration is essential for confronting healthcare disparities. Organizations such as the Global Fund and Doctors Without Borders (MSF) diligently deliver vital healthcare services in resource-limited environments, concentrating on the management of infectious diseases such as HIV/AIDS, malaria, and tuberculosis, which predominantly impact impoverished areas globally. Moreover, global health financing is essential in mitigating healthcare inequities. International aid and development support from nations and entities such as the World Bank and the United Nations have furnished essential financing to enhance healthcare systems in LMICs (Beroukhim et al., 2022).

There is an increasing movement for nations to adopt sustainable funding models that emphasize the development of self-sufficient health systems capable of meeting national healthcare demands independently of foreign assistance. A crucial element of global healthcare fairness is the formulation of worldwide care standards. International efforts to delineate essential health services and establish quality norms can facilitate universal access to fundamental healthcare services for all individuals, irrespective of their location. The WHO's UHC objectives serve as a fundamental foundation for accomplishing this, offering a blueprint for nations to guarantee that health services are available, accessible, and cheap for all individuals (Bayeh, Tsehay, & Negash, 2023; Imperato et al., 2011; Somberg, 2009).

1.1.7 Conclusion

Global healthcare delivery systems are contending with a multitude of intricate and interrelated difficulties, exacerbated by crises such as the COVID-19 pandemic and the persistent threat of climate change. In this chapter we have outlined why hurdles to effective healthcare delivery, including inequitable access, manpower shortages, financial limits, and outmoded technologies, significantly hinder the attainment of UHC. The differences in healthcare access, particularly for marginalized areas, where economic, social, and cultural barriers frequently hinder individuals from obtaining timely and sufficient care have been demonstrated.

The issues are exacerbated by the inadequately funded healthcare systems in LMICs, where fundamental healthcare facilities and medical personnel are frequently lacking. The COVID-19 pandemic highlighted the susceptibility of healthcare systems to abrupt increases in demand, exposing significant deficiencies in preparedness, resource distribution, and coordination.

Moreover, workforce challenges—such as staffing deficiencies, employee burnout, and training inadequacies—have escalated to a critical level in numerous regions globally, especially in high-stress healthcare settings such as hospitals and emergency care facilities. The emigration of proficient HCPs from low-income countries to affluent nations intensifies these issues, resulting in a global disparity in the allocation of healthcare personnel. Retention of healthcare personnel and provision of sufficient mental health assistance, particularly during emergencies, have emerged as urgent priorities for both governments and healthcare organizations.

Financial sustainability continues to be a significant challenge, as escalating healthcare expenditures, resource misallocation, and ineffective insurance schemes exacerbate the disparity in healthcare access. Although several nations have progressed in implementing universal healthcare, others remain mired in disjointed insurance frameworks, rendering care costly for significant portions of the populace. Innovative financial mechanisms, including PPPs, pay-for-performance models, and more fair insurance frameworks, are essential to guarantee that healthcare stays accessible to all.

Notwithstanding these challenges, technological advancements such as AI, precision medicine, and telemedicine provide formidable instruments to revolutionize healthcare delivery. AI is improving diagnostic precision, allowing for early disease identification, and supporting individualized treatment strategies. Telemedicine has demonstrated significant value in accessing rural and underserved people, particularly during the COVID-19 pandemic, and is expected to further enhance its role in regular treatment, mental health services, and chronic disease management. The incorporation of these technologies into healthcare systems necessitates comprehensive steps to tackle data privacy issues, cybersecurity threats, and the digital divide to guarantee fair access to these advancements.

The future of healthcare delivery will rely on technical improvements, thorough policy reforms, and global collaboration. Policymakers must emphasize the development of robust healthcare systems, especially following global health crises. The significance of equitable healthcare policy is paramount—health systems must be structured to deliver complete care for everyone, irrespective of socioeconomic status or geographic location. Moreover, healthcare systems must adjust to the enduring impacts of climate change, guaranteeing their resilience against environmental stressors while maintaining care delivery under adverse situations.

Finally, tackling global healthcare inequities via international collaboration is essential. The COVID-19 pandemic highlighted the necessity for cooperative initiatives to address global health challenges, including the equitable distribution of vaccines via platforms such as COVAX. Comparable international frameworks ought to be developed to mitigate healthcare disparities, enhance cross-border cooperation during health emergencies, and establish universal standards for vital healthcare services. Fundamentally, although the obstacles to healthcare delivery are considerable, they are not insuperable. Investing in innovation, revising legislation, and promoting collaboration can enable the development of healthcare systems that are more robust, inclusive, sustainable, and equitable. The necessity for transformation is evident, and the way forward requires a collaborative endeavor to establish healthcare systems capable of addressing the needs of future generations while ensuring universal access to care.

REFERENCES

Abrams, H. R., Durbin, S., Huang, C. X., Johnson, S. F., Nayak, R. K., Zahner, G. J., & Peppercorn, J. (2021). Financial toxicity in cancer care: Origins, impact, and solutions. *Translational Behavioral Medicine, 11*(11), 2043–2054. doi:10.1093/tbm/ibab091

Adebayo, C. T., Walker, K., Hawkins, M., Olukotun, O., Shaw, L., Sahlstein Parcell, E., … Mkandawire-Valhmu, L. (2020). Race and blackness: A thematic review of communication challenges confronting the black community within the U.S. Health Care System. *Journal of Transcultural Nursing, 31*(4), 397–405. doi:10.1177/1043659619889111

AlJohani, A., Karuppiah, K., Al Mutairi, A., & Al Mutair, A. (2021). Narrative review of infection control knowledge and attitude among healthcare workers. *Journal of Epidemiology and Global Health, 11*(1), 20–25. doi:10.2991/jegh.k.201101.001

Almalki, M., Fitzgerald, G., & Clark, M. (2011). Health care system in Saudi Arabia: An overview. *Eastern Mediterranean Health Journal, 17*(10), 784–793. doi:10.26719/2011.17.10.784

Altaf Dar, M., Maqbool, M., Ara, I., & Zehravi, M. (2023). The intersection of technology and mental health: Enhancing access and care. *International Journal of Adolescent Medicine and Health, 35*(5), 423–428. doi:10.1515/ijamh-2023-0113

Aneja, J., & Arora, S. (2021). Telemedicine and ethics: Opportunities in India. *Indian Journal of Medical Ethics, Vi*(4), 314–320. doi:10.20529/ijme.2021.042

Ayati, N., Afzali, M., Hasanzad, M., Kebriaeezadeh, A., Rajabzadeh, A., & Nikfar, S. (2021). Pharmacogenomics implementation and hurdles to overcome; in the context of a developing country. *Iranian Journal of Pharmaceutical Sciences, 20*(4), 92–106. doi:10.22037/ijpr.2021.114899.15091

Ban, S., Lee, H., Chen, J., Kim, H. S., Hu, Y., Cho, S. J., & Yeo, W. H. (2024). Recent advances in implantable sensors and electronics using printable materials for advanced healthcare. *Biosensors and Bioelectronics, 257*, 116302. doi:10.1016/j.bios.2024.116302

Barry, M. J., & Edgman-Levitan, S. (2012). Shared decision making--pinnacle of patient-centered care. *New England Journal of Medicine, 366*(9), 780–781. doi:10.1056/NEJMp1109283

Bayeh, Y., Tsehay, C. T., & Negash, W. D. (2023). Health system responsiveness and associated factors for delivery care in public health facilities, Dessie City Administration, South Wollo zone, Ethiopia: Cross-sectional study design. *BMJ Open, 13*(7), e069655. doi:10.1136/bmjopen-2022-069655

Benedetto, U., Goodwin, A., Kendall, S., Uppal, R., & Akowuah, E. (2020). A nationwide survey of UK cardiac surgeons' view on clinical decision making during the coronavirus disease 2019 (COVID-19) pandemic. *Journal of Thoracic and Cardiovascular Surgery, 160*(4), 968–973. doi:10.1016/j.jtcvs.2020.05.016

Beroukhim, G., Mahabamunuge, J., & Pal, L. (2022). Racial disparities in access to reproductive health and fertility care in the United States. *Current Opinion in Obstetrics and Gynecology, 34*(3), 138–146. doi:10.1097/gco.0000000000000780

Beswick, A. D., Rees, K., Griebsch, I., Taylor, F. C., Burke, M., West, R. R., … Ebrahim, S. (2004). Provision, uptake and cost of cardiac rehabilitation programmes: Improving services to under-represented groups. *Health Technology Assessment, 8*(41), iii–iv, ix–x, 1–152. doi:10.3310/hta8410

Blinder, V. S. (2022). Pain, financial hardship, and employment in cancer survivors. *Journal of Clinical Oncology, 40*(1), 1–4. doi:10.1200/jco.21.01812

Bogler, O., Liu, J., Cadesky, B., & Bell, C. M. (2021). Quality of care and outcomes in internal medicine patients bedspaced to noninternal medicine units. *Medicine (Baltimore), 100*(18), e25737. doi:10.1097/md.0000000000025737

Bowling, A., & Bond, M. (2001). A national evaluation of specialists' clinics in primary care settings. *British Journal of General Practice, 51*(465), 264–269.

Brown, A. (2020). Communication and leadership in healthcare quality governance. *Journal of Health Organization and Management, 34*(2), 144–161. doi:10.1108/jhom-07-2019-0194

Burkle, F. M., Bradt, D. A., Green, J., & Ryan, B. J. (2021). Global public health database support to population-based management of pandemics and global public health crises, Part II: The database. *Prehospital and Disaster Medicine, 36*(1), 105–110. doi:10.1017/s1049023x20001363

Burkle, F. M., Bradt, D. A., & Ryan, B. J. (2021). Global public health database support to population-based management of pandemics and global public health crises, Part I: The concept. *Prehospital and Disaster Medicine, 36*(1), 95–104. doi:10.1017/s1049023x20001351

Cai, W., Gao, R., Jing, Q., Wang, C., Hou, N., Liu, W., … Sun, X. (2022). Doctor of public health-crisis management and COVID-19 prevention and control: A case study in China. *Frontiers in Public Health, 10*, 814632. doi:10.3389/fpubh.2022.814632

Carbone, R., Ferrari, S., Callegarin, S., Casotti, F., Turina, L., Artioli, G., & Bonacaro, A. (2022). Peer support between healthcare workers in hospital and out-of-hospital settings: A scoping review. *Acta Bio-Medica: Atenei Parmensis, 93*(5), e2022308. doi:10.23750/abm.v93i5.13729

Choi, S. (2023). Enhancing nursing education to bolster nurse governance: Insights from nurse managers. *Frontiers in Medicine (Lausanne), 10*, 1254428. doi:10.3389/fmed.2023.1254428

Chung, C., McKenna, L., & Cooper, S. J. (2020). Patients' experiences of acute deterioration: A scoping review. *International Journal of Nursing Studies, 101*, 103404. doi:10.1016/j.ijnurstu.2019.103404

Correia, T., & Willis, K. (2022). Applying critical realism to the COVID-19 pandemic to improve management of future public health crises. *International Journal of Health Planning and Management, 37*(2), 599–603. doi:10.1002/hpm.3376

Dar, M. A., Maqbool, M., & Ara, I. (2023). The PCOS puzzle: Putting the pieces together for optimal care. *International Journal of Adolescent Medicine and Health, 35*(4), 299–311. doi:10.1515/ijamh-2023-0102

da Silva, P. R., Jr., Porto, P., Rocha, M. C., Tamaki, E. R., Corrêa, M. G., Fernandez, M., … Pimenta, D. N. (2023). Women and working in healthcare during the Covid-19 pandemic in Brazil: Bullying of colleagues. *Global Health, 19*(1), 10. doi:10.1186/s12992-023-00911-2

Dash, S., Aarthy, R., & Mohan, V. (2021). Telemedicine during COVID-19 in India-a new policy and its challenges. *Journal of Public Health Policy, 42*(3), 501–509. doi:10.1057/s41271-021-00287-w

Dennett, E. J., Janjua, S., Stovold, E., Harrison, S. L., McDonnell, M. J., & Holland, A. E. (2021). Tailored or adapted interventions for adults with chronic obstructive pulmonary disease and at least one other long-term condition: A mixed methods review. *Cochrane Database of Systematic Reviews, 7*(7), Cd013384. doi:10.1002/14651858.CD013384.pub2

Dubey, S., Biswas, P., Ghosh, R., Chatterjee, S., Dubey, M. J., Chatterjee, S., … Lavie, C. J. (2020). Psychosocial impact of COVID-19. *Diabetes & Metabolic Syndrome, 14*(5), 779–788. doi:10.1016/j.dsx.2020.05.035

Ehsan, A. N., Wu, C. A., Minasian, A., Singh, T., Bass, M., Pace, L., … Ranganathan, K. (2023). Financial toxicity among patients with breast cancer worldwide: A systematic review and meta-analysis. *JAMA Network Open, 6*(2), e2255388. doi:10.1001/jamanetworkopen.2022.55388

Eisman, A. B., Kim, B., Salloum, R. G., Shuman, C. J., & Glasgow, R. E. (2022). Advancing rapid adaptation for urgent public health crises: Using implementation science to facilitate effective and efficient responses. *Frontiers in Public Health, 10*, 959567. doi:10.3389/fpubh.2022.959567

Fennell, M. L., & Flood, A. B. (1998). Key challenges in studying organizational issues in the delivery of healthcare to older Americans. *Health Services Research, 33*(2 Pt Ii), 424–433.

Forriol, F., & Vaquero, J. (2012). The Spanish health care system: Issues and challenges. *Injury, 43*(Suppl 2), S1–S2. doi:10.1016/s0020-1383(13)70171-2

Franco, C. M., Lima, J. G., & Giovanella, L. (2021). Primary healthcare in rural areas: Access, organization, and health workforce in an integrative literature review. *Cadernos de Saúde Publica, 37*(7), e00310520. doi:10.1590/0102-311x00310520

Ganapathy, K., Nukala, L., Premanand, S., Tamilmaran, P., Aggarwal, P., Saksena, S., & BrindhaDevi, S. P. (2020). Telemedicine in camp mode while screening for noncommunicable diseases: A preliminary report from India. *Telemedicine Journal and e-Health, 26*(1), 42–50. doi:10.1089/tmj.2018.0300

Garnelo, L., Parente, R. C. P., Puchiarelli, M. L. R., Correia, P. C., Torres, M. V., & Herkrath, F. J. (2020). Barriers to access and organization of primary health care services for rural riverside populations in the Amazon. *International Journal for Equity in Health, 19*(1), 54. doi:10.1186/s12939-020-01171-x

Gautam, M., Thakrar, A., Akinyemi, E., & Mahr, G. (2020). Current and future challenges in the delivery of mental healthcare during COVID-19. *SN Comprehensive Clinical Medicine, 2*(7), 865–870. doi:10.1007/s42399-020-00348-3

Gola, M., Brambilla, A., Barach, P., Signorelli, C., & Capolongo, S. (2020). Educational challenges in healthcare design: Training multidisciplinary professionals for future hospitals and healthcare. *Annali di Igiene, 32*(5), 549–566. doi:10.7416/ai.2020.2375

Gruen, R. L., Weeramanthri, T. S., Knight, S. E., & Bailie, R. S. (2004). Specialist outreach clinics in primary care and rural hospital settings. *Cochrane Database of Systematic Reviews,* 2003(1), Cd003798. doi:10.1002/14651858.CD003798.pub2

Guttman, O. T., Lazzara, E. H., Keebler, J. R., Webster, K. L. W., Gisick, L. M., & Baker, A. L. (2021). Dissecting communication barriers in healthcare: A path to enhancing communication resiliency, reliability, and patient safety. *Journal of Patient Safety, 17*(8), e1465–e1471. doi:10.1097/pts.0000000000000541

Gwyther, H., van Velsen, L., Shaw, R. L., D'Avanzo, B., Bujnowska-Fedak, M., Kurpas, D., … Holland, C. (2019). The use of technology in the context of frailty screening and management interventions: A study of stakeholders' perspectives. *BMC Medical Informatics and Decision Making, 19*(1), 110. doi:10.1186/s12911-019-0828-6

Ham, C. (2020a). The challenges facing the NHS in England in 2021. *BMJ, 371*, m4973. doi:10.1136/bmj.m4973

Hayoun, Y., & Gannot, I. (2025). Healthcare delivery in the arctic-telehealth prospects. *InternationalJournalofCircumpolarHealth,84*(1),2438429.doi:10.1080/22423982.2024.2438429

Henneker, K. E., & Reed, K. (2012). Knowing the people planning: Measuring change in mental health services. *Australian Health Review, 36*(2), 213–217. doi:10.1071/ah10871

Hersh, W. R., Wallace, J. A., Patterson, P. K., Shapiro, S. E., Kraemer, D. F., Eilers, G. M., … Helfand, M. (2001). Telemedicine for the Medicare population: Pediatric, obstetric, and clinician-indirect home interventions. *Evidence Report/Technology Assessment, 2001* (24 Suppl), 1–32.

Imperato, P. J., LaRosa, J. H., Kavaler, F., Benker, K., & Schechter, L. (2011). The establishment of the School of Public Health at the State University of New York, Downstate Medical Center: The first nationally accredited school of public health in a public university in New York City. *Journal of Community Health, 36*(1), 1–13. doi:10.1007/s10900-010-9330-x

Jalal, M., Bardhan, K. D., Sanders, D., & Illing, J. (2019). International: Overseas doctors of the NHS: Migration, transition, challenges and towards resolution. *Future Healthcare Journal, 6*(1), 76–81. doi:10.7861/futurehosp.6-1-76

Jalal, M., Schirwani, S., & Bardhan, K. D. (2021). The imbalance in medico-legal cover awareness and uptake between overseas junior doctors and local graduates in the NHS. *Cureus, 13*(2), e13336. doi:10.7759/cureus.13336

James, L., McPhail, H., Foisey, L., Donelle, L., Bauer, M., & Kothari, A. (2023). Exploring communication by public health leaders and organizations during the pandemic: A content analysis of COVID-related tweets. *Canadian Journal of Public Health. Revue Canadienne de Santé Publique, 114*(4), 563–583. doi:10.17269/s41997-023-00783-4

Johnson, D., Cahill, M., Choate, S., Roelfs, D., & Walsh, S. E. (2021). The Influence of public health faculty on college and university plans during the COVID-19 pandemic. *Frontiers Public Health, 9*, 745232. doi:10.3389/fpubh.2021.745232

Johnson, K. B., Wei, W. Q., Weeraratne, D., Frisse, M. E., Misulis, K., Rhee, K., … Snowdon, J. L. (2021). Precision medicine, AI, and the future of personalized health care. *Clinical and Translational Science, 14*(1), 86–93. doi:10.1111/cts.12884

Jones, P., Chalmers, L., Wells, S., Ameratunga, S., Carswell, P., Ashton, T., … Tenbensel, T. (2012). Implementing performance improvement in New Zealand emergency departments: The six hour time target policy national research project protocol. *BMC Health Services Research, 12*, 45. doi:10.1186/1472-6963-12-45

Kadakia, A., Catillon, M., Fan, Q., Williams, G. R., Marden, J. R., Anderson, A., … Dembek, C. (2022). The economic burden of schizophrenia in the United States. *Journal of Clinical Psychiatry, 83*(6). doi:10.4088/JCP.22m14458

Kamel Boulos, M. N., Wilson, J. T., & Clauson, K. A. (2018). Geospatial blockchain: Promises, challenges, and scenarios in health and healthcare. *International Journal of Health Geographics, 17*(1), 25. doi:10.1186/s12942-018-0144-x

Kelly, K. (1985). Nurse practitioner challenges to the orthodox structure of health care delivery: Regulation and restraints on trade. *American Journal of Law and Medicine, 11*(2), 195–225.

Khan, Y., Hussain, M. S., Ramalingam, P. S., Fatima, R., Maqbool, M., Ashique, S., … Gupta, G. (2025). Exploring extracellular RNA as drivers of chemotherapy resistance in cancer. *Molecular Biology Reports, 52*(1), 142. doi:10.1007/s11033-025-10263-2

Kurpas, D., Gwyther, H., Szwamel, K., Shaw, R. L., D'Avanzo, B., Holland, C. A., & Bujnowska-Fedak, M. M. (2018). Patient-centred access to health care: A framework analysis of the care interface for frail older adults. *BMC Geriatrics, 18*(1), 273. doi:10.1186/s12877-018-0960-7

Lamb, C. C., & Wang, Y. (2020). Physician characteristics that influence patient participation in the treatment of primary immunodeficiency. *Patient Education and Counseling, 103*(11), 2280–2289. doi:10.1016/j.pec.2020.05.021

Leightley, D., & Murphy, D. (2023). Personalised digital technology for mental health in the armed forces: The potential, the hype and the dangers. *BMJ Military Health, 169*(1), 406–408. doi:10.1136/military-2022-002279

Levesque, J. F., Harris, M. F., & Russell, G. (2013). Patient-centred access to health care: Conceptualising access at the interface of health systems and populations. *International Journal for Equity in Health, 12*, 18. doi:10.1186/1475-9276-12-18

Longo, C. J., Fitch, M. I., Banfield, L., Hanly, P., Yabroff, K. R., & Sharp, L. (2020). Financial toxicity associated with a cancer diagnosis in publicly funded healthcare countries: A systematic review. *Supportive Care in Cancer, 28*(10), 4645–4665. doi:10.1007/s00520-020-05620-9

Malik, M., Prescott, K., Khalid, M., Hashmi, A., & Kiani, A. (2021). Expectations and experiences of women regarding maternal healthcare services in Pakistan: Challenges and lessons to be learnt. *Journal of Pharmaceutical Policy and Practice, 14*(1), 108. doi:10.1186/s40545-021-00392-x

Maniruzzaman, M., Islam, M. M., Ali, M. H., Mukerjee, N., Maitra, S., Kamal, M. A., … Rahman, M. H. (2022). COVID-19 diagnostic methods in developing countries. *Environmental Science and Pollution Research International, 29*(34), 51384–51397. doi:10.1007/s11356-022-21041-z

Maqbool, M., Bekele, F., & Fekadu, G. (2022). Treatment strategies against triple-negative breast cancer: An updated review. *Breast Cancer (Dove Medical Press), 14*, 15–24. doi:10.2147/bctt.S348060

Maqbool, M., Fekadu, G., Jiang, X., Bekele, F., Tolossa, T., Turi, E., … Fanta, K. (2021). An up to date on clinical prospects and management of osteoarthritis. *Annals of Medicine and Surgery (London), 72*, 103077. doi:10.1016/j.amsu.2021.103077

Maqbool, R., Maqbool, M., Zehravi, M., & Ara, I. (2021a). Acute neurological conditions during pregnancy and their management: A review. *International Journal of Adolescent Medicine and Health, 33*(6), 357–366. doi:10.1515/ijamh-2021-0084

Maqbool, R., Maqbool, M., Zehravi, M., & Ara, I. (2021b). Menstrual distress in females of reproductive age: A literature review. *International Journal of Adolescent Medicine and Health, 34*(2), 11–17. doi:10.1515/ijamh-2021-0081

Marques, L., Bartuska, A. D., Cohen, J. N., & Youn, S. J. (2020). Three steps to flatten the mental health need curve amid the COVID-19 pandemic. *Depression and Anxiety, 37*(5), 405–406. doi:10.1002/da.23031

McKinney, J., Kelm, N., Windsor, B., & Keyser, L. E. (2024). Addressing health care access disparities through a public health approach to physical therapist practice. *Physical Therapy, 104*(10). doi:10.1093/ptj/pzae136

Mefford, M. T., Li, B. H., Qian, L., Reading, S. R., Harrison, T. N., Scott, R. D., … Reynolds, K. (2020). Sex-specific trends in acute myocardial infarction within an integrated healthcare network, 2000 through 2014. *Circulation, 141*(7), 509–519. doi:10.1161/circulationaha.119.044738

Mefford, M. T., Zhuang, Z., Liang, Z., Chen, W., Koyama, S. Y., Taitano, M. T., … Reynolds, K. (2021). Temporal trends in heart failure mortality in an integrated healthcare delivery system, California, and the US, 2001–2017. *BMC Cardiovascular Disorders, 21*(1), 261. doi:10.1186/s12872-021-02075-6

Merner, B., Schonfeld, L., Virgona, A., Lowe, D., Walsh, L., Wardrope, C., … Hill, S. (2023). Consumers' and health providers' views and perceptions of partnering to improve health services design, delivery and evaluation: A co-produced qualitative evidence synthesis. *Cochrane Database of Systematic Reviews, 3*(3), Cd013274. doi:10.1002/14651858.CD013274.pub2

Mitton, C., Dionne, F., Masucci, L., Wong, S., & Law, S. (2011). Innovations in health service organization and delivery in northern rural and remote regions: A review of the literature. *International Journal of Circumpolar Health, 70*(5), 460–472. doi:10.3402/ijch.v70i5.17859

Mouawad, N. J., Woo, K., Malgor, R. D., Wohlauer, M. V., Johnson, A. P., Cuff, R. F., … Shalhub, S. (2021). The impact of the COVID-19 pandemic on vascular surgery practice in the United States. *Journal of Vascular Surgery, 73*(3), 772–779.e774. doi:10.1016/j.jvs.2020.08.036

Mubin, N., Bin Abdul Baten, R., Jahan, S., Zohora, F. T., Chowdhury, N. M., & Faruque, G. M. (2021). Cancer related knowledge, attitude, and practice among community health care providers and health assistants in rural Bangladesh. *BMC Health Services Research, 21*(1), 191. doi:10.1186/s12913-021-06202-z

Myhre, S., Habtemariam, M. K., Heymann, D. L., Ottersen, T., Stoltenberg, C., Ventura, D. F. L., … Bergh, A. (2022). Bridging global health actors and agendas: The role of national public health institutes. *Journal of Public Health Policy, 43*(2), 251–265. doi:10.1057/s41271-022-00342-0

Nandhra, S., & Benson, R. A. (2022). The persistent challenges faced by vascular surgery services during the UK coronavirus pandemic: A snapshot qualitative survey. *Annals of the Royal College of Surgeons of England, 104*(5), 385–388. doi:10.1308/rcsann.2021.0202

Nath, S., Mishra, B. R., Padhy, S. K., & Ranjan, R. (2020). Meeting the unmet mental health needs during COVID-19: Where does telemedicine stands during these times in India? *Psychiatria Danubina, 32*(3–4), 594–595.

Ng, J. Y., Kim, M., & Suri, A. (2022). Exploration of facilitators and barriers to the regulatory frameworks of dietary and herbal supplements: A scoping review. *Journal of Pharmaceutical Policy and Practice, 15*(1), 55. doi:10.1186/s40545-022-00447-7

Norcross, J. C., & Wampold, B. E. (2011). Evidence-based therapy relationships: Research conclusions and clinical practices. *Psychotherapy (Chic), 48*(1), 98–102. doi:10.1037/a0022161

Northridge, M. E., Kumar, A., & Kaur, R. (2020). Disparities in access to oral health care. *Annual Review of Public Health, 41*, 513–535. doi:10.1146/annurev-publhealth-040119-094318

O'Sullivan, B., McGrail, M., & Russell, D. (2017). Rural specialists: The nature of their work and professional satisfaction by geographical location of work. *Australian Journal of Rural Health, 25*(6), 338–346. doi:10.1111/ajr.12354

Ostini, R., McGrail, M. R., Kondalsamy-Chennakesavan, S., Hill, P., O'Sullivan, B., Selvey, L. A., … Strasser, S. (2021). Building a sustainable rural physician workforce. *Medical Journal of Australia, 215*(Suppl 1), S5–s33. doi:10.5694/mja2.51122

Oza, S., Chen, F., Selser, V., Clougherty, M. M., Dale, K. D., Iberg Johnson, J., … Bourdeaux, M. (2023). Community-based outbreak investigation and response: Enhancing preparedness, public health capacity, and equity. *Health Affairs, 42*(3), 349–356. doi:10.1377/hlthaff.2022.01257

Pastorino, R., De Vito, C., Migliara, G., Glocker, K., Binenbaum, I., Ricciardi, W., & Boccia, S. (2019). Benefits and challenges of Big Data in healthcare: An overview of the European initiatives. *European Journal of Public Health, 29*(Supplement_3), 23–27. doi:10.1093/eurpub/ckz168

Peri, S. S., Bagchi, A. D., & Baveja, A. (2022). A systematic review of the effectiveness of telemedicine in reproductive and neonatal health in rural and low-income areas in India. *Telemedicine Journal and e-Health, 28*(9), 1251–1260. doi:10.1089/tmj.2021.0481

Peters, G. M., Kooij, L., Lenferink, A., van Harten, W. H., & Doggen, C. J. M. (2021). The effect of telehealth on hospital services use: Systematic review and meta-analysis. *Journal of Medical Internet Research, 23*(9), e25195. doi:10.2196/25195

Prince, M. A. (2023). The nation's promise of care. *Professional Case Management, 28*(3), 95–97. doi:10.1097/ncm.0000000000000648

Priyanka, T. R., Kumar, S., & Kamaraj, R. (2024). A comparative analysis of the regulatory framework and collaborative environment for pediatric medical device development in Japan and the United States: Identifying challenges, support mechanisms, and emerging opportunities. *Cureus, 16*(9), e68583. doi:10.7759/cureus.68583

Purkey, E., & MacKenzie, M. (2019). Experience of healthcare among the homeless and vulnerably housed a qualitative study: Opportunities for equity-oriented health care. *International Journal for Equity in Health, 18*(1), 101. doi:10.1186/s12939-019-1004-4

Ramasamy, K., Mishra, C., Kannan, N. B., Namperumalsamy, P., & Sen, S. (2021). Telemedicine in diabetic retinopathy screening in India. *Indian Journal of Ophthalmology, 69*(11), 2977–2986. doi:10.4103/ijo.IJO_1442_21

Reddy, S. (2024). Generative AI in healthcare: An implementation science informed translational path on application, integration and governance. *Implementation Science, 19*(1), 27. doi:10.1186/s13012-024-01357-9

Rubel, A. J., & Garro, L. C. (1992). Social and cultural factors in the successful control of tuberculosis. *Public Health Reports, 107*(6), 626–636.

Sangaleti, C., Schveitzer, M. C., Peduzzi, M., Zoboli, E., & Soares, C. B. (2017). Experiences and shared meaning of teamwork and interprofessional collaboration among health care professionals in primary health care settings: A systematic review. *JBI Database of Systematic Reviews and Implementation Reports, 15*(11), 2723–2788. doi:10.11124/jbisrir-2016-003016

Shinfuku, N. (1998). Mental health services in Asia: International perspective and challenge for the coming years. *Psychiatry and Clinical Neurosciences, 52*(3), 269–274. doi:10.1046/j.1440-1819.1998.00400.x

Sloan, T., Fitzgerald, A., Hayes, K. J., Radnor, Z., Robinson, S., & Sohal, A. (2014). Lean in healthcare-- history and recent developments. *Journal of Health Organization and Management, 28*(2), 130–134. doi:10.1108/jhom-04-2014-0064

Smith, G. L., Banegas, M. P., Acquati, C., Chang, S., Chino, F., Conti, R. M., … Yabroff, K. R. (2022). Navigating financial toxicity in patients with cancer: A multidisciplinary management approach. *CA: A Cancer Journal for Clinicians, 72*(5), 437–453. doi:10.3322/caac.21730

Smith, G. L., Mendoza, T. R., Lowenstein, L. M., & Shih, Y. T. (2021). Financial hardship in survivorship care delivery. *Journal of the National Cancer Institute. Monographs, 2021*(57), 10–14. doi:10.1093/jncimonographs/lgaa012

Sohal, T., Sohal, P., King-Shier, K. M., & Khan, N. A. (2015). Barriers and facilitators for type-2 diabetes management in south Asians: A systematic review. *PLoS ONE, 10*(9), e0136202. doi:10.1371/journal.pone.0136202

Somberg, J. (2009). Health care reform. *American Journal of Therapeutics, 16*(4), 281–282. doi:10.1097/MJT.0b013e3181b3a331

St Clair, N. E., Pitt, M. B., Bakeera-Kitaka, S., McCall, N., Lukolyo, H., Arnold, L. D., … Butteris, S. (2017). Global health: Preparation for working in resource-limited settings. *Pediatrics, 140*(5). doi:10.1542/peds.2016-3783

Sugand, K., Park, C., Aframian, A., Gupte, C. M., & Sarraf, K. M. (2024). Policy and practice review consensus statements and clinical guidelines on managing pediatric trauma and orthopedics during the COVID-19 pandemic: A systematic review on the global response for future pandemics and public health crises. *Frontiers in Pediatrics, 12*, 1453574. doi:10.3389/fped.2024.1453574

Sun, S., Chen, J., Li, H., Lou, Y., Chen, L., & Lv, B. (2023). Patients' perspectives on irritable bowel syndrome: A qualitative analysis based on social media in China. *Quality of Life Research, 32*(9), 2561–2571. doi:10.1007/s11136-023-03417-x

Sweet, M. A., Williams, M., Armstrong, R., Mohamed, J., Finlay, S. M., & Coopes, A. (2020). Converging crises: Public interest journalism, the pandemic and public health. *Public Health Research and Practice, 30*(4). doi:10.17061/phrp3042029

Talati, A. N., Lappen, J. R., Bondurant-Sullivan, A., Cossler, N. J., Wieczorek, M., & Gecsi, K. S. (2018). Starting health disparities education during resident orientation: Our patients, our community. *Obstetrics and Gynecology, 132*(5), 1153–1157. doi:10.1097/aog.0000000000002911

Tepper, M. C., Ward, M. C., Aldis, R., Lanca, M., Wang, P. S., & Fulwiler, C. E. (2022). Toward population health: Using a learning behavioral health system and measurement-based care to improve access, care, outcomes, and disparities. *Community Mental Health Journal, 58*(8), 1428–1436. doi:10.1007/s10597-022-00957-3

Terkola, R., Antoñanzas, F., & Postma, M. (2019). Stakeholder opinions on value in healthcare. *European Journal of Hospital Pharmacy, 26*(2), 79–84. doi:10.1136/ejhpharm-2017-001295

Tran, C. L., Ehrmann, B. J., Messer, K. L., Herreshoff, E., Kroeker, A., Wickman, L., … Gipson, D. S. (2012). Recent trends in healthcare utilization among children and adolescents with hypertension in the United States. *Hypertension, 60*(2), 296–302. doi:10.1161/hypertensionaha.111.188813

Van Nguyen, H., Lan Nguyen, H., Thi Minh Dao, A., Van Nguyen, T., The Nguyen, P., Mai Le, P., … Debattista, J. (2022). The COVID-19 pandemic in Australia: Public health responses, opportunities and challenges. *International Journal of Health Planning and Management, 37*(1), 5–13. doi:10.1002/hpm.3326

Venkataraman, A., Fatma, N., Edirippulige, S., & Ramamohan, V. (2024). Facilitators and barriers for telemedicine systems in India from multiple stakeholder perspectives and settings: A systematic review. *Telemedicine Journal and e-Health, 30*(5), 1341–1356. doi:10.1089/tmj.2023.0297

von Gerich, H., Moen, H., Block, L. J., Chu, C. H., DeForest, H., Hobensack, M., … Peltonen, L. M. (2022). Artificial Intelligence -based technologies in nursing: A scoping literature review of the evidence. *International Journal of Nursing Studies, 127*, 104153. doi:10.1016/j.ijnurstu.2021.104153

Voumard, R., Rubli Truchard, E., Benaroyo, L., Borasio, G. D., Büla, C., & Jox, R. J. (2018). Geriatric palliative care: A view of its concept, challenges and strategies. *BMC Geriatrics, 18*(1), 220. doi:10.1186/s12877-018-0914-0

Wang, C., Rao, K., Wu, S., & Liu, Q. (2013). Health care in China: Improvement, challenges, and reform. *Chest, 143*(2), 524–531. doi:10.1378/chest.12-1839

Waterson, P. (2021). Promoting systemic incident analysis in healthcare-key challenges and ways forwards. *International Journal for Quality in Health Care, 33*(4). doi:10.1093/intqhc/mzab139

Watson, D. P., Staton, M. D., Grella, C. E., Scott, C. K., & Dennis, M. L. (2022). Navigating intersecting public health crises: A qualitative study of people with opioid use disorders' experiences during the COVID-19 pandemic. *Substance Abuse Treatment, Prevention, and Policy, 17*(1), 22. doi:10.1186/s13011-022-00449-3

White, E. M., Kosar, C. M., Rahman, M., & Mor, V. (2020). Trends in hospitals and skilled nursing facilities sharing medical providers, 2008–16. *Health Affairs, 39*(8), 1312–1320. doi:10.1377/hlthaff.2019.01502

Whiteford, H. (2017). Mental health services research in Australia. *Australian and New Zealand Journal of Psychiatry, 51*(11), 1075–1076. doi:10.1177/0004867417738413

Wu, J., & Moss, H. (2023). Financial toxicity in the post-health reform era. *Journal of the American College of Radiology, 20*(1), 10–17. doi:10.1016/j.jacr.2022.09.036

Xie, Y., Lu, L., Gao, F., He, S. J., Zhao, H. J., Fang, Y., … Dong, Z. (2021). Integration of artificial intelligence, blockchain, and wearable technology for chronic disease management: A new paradigm in smart healthcare. *Current Medical Science, 41*(6), 1123–1133. doi:10.1007/s11596-021-2485-0

Zehravi, M., Maqbool, M., & Ara, I. (2021a). Correlation between obesity, gestational diabetes mellitus, and pregnancy outcomes: An overview. *International Journal of Adolescent Medicine and Health, 33*(6), 339–345. doi:10.1515/ijamh-2021-0058

Zehravi, M., Maqbool, M., & Ara, I. (2021b). Polycystic ovary syndrome and infertility: An update. *International Journal of Adolescent Medicine and Health, 34*(2), 1–9. doi:10.1515/ijamh-2021-0073

Zehravi, M., Maqbool, M., & Ara, I. (2023a). Teenage menstrual dysfunction: An overview. *International Journal of Adolescent Medicine and Health, 35*(1), 15–19. doi:10.1515/ijamh-2022-0018

Zehravi, M., Maqbool, M., & Ara, I. (2023b). Unfolding the mystery of premenstrual syndrome (PMS): An overview. *International Journal of Adolescent Medicine and Health, 35*(1), 9–13. doi:10.1515/ijamh-2022-0023

Zeng, Q., Li, N., Pan, X. F., Chen, L., & Pan, A. (2021). Clinical management and treatment of obesity in China. *Lancet Diabetes Endocrinology, 9*(6), 393–405. doi:10.1016/s2213-8587(21)00047-4

Zhao, X., Liu, L., Hu, C., Chen, F., & Sun, X. (2017). Necessity and feasibility of improving mental health services in China: A systematic qualitative review. *International Journal of Health Planning and Management, 32*(3), 363–371. doi:10.1002/hpm.2437

2 Healthcare Innovation as a Complex Adaptive System

Tasnia Nabil and Julia Aman

2.1 INTRODUCTION

Imagine a flock of birds swooping and swirling through the sky in perfect harmony. There is no leader dictating their path, yet the flock moves as one, adapting in real time to changes in directions or threats from predators. This mesmerizing dance is a glimpse into the world of Complex Adaptive Systems (CASs). A CAS is like a living, breathing ecosystem with a network of diverse agents—whether it be birds in flight, cells in a body, or stakeholders in a healthcare system—that interact with each other and adapt to their environment based on feedback and external conditions. These interactions are not linear or predictable; instead, they give rise to new patterns and behaviors that cannot be understood by examining the individual components alone (Holland, 2006).

In a CAS, the whole is greater than the sum of its parts. Take an ant colony for example—each ant is an agent that operates based on local information and simple rules, like following pheromone trails or responding to environmental cues. There is no central command dictating the colony's actions, yet collectively, ants construct intricate nests, efficiently forage for food, and defend their colony against threats. This emergent intelligence arises from the interactions among individual ants, illustrating how complex behaviors can develop from simple components (Mitchell, 2009). Similarly, in complex systems like healthcare, the interactions of various stakeholders—patients, providers, and administrators—lead to outcomes and patterns that cannot be predicted by looking at any part of the system.

Understanding CAS requires embracing complexity and uncertainty, looking beyond simple solutions and investigating the intricate web of interactions that drive system-wide behavior. The innovation pipeline can be considered a CAS, as there are many factors that need to be considered as a system for implementation in healthcare. This perspective encourages interdisciplinary collaboration across medical, engineering, social and policy fields, breaking down silos that hinder progress.

2.1.1 Healthcare as a CAS

A healthcare system is much like a rainforest—an intricate ecosystem where countless species of plants, animals, fungi, and microorganisms coexist, compete, and collaborate in an ever-changing environment. The removal of one species can ripple

DOI: 10.1201/9781003513834-2

through the ecosystem, affecting others in unexpected ways. Similarly, within a hospital, diverse agents—from doctors treating patients to those handling the procurement of medical supplies and insurance reimbursements—interact dynamically to keep the system afloat. A seemingly small policy change can reverberate throughout the system, reshaping the culture of care.

At the core of healthcare's complexity lies a vast network of interconnected agents, including patients, healthcare providers, policymakers, technology innovators, and social determinants of health. These agents interact in multifaceted ways, often revealing their impact only when viewed from a broader perspective. For example, managing chronic diseases like diabetes or heart failure requires coordinated care across multiple disciplines. A heart failure clinic, for instance, may bring together physicians, nurses, dietitians, pharmacists, and social workers to develop comprehensive care plans tailored to each patient. Studies have shown that such multidisciplinary approaches can significantly reduce hospital readmissions and improve quality of life for patients (Strömberg, 2005).

Today's healthcare challenges, such as chronic diseases, are rarely isolated medical issues; they are deeply influenced by genetics, patient behavior, environmental factors, and socio-economic status. For example, a patient's ability to manage diabetes effectively may depend on coordinated efforts from nutritionists for dietary education, pharmacists for medication adherence, IT specialists for technological support, and behavioral scientists for promoting lifestyle changes. This interconnectedness makes healthcare a CAS, where the actions of one agent can ripple through the system, impacting others in both predictable and unpredictable ways.

Case Study 2.1: Introduction of a New Electronic Health Record (EHR) System

In 2009, the Health Information Technology for Economic and Clinical Health Act incentivized healthcare providers in the United States to adopt digital records (Blumenthal and Tavenner, 2010). Despite being well into the Information Age, the transition from paper to digital records was a drastic change for many agents involved. The concept of EHRs promised improved efficiency and patient outcomes and held potential for integrating future technologies such as remote patient monitoring (RPM) records and incorporating artificial intelligence (AI) tools. However, the implementation of this innovation revealed challenges such as workflow disruptions, increased provider workload, and interoperability issues (Boonstra and Broekhuis, 2010).

The introduction of EHRs is a compelling example of healthcare functioning as a CAS, where interconnected agents such as hospital procurement teams, clinicians, administrators, IT staff, insurance companies, regulatory bodies, and patients interact dynamically. Hospital procurement evaluates vendors based on cost, functionality, and compliance with data privacy standards like the Health Insurance Portability and Accountability Act (HIPAA) in the United States. Clinicians and nurses must adapt to new workflows, initially experiencing slowed patient care as they learn the system. Administrators monitor financial impacts and training costs, while IT staff work to integrate the EHR with existing systems. Insurance companies may also be affected if the new EHR changes billing codes or documentation practices, potentially impacting reimbursements. Regulatory bodies might update compliance requirements related to electronic records, influencing how data is captured and reported. Patients, as key agents, experience a shift in their interaction with healthcare, such as gaining access to online portals for appointments and test results.

The EHR transition highlights the ripple effects of innovation in a CAS, where the actions of one agent influence the actions of others in often unpredictable ways. This case study illustrates how healthcare has already adopted the CAS perspective, as the implementation of EHRs reflects the system's inherent interdependencies and feedback loops. As innovations like remote monitoring and AI tools continue to build on this foundation, the importance of understanding and leveraging the CAS framework remains central to navigating the challenges and opportunities of healthcare transformation.

2.1.2 Framework for Decision-Making in Healthcare

In the healthcare sector, decision-making frameworks are integral to guiding policy, practice, and innovation. As a CAS, the dynamic interactions between agents and non-linear processes demand frameworks that account for complexity and adaptability, with various structured approaches to risk management, patient-centric care, and operational efficiency. Lean Six Sigma is a widely adopted framework that combines Lean principles with Six Sigma methodologies to enhance process efficiency, reduce errors, and improve patient outcomes. Principles of Lean Manufacturing have been applied in the healthcare industry to address the 7.5% projected annual growth in national health expenditures in the United States (NEJM Catalyst, 2018; Centers for Medicare and Medicaid Services, 2022) by focusing on eliminating waste. Six Sigma methodologies are data-driven and focus on eliminating defects and reducing variability in processes, which directly benefits patient care by improving factors like diagnostic accuracy, reducing wait times, and enhancing patient satisfaction. Lean Six Sigma employs tools like DMAIC (Define, Measure, Analyze, Improve, Control) to streamline operations and optimize resource utilization. Taking a different perspective, the IDEA Ethical Decision-Making Framework provides a robust method for resolving ethical dilemmas and incorporating fairness and accountability, which are critical in addressing sensitive healthcare decisions (Levenson, 2023). Another instance is Health Canada's Decision-Making (Canada, 2024) Framework focusing on identifying, assessing, and managing health risks through a systematic process, ensuring evidence-based and transparent decision-making.

In this chapter, the Cynefin Framework and Kotter Change Management Model are highlighted as particularly valuable for analyzing and implementing innovation within healthcare systems understood as CAS. The Cynefin Framework, developed by David Snowden, excels at navigating the inherent complexity of CAS by categorizing problems into domains—simple, complicated, complex, chaotic, and disorder. This categorization enables healthcare leaders to adopt context-specific strategies, such as iterative experimentation in complex domains or decisive action in chaotic ones, which is essential for adapting to emergent challenges and unpredictable dynamics in healthcare (Snowden and Boone, 2007). The Kotter Model, developed by John Kotter, addresses the human and organizational dimensions of change, which are critical in CAS where the behavior of individual agents and networks influences system-wide outcomes (Kotter, 1996). Its eight-step process—from creating urgency to embedding change—facilitates structured transformation, fostering alignment and coherence within adaptive systems.

These frameworks address key features of CAS in healthcare innovation. TheCynefin Framework provides a strategic understanding of the complexities involved, guiding adaptive decision-making, while Kotter's model ensures the structured adoption of change, fostering stakeholder buy-in and sustainability. When complemented by operational frameworks like Lean Six Sigma, which optimizes processes and resource allocation, these models form a holistic toolkit for addressing the intricate and often unpredictable challenges of healthcare innovation.

2.1.2.1 Introduction to the Cynefin Framework

The Cynefin Framework, as seen in Figure 2.1, divides situations into four primary domains: Clear, Complicated, Complex, and Chaos. Each of these is characterized by distinct cause-and-effect relationships and decision-making approaches. Understanding these domains and their inherent constraints is essential for effective problem-solving in CAS like healthcare.

The Clear Domain represents situations with obvious cause-and-effect relationships. The path from problem to solution is evident, and best practices are established. Decision-making here involved sensing the situation, categorizing it, and responding with predetermined procedures. The constraints are rigid constraints—strict rules and protocols that must be followed to achieve the desired outcome. For example, suppose you are driving a car to the mall. As a new driver, you learned the rules of the road and adhere to them as best as you can. Deviating from the instructions is unnecessary.

The Complicated Domain encompasses scenarios where cause-and-effect relationships exist but are not evident to everyone. These situations require analysis and

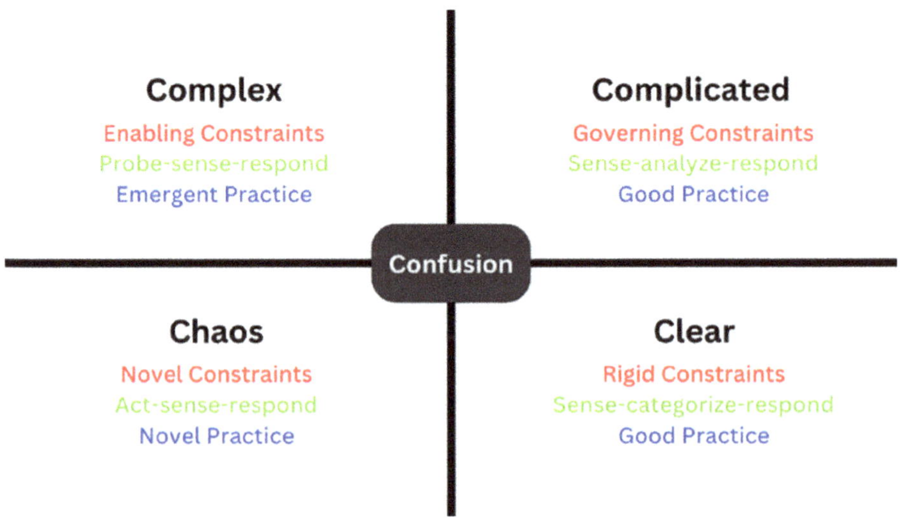

FIGURE 2.1 The Cynefin Framework.

expertise. Decision-makers must sense the issue, analyze it with the help of specialists, and respond accordingly. The constraints here are governing constraints—established rules and processes that necessitate specialized knowledge to interpret and apply effectively. Suppose you are at the mall trying to parallel park on a busy street. A new driver may not know how to do it, but as a seasoned driver, you recall the steps and assess the narrow parking space. Taking the zooming cars passing by and the car honking at you from behind into consideration, you take measures to (hopefully) park successfully.

In the Complex Domain, cause-and-effect relationships are obscured and usually can be understood in hindsight. Patterns and solutions emerge over time through experimentation and observation. Decision-making here involves probing the environment, sensing how the system responds, and adapting accordingly. The constraints are enabling constraints, which provide a flexible framework that guides action while allowing for innovation and adaptation. Let's say you go for a vacation in a foreign country where you are not familiar with the geography or rules of the road, and you don't have Google Maps to guide you. You need to probe your environment, trying to combine external cues like road signs and directions from strangers with your internal inferences from navigating the roads back at home. After some trial and error, and potentially a few detours, you manage to make it to your destination.

The Chaos Domain represents situations of high turbulence with unpredictable relationships. Immediate action is necessary to establish order, as there is often no time to think and analyze the situation. Here, the steps are to act decisively, sense the results of the action, and respond to stabilize the situation. The constraints are novel constraints—there are no existing rules or guidelines, and the only way to prepare is to expect the unexpected. New approaches must be invented on the spot to manage the crisis. A situation in the Chaos Domain tends to be the worst-case scenario, such as your car bursting into flames after crashing into an oncoming truck. You don't have time to pause and analyze the situation—you need to act fast and get yourself out of there before you burn to death. In that sense, the Chaos Domain is like a fire you are trying to put out.

By using the Cynefin Framework, healthcare leaders can categorize challenges, informing their approach to technology implementation. In the Clear and Complicated Domains, established technologies and processes can be implemented with standard project management techniques. Examples of this are implementing standardized e-prescription software. The outcomes are predictable, as the software streamlines the prescription process and reduces handwriting errors. There are already established protocols governing e-prescriptions, and it is easily integrated into EHR systems, meaning staff training is minimal and usage instructions are relatively straightforward. Rigid constraints apply, as there are strict compliance requirements with regulations like HIPAA.

New technologies in the Complex Domain address unprecedented challenges that require experimentation and adaptive strategies. Deploying an AI software for diagnostic support in radiology is considered complex. There are unpredictable outcomes, as the impact of AI on diagnostic accuracy and workflow efficiency is uncertain and variable depending on the user. New protocols develop as clinicians learn to integrate AI insights into their decision-making processes, and pilot programs are initiated to test the AI tool's effectiveness, with iterative adjustments based on feedback. Enabling constraints here guide the experimentation, such as ethical considerations, data privacy regulations, and the need for clinician oversight, while allowing for flexibility for innovation.

A prime example for the Chaotic Domain is the COVID-19 pandemic, where novel solutions were needed without the benefit of prior experiences to depend on. The switch to telehealth platforms and rapid rollout of vaccines required immediate action with little time to develop policies or best practices beforehand.

Case Study 2.2: Implementing a Nationwide Telehealth Platform during the COVID-19 Pandemic

The COVID-19 pandemic posed unprecedented challenges to healthcare systems worldwide. One critical problem was ensuring continuous access to medical care while minimizing the risk of virus transmission. The sudden need for remote healthcare solutions accelerated the adoption of telehealth services across the globe. Countries like India, Brazil, and Sri Lanka rapidly developed legal frameworks and guidelines to facilitate telemedicine services. The United Kingdom transitioned a significant portion of healthcare providers to conduct consultations on telehealth platforms (Basu et al., 2021). The United States expanded telehealth access through legislative changes, such as the CARES Act, which relaxed Medicare restrictions. Additionally, countries like Australia and Canada scaled up telehealth services to ensure continued access to primary healthcare (OECD, 2023).

This case study examines the implementation of a nationwide telehealth platform within 6 months across the United States as an example, utilizing the Cynefin Framework and its four phases of problem-solving: assess, adapt, experiment, and transcend.

2.1.2.2 Step 1: Assess the Problem

Problem Identification: Implementing a nationwide telehealth platform in the United States to provide remote medical consultations, ensuring that patients could access healthcare services safely during the pandemic.

SMART Problem Framework:

- **Specific**: Deploy a secure and user-friendly telehealth platform accessible to all citizens.
- **Measurable**: Achieve at least 70% adoption among healthcare providers and serve 50 million virtual consultations within 6 months.
- **Achievable**: Leverage existing technologies and infrastructure with government support.
- **Relevant**: Reduce the risk of COVID-19 transmission by minimizing in-person visits.
- **Time-Bound**: Complete implementation and reach adoption targets within 6 months.

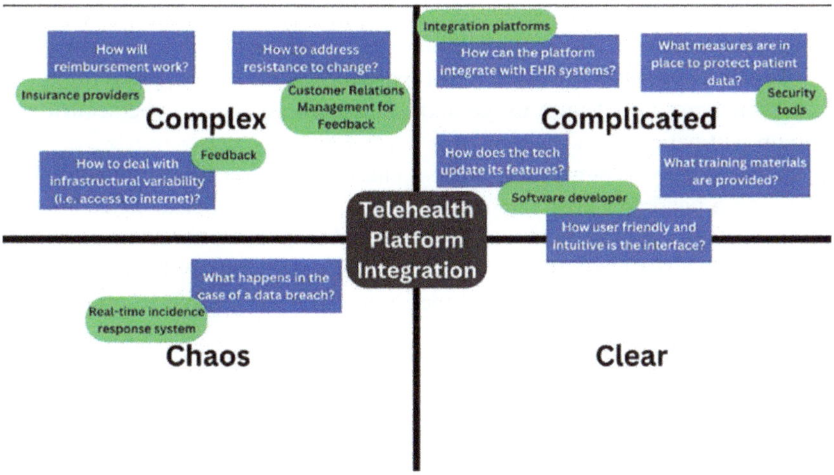

FIGURE 2.2 Cynefin Framework for telehealth platform integration.

2.1.2.3 Step 2: Adapt to Decision Elements

Figure 2.2 highlights a Cynefin Framework for the proposed telehealth platform integration. Key questions are highlighted in blue rectangles. Due to the complex nature of the COVID-19 pandemic, there are not many situations where there is one clear-cut answer. Most of these questions lie within the Complicated/Complex/Chaos domains. The green boxes highlight tools that can be used to help answer these questions. The matter of user interface and features require the expertise of the software developer. Decisions like how to address resistance to change and how to implement within different infrastructures are not easily predictable and require multiple trials to see what the best answer is. In the case of a sudden data breach, novel practices are required and are critical to act on.

2.1.2.4 Step 3: Experiment

To navigate the complexities and uncertainties, parallel experiments were conducted. Pilot programs in diverse regions were deployed, focusing on implementing telehealth in urban areas with high internet penetration to test scalability, and introducing it in rural areas to address accessibility challenges. Various technology platforms were also investigated. Platform A was a commercially available telehealth solution, and Platform B was an open-source platform customized to local needs. Various training approaches were also taken, observing the efficacy of self-paced online modules or live virtual workshops. Throughout all this, feedback was constantly monitored, tracking uptake rates and demographic data. Analyzing the results from these various methods allowed for refinement of approaches and scale successful models.

2.1.2.5 Step 4: Transcend

Based on the outcome of the experiments, successful strategies were formalized and implemented. The expansion of successful platforms led to the scaled deployment nationwide with necessary customizations taken from feedback. This also introduced policy reforms as new regulations came out to support telehealth reimbursement permanently, along with established guidelines for telehealth practice standards. The results also invested in infrastructure such as upgrading digital tools to support increased telehealth usage and implementing robust cybersecurity measures to protect patient data.

By applying the Cynefin Framework, a chaotic situation like telemedicine platforms during a pandemic was able to be deconstructed in order to efficiently find a solution. This approach allowed for flexibility and responsive adjustments by laying everything out on the table as is, ultimately leading to a successful telehealth platform deployment effort that addressed the immediate crisis while strengthening the healthcare system for future challenges.

2.2 MULTIDISCIPLINARY APPROACH TO PATIENT-CENTRIC INNOVATION

2.2.1 The Necessity of Multidisciplinary Collaboration in CAS

Imagine trying to solve a thousand-piece jigsaw puzzle with only a handful of pieces—you might get a fragment of the picture, but the complete image remains a mystery. Similarly, healthcare challenges are multifaceted puzzles that cannot be solved through a singular lens. They encompass biological, technological, psychological, social, and economic dimensions that intertwine and influence one another within a CAS. When disciplines operate in silos, solutions often address symptoms rather than root causes. For example, prescribing medication for hypertension without considering a patient's access to healthy food or space for exercise may yield limited long-term benefits. The CAS nature of healthcare demands a wholistic approach where multiple perspectives converge to address these complex challenges.

Multidisciplinary collaboration fosters an environment where ideas cross-pollinate, leading to breakthroughs that no single expert could achieve alone. This synergy leverages the strengths of each discipline:

- **Clinicians** bring medical knowledge and patient care experience.
- **Engineers** contribute problem-solving skills and technological innovation.
- **IT Specialists** offer expertise in data management and digital solutions.
- **Behavioral Scientists** provide insights into human behavior and motivation.
- **Health Economists** analyze cost-effectiveness and resource allocation.

Consider the development of the KardiaMobile, a portable single-lead electrocardiogram (ECG) that enables tracking heart rhythms from the comfort of your home. This innovation was revolutionary to cardiologists and patients alike as heart rhythm irregularities such as arrhythmias occur at unpredictable moments, which is not always when the patient is seeing the doctor in clinic. This leads to missing key ECG data needed for diagnoses. This device resulted from the collaboration between many key agents. Cardiologists identified the need for continuous monitoring in patients with arrhythmias. Electrical, mechanical, and biomedical engineers designed the compact device that gives high-accuracy readings. IT professionals developed secure platforms for data transmission and analysis. Data scientists are actively working on developing algorithms to detect anomalies and alert healthcare providers. And most importantly, patient advocates ensured the device was user-friendly and addressed patient concerns. This collaborative effort resulted in a patient-centric solution that improved early detection of cardiac events, enhanced patient engagement, and reduced hospital admissions.

Diversity within teams catalyzes innovation as various perspectives yield different approaches, questioning assumptions, exploring unconventional ideas, and mitigating groupthink. This is particularly valuable in a CAS where adaptability is key to navigating complexity. For example, chronic pain management has been historically challenging, often leading to an over-reliance on opioids (Gatchel et al., 2014). A multidisciplinary team comprising physicians, physical therapists, psychologists, and alternative medicine practitioners collaborated to develop integrative pain management programs. These programs combined medical treatments with physical therapy, cognitive-behavioral therapy, and mindfulness practices. The result was a more effective, holistic approach that reduced opioid dependency and improved patient quality of life.

Patient-centric care is fundamental to effective healthcare delivery within CAS because it focuses on tailoring medical interventions to the individual needs, preferences, and values of patients, thereby enhancing clinical outcomes and patient satisfaction. Technically, this approach involves multidisciplinary teams collaborating to engage patients as active participants in their own care, promoting shared decision-making and personalized treatment plans. For instance, a case study on diabetes management showed that when patients received individualized education and support from a team comprising physicians, nurses, dietitians, and educators, there was a significant improvement in glycemic control and a reduction in diabetes-related complications (Trento et al., 2004). Another example is in oncology care, where incorporating patient preferences and psychosocial support into treatment planning led to better adherence to therapy and improved quality of life for cancer patients (Jacobsen and Jim, 2008). These cases underscore that patient-centric care enhances the effectiveness of healthcare.

2.2.2 Innovation Diffusion and Adoption Readiness in Patient-Centric Innovation

2.2.2.1 The Diffusion of Innovations Theory in Healthcare

Understanding how innovations spread and are adopted in CAS is crucial for driving patient-centric advancements. The **Diffusion of Innovations** Theory, developed by Everett M. Rogers, provides a framework for understanding how new technologies spread within a social system over time (Rogers, 2003). The theory delineates five categories of adopters: innovators, early adopters, early majority, late majority, and laggards (as seen in Figure 2.3).

This model also applies to healthcare, where new technologies and practices are adopted by different stakeholders at different points in the innovation pipeline. Innovators might be cutting-edge research hospitals or clinician scientists developing

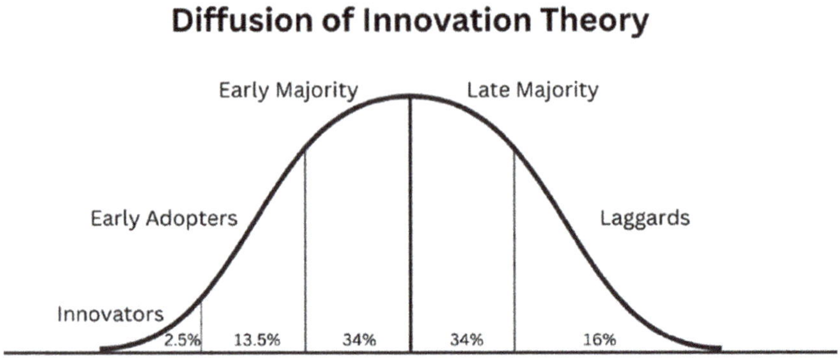

FIGURE 2.3 Diffusion of innovation curve as theorized by Everett Rogers.

novel treatments. Early adopters often include leading healthcare institutions that have a robust research and development arm, influencing others through demonstrated successes. There is a certain risk associated with adopting technology early, but early adopters either believe in the positive outcomes or have fiscal room to experiment. Early majority represents the bulk of healthcare providers who adopt innovations after seeing them work effectively elsewhere. Late majority tend to require significant evidence before implementation and may adopt due to regulatory changes or market pressures. Laggards are those resistant to change, possibly due to resource constraints or entrenched practices.

The adoption of EHRs exemplifies the Diffusion of Innovations Theory. Early adopters like Kaiser Permanente embraced EHRs in the early 2000s, driven by robust access to resources and alignment with strategic goals. These organizations showcased the benefits of EHRs, setting the benchmark for others to follow. In contrast, late adopters, including small private practices and rural hospitals, faced significant barriers such as financial constraints, technical compatibility challenges, and resistance to change. Their adoption of EHRs occurred much later, often initiated by policy interventions like the HITECH Act of 2009, which provided financial initiatives and support mechanisms to help implementation. This diffusion pattern highlights the need for tailored strategies to address the specific challenges of different adopter categories.

2.2.2.2 Factors Influencing Adoption Readiness

Rogers identified five key attributes that influence the rate of adoption for innovations: relative advantage; compatibility; complexity; trialability; and observability (Rogers, 2003). Relative advantage is when stakeholders see clear benefits—such as improved patient outcomes or cost savings—they are more likely to adopt the innovation. Compatibility assesses how the innovation aligns with current workflows. Complexity involves the perceived difficulty of using the innovation—typically more user-friendly innovations are adopted more rapidly. Trialability is the extent to which an innovation can be tested on a limited basis. Trial runs reduce uncertainty and build confidence among the potential adopters and end users. Observability is the visibility of the innovation's results. When positive outcomes are apparent to others, such as reduced hospital admissions, adoption is accelerated.

Technology Readiness Levels (TRLs) is a scale developed by NASA to measure the maturity of a technology, ranging from basic principles observed (TRL 1) to proven operational use (TRL 9). Minimum Viable Products (MVPs) are products with enough features to attract an early adopter, and tends to be around TRL 4–5, where proof-of-concept studies have taken place. Innovations tend to be at TRL 6 or higher when looking at getting adopted, because there is a validated prototype at this point. However, high TRLs alone are insufficient in healthcare implementation because they focus primarily on technological development without accounting for adoption factors.

Adoption Readiness Levels (ARLs) complement TRLs by evaluating how prepared an innovation is for integration into real-world settings. ARLs provide a framework for determining whether an innovation is ready to be integrated into real-world healthcare settings. This includes evaluating factors like stakeholder engagement, regulatory compliance, clinical workflow integration, and training requirements for healthcare professionals. In the context of patient-centric innovation, ARLs are particularly important because they ensure that innovations not only function technically but also align with patient needs, preferences, and healthcare delivery processes. For example, a new digital health tool may reach TRL 9, indicating technological maturity ready for commercial deployment. However, without assessing ARL factors like compatibility with existing clinical workflows, training requirements for staff, and acceptance by patients, the device may fail to achieve widespread adoption. Therefore, incorporating ARLs into the innovation process addresses the socio-technical dimensions crucial for implementation in a CAS.

2.2.3 Tools for Managing Multidisciplinary Collaboration

In healthcare innovation, balancing diverse viewpoints of all the different agents involved is daunting. Effective tools are necessary to ensure that the collaborative efforts of clinicians, engineers, administrators, patients, and policymakers align with the broader goal of patient-centric innovation.

2.2.3.1 Stakeholder Analysis and the Power-Interest Grid

Imagine you decide to build a house without consulting the architect, the contractor, or the people who will live in it. You may lay a strong foundation, but without input from those who understand the technical design or the daily needs of future residents, you risk constructing something that doesn't work for anyone. In healthcare innovation, **stakeholder analysis** functions much like assembling the right team of experts before the building begins—ensuring that every voice is heard and every critical angle is considered. Stakeholder analysis is the process of identifying the key players who will be impacted by or can influence an innovation. Each stakeholder has a distinct role to play: clinicians interact with the technology in their daily workflows, IT professionals ensure seamless integration with existing systems, administrators and procurement officers focus on financial viability and operational efficiency. Additionally, regulatory bodies safeguard compliance with Food and Health Administration (FDA) or Health Canada standards. Even patient advocates and community leaders play a role in shaping the innovation's implementation to meet broader public health needs. It's more than just asking, "Who will use this?"

In healthcare, the **end user** is not always the patient. For example, in the adoption of a new clinical decision support tool, the end user may be a nurse or physician who interacts with the system directly, while the patient benefits indirectly through improved care outcomes. This process ensures that innovators don't move forward blindly; instead, engaging the right people early on allows for insights to address potential challenges and champion the change. A useful tool to map where these stakeholders stand on your innovation pipeline is the **Power-Interest Grid**.

The **Power-Interest Grid** is like a roadmap for navigating the relationships that can make or break an innovation (Mendelow, 1991). Picture it as a tool that helps you figure out who's holding the steering wheel and who's just along for the ride. It categorizes stakeholders into four quadrants based on two key factors: their **power**—or ability to influence the success of the project—and their **interest**—or how much they care about its outcome.

In one corner, you've got the **high-power, high-interest** stakeholders—these are the heavy hitters, like senior clinicians or key decision-makers, who need to be closely managed because they can either champion or block the innovation. Then, there are the **high-power, low-interest** players, such as hospital board members. They may not care about the details, but they can still pull the plug if their broader goals aren't met, so it's crucial to keep them satisfied. Next are the **low-power, high-interest** stakeholders, like nurses or patient advocates, who might not hold much formal sway but have valuable insights and can rally support for the innovation. Finally, the **low-power, low-interest** group—think peripheral departments—don't need constant attention but monitoring them ensures no unexpected hurdles pop up later. By mapping stakeholders onto this grid, innovators can find powerful champions for their technology and allocate energy accordingly to focus on the key players.

In a CAS like healthcare, where countless moving parts—people, technologies, and processes—interact in unpredictable ways, stakeholder analysis is not just a helpful step, but a critical foundation for success. By thoroughly understanding who the key players are and mapping their power and interest, innovators can anticipate challenges, align goals, and engage the right people at the right time.

Case Study 2.3: AI-Enabled Veterinary Medical Scribe

Figure 2.4 shows an example of Power-Interest Grid for ScribeNote, a digital tool that uses AI to get veterinary notes done a lot faster. Large veterinary hospitals are an example of a body that would have positive support, as it has the potential to make workflow more efficient, and with high influence, since they may have the resources and funding to implement it faster. Veterinary students who are future-oriented may be more inclined to include AI in their future workflows, but at their student status, they don't have much say in terms of implementation. On the other side, traditional veterinarians may prefer manual note taking because they are used to it, or they don't see a justification in the subscription cost. Finally, community pet owners may be wary of the increase in veterinary care prices that a new AI scribe may introduce, but they don't have the influence on whether it gets implemented or not.

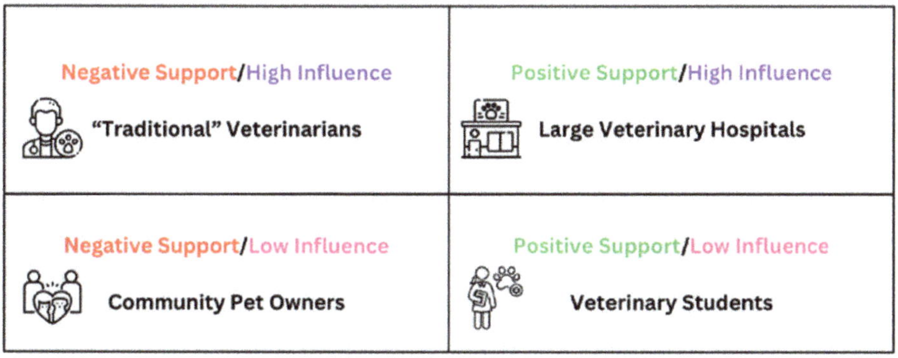

FIGURE 2.4 Example Power-Interest Grid for ScribeNote, an AI veterinary scribe application.

2.2.3.2 Kotter's 8-Step Change Management Framework

Introducing innovation is not just about implementing new technologies—it is also about guiding an entire organization through a change process. John Kotter developed the Kotter's 8-Step Change Management Framework, as seen in Figure 2.5,

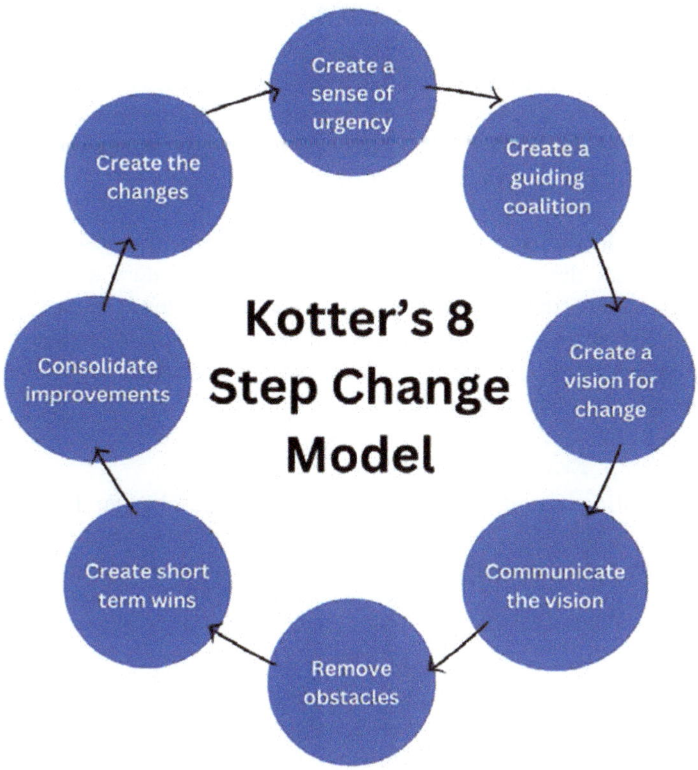

FIGURE 2.5 Kotter's 8-step change model.

which is a structured approach to navigating complex transitions, ensuring that innovations are adopted sustainably across diverse teams (Kotter, 1996). In a healthcare CAS, Kotter's framework offers a pathway to engage multidisciplinary teams, reduce friction, and create a culture of innovation.

2.2.3.2.1 Step 1: Create a Sense of Urgency

In healthcare, the stakes are often high—whether it's improving patient outcomes, addressing inefficiencies, or staying compliant with evolving regulations. Communicating the consequences of inaction, backed up by data, helps mobilize the organization.

- **Example:** Consider the rollout of telemedicine during the COVID-19 pandemic. The urgent need to maintain patient care while minimizing in-person contact created an immediate call to action. Leaders communicated this urgency by emphasizing patient safety, access to care, and the opportunity to innovate healthcare delivery in response to a crisis. By highlighting the pressing nature of the pandemic, organizations could rapidly implement telemedicine solutions that might have otherwise taken years to adopt.

2.2.3.2.2 Step 2: Build a Guiding Coalition

Change cannot happen in isolation; it requires a coalition of influential leaders and stakeholders who are committed to the innovation's success. A multidisciplinary coalition of clinicians, IT specialists, administrators, and patient advocates creates a powerful team to champion the innovation. Having early champions is key to promoting support for the innovation across departments.

- **Example:** In the adoption of a new EHR system, the guiding coalition might include department heads, senior nurses, IT leaders, and compliance officers. Each brings a unique perspective on the system's impact, ensuring that no aspect of care or workflow is overlooked. These leaders can also identify potential pockets of resistance early and work to address concerns before they become barriers to implementation.

2.2.3.2.3 Step 3: Develop a Vision and Strategy

A clear, compelling vision is essential for guiding the change. This vision must explain not only what the innovation is but also why it matters and how it will benefit the organization and, ultimately, the patients. The strategy should outline actionable steps, providing a roadmap for how the organization will achieve its goals.

- **Example:** When introducing a clinical decision support tool that aids in diagnosis, the vision might be to reduce diagnostic errors by 20% within the first year. The strategy would then detail how the tool will be integrated into daily clinical workflows, how staff will be trained, and how the success of the tool will be measured in terms of both clinical outcomes and efficiency improvements.

2.2.3.2.4 Step 4: Communicate the Vision

Even the best vision will falter if it isn't communicated effectively. It's essential to share the vision across all levels of the organization, ensuring that everyone understands the "why" behind the change. Frequent, transparent communication using multiple channels—town hall meetings, newsletters, and even one-on-one conversations—helps keep the vision alive and front of mind.

- **Example:** A hospital implementing a new mobile health app for patient monitoring can communicate its vision by hosting webinars for staff, explaining how the app will empower patients to manage their chronic conditions while providing real-time data to clinicians. Visual aids, case studies, and patient testimonials can be shared through email and intranet platforms to reinforce the benefits of the app, ensuring that everyone is aligned with the innovation's goals.

2.2.3.2.5 Step 5: Empower Broad-Based Action

Empowerment is about removing barriers that prevent teams from taking action. This could involve addressing concerns, streamlining workflows, or providing the necessary resources to ensure success. It's critical to allow team members the flexibility to adapt the innovation to their specific context, enabling them to take ownership of the change.

- **Example:** In the rollout of a new medication administration system, front-line nurses may need additional training, while the pharmacy team might require adjustments to inventory management protocols. By providing these resources and fostering open dialogue, healthcare leaders empower staff to confidently adopt the new system. This empowerment is further enhanced by encouraging feedback, allowing staff to suggest modifications that improve the system's functionality and alignment with their day-to-day operations.

2.2.3.2.6 Step 6: Generate Short-Term Wins

Generating short-term wins is key to building momentum and reducing resistance. Focusing on small, measurable victories, like implementing a pilot program in one department, shows tangible improvements like reduced wait times or fewer errors. Publicly celebrating these wins through newsletters, meetings, or even rewards helps reinforce confidence and encourages broader buy-in from stakeholders.

- **Example:** In the first few months of implementing a new patient portal, tracking and showcasing metrics such as a 30% increase in appointment scheduling efficiency or improved patient satisfaction scores can serve as short-term wins. These successes should be shared in staff meetings, newsletters, and even through personal acknowledgment of those who contributed to making the system work smoothly. Positive feedback from patients who find the portal easy to use can further bolster support among hesitant staff.

2.2.3.2.7 Step 7: Sustain Acceleration

As the innovation gains traction, it's important to keep pushing forward. This means refining the process, addressing any lingering issues, and looking for opportunities to expand the change. It's easy for momentum to slow once initial goals are met, but continuous focus ensures that the change becomes deeply embedded in the organization's culture.

- **Example:** After successfully rolling out an EHR system in one department, leadership might identify other areas where similar digital transformation efforts could drive additional benefits, such as extending the system's use to outpatient care or integrating advanced analytics tools to enhance data-driven decision-making. Continuous feedback loops ensure that the system is refined based on real-world experiences, keeping the innovation dynamic and responsive to new needs.

2.2.3.2.8 Step 8: Institute Change

The final step is making the innovation a permanent part of the organization's fabric. This involves embedding the new practices into organizational policies, creating structures that support the innovation's ongoing use, and continually measuring its effectiveness. The change becomes "institutionalized" when it is no longer viewed as new or temporary but as an integral aspect of how the organization operates.

- **Example:** Once a hospital successfully adopts a telemedicine platform, it should update its operational policies to include telehealth as a standard care option, integrate telemedicine metrics into performance reviews, and continuously monitor patient outcomes to ensure the platform remains effective. This institutionalization process ensures that the innovation is sustained beyond the initial excitement, becoming a routine part of patient care.

Kotter's framework is not just a theoretical model; it is a practical tool that provides clear steps for navigating the complexities of change in healthcare. By following this structured approach, healthcare organizations can drive patient-centric innovations while maintaining the flexibility needed to adapt to the unpredictable challenges inherent in a CAS.

2.2.4 Other Approaches to Innovation Implementation

2.2.4.1 Behavioral Science and Social Innovation in Healthcare

Behavioral science plays a pivotal role in shaping patient-centric innovations by leveraging insights into human behavior to enhance healthcare delivery and outcomes. Human-centered design is where healthcare teams collaborate with behavioral scientists to create solutions tailored to patients' needs and preferences. For example, Project ECHO (Extension for Community Healthcare Outcomes) utilizes a tele-mentoring model to empower healthcare providers in rural areas, thereby improving patient care through continuous learning and support (Arora et al., 2017).

Additionally, behavioral economics principles, such as nudges and incentive structures, are employed to encourage healthier behaviors and improve medication adherence. The Vitality Active Rewards exemplifies this by offering rewards for engaging in healthy activities, resulting in significant improvements in participants' health metrics and reduced healthcare costs. These interdisciplinary approaches foster social innovation and ensure healthcare solutions are effective and aligned with patients' behavioral patterns.

2.2.4.2 Engineering and Architecture Contributions to Patient Care

Designing and implementing infrastructures that promote efficiency and sustainability within healthcare facilities also can enhance patient care. Smart infrastructures in hospitals, such as those implemented at Mackenzie Health hospitals in Canada, integrate Internet of Things (IoT) technologies to enhance patient care. The Cortellucci Vaughan Hospital integrates embedded systems and sensor networks to create a seamless flow of information between medical devices, staff, and patients. This connectivity allows for real-time health monitoring and data sharing.

Sustainable healthcare design is increasingly important as hospitals strive to reduce their environmental footprint while enhancing patient well-being. The Dell Children's Medical Center, the first LEED Platinum-certified hospital, showcases how sustainable architectural practices—such as using energy-efficient systems and incorporating green spaces—can enhance clinical environments by improving air quality, increasing exposure to natural sunlight, and reducing pollutants. These have been shown to benefit patient recovery processes, with a study showing that the inclusion of natural light and outdoor views in hospital design is correlated with shorter hospital stays and improved health outcomes (Totaforti, 2018). These contributions illustrate how multidisciplinary collaboration between engineers, architects, and healthcare professionals can lead to innovative, sustainable, and patient-focused healthcare environments.

2.2.5 AI and IoTs in Healthcare Innovation Implementation

2.2.5.1 AI and IoTs

AI and IoT are emerging technologies reshaping healthcare systems with their increase in efficiency and patient-centricity, introducing new layers of adaptability that healthcare systems have to respond to.

AI applications in healthcare range from diagnostic tools to personalized treatments. Mayo Clinic has developed applications that use machine learning (ML) algorithms to improve early disease detection. For instance, AI-enabled ECGs can predict heart conditions like atrial fibrillation and heart failure, allowing for earlier diagnosis and intervention (Attia et al., 2019). Additionally, AI is being used to facilitate personalized treatment plans by analyzing large datasets to identify unique patient traits and medical histories. Incorporating the latest advances in genetic screening, this can potentially enhance therapy effectiveness and bring a new meaning to patient-centric care (Johnson et al., 2020). An example of a company harnessing this is Tempus, which employs AI to analyze the world's largest collection of clinical and molecular data to provide physicians with insights into treatments and cures (Tempus, 2024). The adaptability of AI-driven personalized medicine will require continuous learning and adjustment. AI is also revolutionizing medical imaging by providing rapid analysis of X-rays and computed tomography (CT) scans, aiding in early detection of diseases like pancreatic cancer (Adams et al., 2020). These models have clinically achieved significant levels of accuracy with above 90% sensitivities and specificities (Attia et al., 2019; Changhez et al., 2024). Integrating these technologies into diagnostic workflows will allow systems to respond dynamically to new information and improve decision-making processes.

Similarly, IoT technologies are revolutionizing the healthcare industry with RPM and wearable technologies. IoT devices enable continuous monitoring of patients' vital signs, providing real-time data that can be analyzed by AI algorithms for early detection of health issues. The medical device market is shifting its focus on the increasing demand for wearable technology. Wearables are electronic devices that are worn on or within the body that can track health metrics and be shared with healthcare providers. In November 2022, 30% of Americans reported using wearables for health monitoring, and over half of the users used it daily (Chandrasekaran et al., 2020). A study demonstrated that 92% of smartwatch users use it for health-related objectives (Friend et al., 2023). Using existing sensors, wearables equipped with AI capabilities can track health metrics and notify users' health risks, such as irregular heartbeats or obstructive sleep apnea (Apple Support (CA), 2024).

The integration of AI and IoT into healthcare highlights how the intricate web of multiple interacting agents and layers of feedback loops continuously shape outcomes. RPM technologies, including wearables, present extensive and intricate patient data, which will continue to transform the flow of information, introducing both opportunities and challenges. For example, devices like continuous glucose monitors and smartwatches provide patients with real-time insights into their health. Sharing these insights with the users' healthcare providers gives a holistic representation of the users' condition, compared to siloed readings conducted in the clinic. The latter is not always representative of what is really going on with the patient in non-ambulatory settings. This increases engagement and enables healthcare systems to adapt dynamically to patient needs. This increased connectivity requires a vast network of agents, including patients, clinicians, data scientists, developers, and regulatory bodies, each playing a pivotal role in ensuring these technologies are used effectively and ethically. Companies like Rad AI exemplify how AI can streamline medical workflows, such as reducing the burden on radiologists by automating imaging analysis. However, there are many logistical considerations that need to be considered before implementation. Integrating additional data into EHR systems will need to be seamless for both the patient to upload their information and for the physicians and nurses to access it.

Additionally, patient data privacy concerns are crucial to mitigate with sufficient cybersecurity measures, ensuring that the technology follows acts such as the HIPAA in the United States and Personal Information Protection and Electronic Documents Act (PIPEDA) in Canada. Additionally, ensuring accuracy is a major concern to ensure patients are not receiving false positives or false negatives. Moreover, while AI enables personalized medicine, these technologies require rigorous medical oversight to ensure they remain evidence-based and clinically validated. In a CAS, the interaction between AI systems and healthcare agents can create emergent behaviors, ranging from improved diagnostic accuracies to unforeseen ethical dilemmas. An issue with AI-enabled diagnostics is the "Black Box Problem," where the inputs and outputs of the AI model can be seen but the intricacies of the model, or the basis of how an AI came to diagnostic conclusion, is not always known (Xu and Michael, 2023). This can be unsettling for clinicians to fully trust. This further emphasizes the need for adaptability and collaboration across all stakeholders as well as increased ethical oversight on the training, development, and deployment of such AI models.

The IoT's role in RPM adds another layer of complexity. RPM devices feed data into AI models that continuously learn and adapt, enabling predictive analytics that can anticipate patient deterioration or recommend early interventions. These systems require a robust infrastructure to manage the massive influx of data and to integrate insights into clinical workflows seamlessly. Additionally, the sheer number of agents involved—from device manufacturers and healthcare providers to patients and regulatory bodies—creates a dynamic, interconnected system where small changes, such as a software update or a policy shift, can have cascading effects across the ecosystem. By enabling these feedback loops and fostering adaptability, AI and IoT technologies both exemplify and enhance healthcare's function as a CAS.

2.2.5.2 Blockchain Technology in Healthcare Innovation Implementation

Blockchain technology has the potential to revolutionize healthcare by ensuring secure, transparent, and decentralized management of medical information and supply chain processes. Its decentralized ledger system offers a tamper-proof method for storing sensitive medical records, enhancing data integrity and patient privacy. Patients gain greater control over their health data, allowing them to share specific information with healthcare providers as needed, fostering trust and transparency. Platforms like MedRec, a mobile app that tracks the user's health data, demonstrate how blockchain can streamline EHR management, ensuring interoperability and seamless data sharing across healthcare systems while maintaining strict privacy standards.

When combined with IoT, blockchain further transforms complementary medical supply chains. IoT-enabled sensors can monitor and transmit real-time data about environmental conditions, such as temperature and humidity, for sensitive products like vaccines and biologics. This data, recorded on blockchain, ensures complete traceability and accountability throughout the supply chain, preventing issues like counterfeit medications and improper handling. Smart contracts—automated protocols embedded in blockchain—can streamline processes by triggering payments or updates upon meeting predefined conditions, reducing inefficiencies and errors. In the context of CAS, blockchain and IoT introduce adaptability and transparency into healthcare systems, where diverse agents such as suppliers, providers, and regulators interact dynamically. Together, they create an integrated ecosystem that enhances efficiency, ensures data integration, and builds resilience in healthcare supply chains, paving the way for more secure and transparent healthcare delivery systems.

2.3 FINAL THOUGHTS

Healthcare systems are not static entities but dynamic, interconnected ecosystems that exemplify the principles of CAS. This chapter has demonstrated that successfully navigating healthcare's complexity requires embracing its inherent unpredictability, leveraging multidisciplinary approaches, and implementing frameworks that translate systemic challenges into actionable solutions. Through the exploration of frameworks such as the Cynefin Framework and Kotter's Change Management Model, we have shown how structured methodologies can enable healthcare leaders to categorize complexity, foster innovation, and manage transformative change. Moreover, case studies on the deployment of telemedicine during the COVID-19 pandemic and the integration of AI in diagnostics illustrate both the promise and pitfalls of introducing innovations into such intricate systems.

The rise of telemedicine highlighted the potential of **decentralized healthcare models** to expand access and enhance patient outcomes, particularly in underserved regions. However, its rapid implementation also revealed challenges such as disparities in access to technology and the need for robust digital infrastructure. Similarly, AI in diagnostics offers unprecedented opportunities for accuracy and efficiency but raises questions around bias, interoperability, and the ethical implications of automated decision-making. These case studies underscore a critical lesson: healthcare innovation must be viewed not as isolated technological advancements but as interventions that ripple through a network of stakeholders, influencing policies, workflows, and, ultimately, patient care.

To navigate these ongoing challenges, this chapter underscores the need for systematic, stakeholder-driven approaches that align with CAS principles. Policymakers must craft regulations that balance innovation with patient safety, fostering environments where emerging technologies can integrate seamlessly into existing systems. Practitioners should adopt iterative pilot testing and adaptive learning processes, ensuring that innovations are rigorously evaluated in real-world settings before scaling. Additionally, interdisciplinary collaboration must remain central, drawing on expertise from clinicians, technologists, behavioral scientists, and policymakers to address barriers such as interoperability, training, and equity in care delivery.

The role of leadership in this process cannot be overstated. As healthcare continues to evolve, leaders must act as facilitators who can bridge diverse perspectives, anticipate resistance, and champion a culture of continuous learning and adaptation. Ethical considerations must also remain at the forefront, particularly in the integration of AI, where transparency, accountability, and inclusivity are integral. By fostering trust and prioritizing the equitable distribution of benefits, healthcare systems can avoid exacerbating disparities while leveraging technology to its fullest potential.

Ultimately, the transformation of healthcare infrastructure lies in the recognition that complexity is not a barrier but a strength. This chapter invites practitioners, policymakers, and researchers to take actionable steps to build systems that not only adapt to today's challenges but are agile enough to address the uncertainties of tomorrow. The future of healthcare will not be defined by technology alone but by the ability of its stakeholders to collaborate, innovate, and evolve—ensuring that the systems we design today will sustain equitable care for generations to come.

REFERENCES

Adams, S. J., Robert, Yi, X., & Babyn, P. (2020). Artificial intelligence solutions for analysis of X-ray images. *Canadian Association of Radiologists Journal*, *72*(1), 60–72. https://doi.org/10.1177/0846537120941671

Apple Support (CA). (2024). Sleep apnea notifications on your Apple watch. https://support.apple.com/en-ca/120031

Arora, S., Kalishman, S. G., Thornton, K. A., Komaromy, M. S., Katzman, J. G., Struminger, B. B., Rayburn, W. F., & Bradford, A. M. (2017). Project ECHO: A telementoring network model for continuing professional development. *Journal of Continuing Education in the Health Professions, 37*(4), 239–244. https://doi.org/10.1097/ceh.0000000000000172

Attia, Z. I., Noseworthy, P. A., Lopez-Jimenez, F., Asirvatham, S. J., Deshmukh, A. J., Gersh, B. J., Carter, R. E., Yao, X., Rabinstein, A. A., Erickson, B. J., Kapa, S., & Friedman, P. A. (2019). An artificial intelligence-enabled ECG algorithm for the identification of patients with atrial fibrillation during sinus rhythm: A retrospective analysis of outcome prediction. *Lancet*, *394*(10201), 861–867. https://doi.org/10.1016/s0140-6736(19)31721-0

Basu, A., Kuziemsky, C., de Araújo Novaes, M., Kleber, A., Sales, F., Al-Shorbaji, N., Flórez-Arango, J. F., Gogia, S. B., Ho, K., Hunter, I., Iyengar, S., John, O., John, S., Kulatunga, G., Rajput, V. K., Ranatunga, P., & Udayasankaran, J. G. (2021). Telehealth and the COVID-19 pandemic: International perspectives and a health systems framework for telehealth implementation to support critical response. *Yearbook of Medical Informatics*, *30*(01), 126–133. https://doi.org/10.1055/s-0041-1726484

Blumenthal, D., & Tavenner, M. (2010). The "meaningful use" regulation for electronic health records. *New England Journal of Medicine, 363*(6), 501–504.

Boonstra, A., & Broekhuis, M. (2010). Barriers to the acceptance of electronic medical records by physicians: From systematic review to taxonomy and interventions. *BMC Health Services Research, 10*(1), 231.

Canada, H. (2024). Decision making framework. https://www.canada.ca/en/health-canada/services/science-research/science-advice-decision-making/decision-making-framework-science-research.html?

Centers for Medicare and Medicaid Services. (2022). NHE fact sheet. CMS. https://www.cms.gov/data-research/statistics-trends-and-reports/national-health-expenditure-data/nhe-fact-sheet

Chandrasekaran, R., Katthula, V., & Moustakas, E. (2020). Patterns of use and key predictors for the use of wearable health care devices by US adults: Insights from a National Survey. *Journal of Medical Internet Research*, *22*(10), e22443. https://doi.org/10.2196/22443

Changhez, J., James, S., Jamala, F., Khan, S., Khan, M. Z., Gul, S., & Zainab, I. (2024). Evaluating the efficacy and accuracy of ai-assisted diagnostic techniques in endometrial carcinoma: A systematic review. *Cureus*. https://doi.org/10.7759/cureus.60973

Friend, S. H., Ginsburg, G. S., & Picard, R. W. (2023). Wearable digital health technology. *New England Journal of Medicine*, *389*(22), 2100–2101. https://doi.org/10.1056/nejme2303219

Gatchel, R. J., McGeary, D. D., McGeary, C. A., & Lippe, B. (2014). Interdisciplinary chronic pain management: Past, present, and future. *American Psychologist, 69*(2), 119–130.

Holland, J. H. (2006). Studying complex adaptive systems. *Journal of Systems Science and Complexity, 19*(1), 1–8.

Jacobsen, P. B., & Jim, H. S. (2008). Psychosocial interventions for anxiety and depression in adult cancer patients: Achievements and challenges. *CA: A Cancer Journal for Clinicians, 58*(4), 214–230.

Johnson, K. B., Wei, W., Dilhan Weeraratne, Frisse, M. E., Misulis, K., Rhee, K., Zhao, J., & Snowdon, J. L. (2020). Precision medicine, AI, and the future of personalized health care. *Clinical and Translational Science*, *14*(1), 86–93. https://doi.org/10.1111/cts.12884

Kotter, J. (1996). John Kotter's eight step change model. https://portal.ct.gov/-/media/SDE/Turnaround/School-Improvement-Resources/Kotters_model.pdf

Levenson, S. A. (2023). The health care decision-making process framework. Maryland Medicine: MM: A publication of MEDCHI. *Maryland State Medical Society*, *11*(1). https://pubmed.ncbi.nlm.nih.gov/21140861/

Mendelow, A. (1991). Stakeholder mapping. In: *Proceedings of the 2nd International Conference on Information Systems* (pp. 10–24). Cambridge, MA: ACM.

Mitchell, M. (2009). *Complexity: A Guided Tour*. Oxford: Oxford University Press.

NEJM Catalyst. (2018). What is lean healthcare? https://catalyst.nejm.org/doi/full/10.1056/CAT.18.0193

OCED. (2023). Use of telemedicine has boomed during the COVID-19 pandemic. *OECD Health Policy Studies*. https://doi.org/10.1787/e41e1ce6-en

Rogers, E. M. (2003). *Diffusion of Innovations* (5th ed.). New York: Free Press.

Scribenote|veterinarian AI Scribe App and Software. (2024). https://www.scribenote.com/

SMART Hospital and Innovation—Mackenzie Health. (2022). Mackenzie health. https://www.mackenziehealth.ca/about-us/smart-hospital-and-innovation

Snowden, D. J., & Boone, M. E. (2007). A leader's framework for decision making. *Harvard Business Review, 85*(11), 68–76.

Strömberg, A. (2005). The crucial role of patient education in heart failure. *European Journal of Heart Failure, 7*(3), 363–369. https://doi.org/10.1016/j.ejheart.2005.01.002

Tempus. (2024). AI-enabled precision medicine. *Tempus*. https://www.tempus.com/?srsltid=AfmBOorVeMbZ2aLl1xDPaHbqbPmbaT7otwADLXa0rnhLwvfILI1Ukpwo

Totaforti, S. (2018). Applying the benefits of biophilic theory to hospital design. *City Territory and Architecture, 5*(1). https://doi.org/10.1186/s40410-018-0077-5

Trento, M., Passera, P., Bajardi, M., Tomalino, M., Grassi, G., Miselli, V., & Porta, M. (2004). Lifestyle intervention by group care prevents deterioration of type II diabetes: A 4-year randomized controlled clinical trial. *Diabetologia, 47*(9), 1459–1465.

Xu, H., & Michael, K. (2023). Medical artificial intelligence and the black box problem: A view based on the ethical principle of "do no harm." *Intelligent Medicine*, *4*(1), 52–57. https://doi.org/10.1016/j.imed.2023.08.001

BIBLIOGRAPHIES

Adoption Readiness Levels (ARL): A complement to TRL. (2024). https://www.energy.gov/technologytransitions/adoption-readiness-levels-arl-complement-trl

Centers for Medicare & Medicaid Services (CMS). (2020). Physicians and other clinicians: CMS flexibilities to fight COVID-19. https://www.cms.gov/files/document/physicians-and-other-clinicians-cms-flexibilities-fight-covid-19.pdf

Ephraim, G. (2024). Vitality|vitality active rewards. *Vitality International*. https://vitality.international/about-vitality/vitality-active-rewards.html

Flor, H., Fydrich, T., & Turk, D. C. (1992). Efficacy of multidisciplinary pain treatment centers: A meta-analytic review. *Pain, 49*(2), 221–230.

Free, C., Phillips, G., Galli, L., Watson, L., Felix, L., Edwards, P., … & Haines, A. (2013). The effectiveness of mobile-health technology-based health behaviour change or disease management interventions for health care consumers: A systematic review. *PLOS Medicine, 10*(1), e1001362.

Goldzweig, C. L., Towfigh, A., Paige, N. M., Orshansky, G., Haggstrom, D. A., Beroes, J. M., Miake-Lye, I., & Shekelle, P. G. (2013). Systematic review: Secure messaging between providers and patients, and patients' access to their own medical record. Evidence on Health Outcomes, Satisfaction, Efficiency and Attitudes. VA-ESP Project #05-226, 2012.

Hollander, J. E., & Carr, B. G. (2020). Virtually perfect? Telemedicine for Covid-19. *New England Journal of Medicine, 382*(18), 1679–1681.

Koltowski, L., Balsam, P., Glowczynska, R., Rokicki, J. K., Peller, M., Maksym, J., … Grabowski, M. (2021). Kardia mobile applicability in clinical practice: A comparison of Kardia mobile and standard 12-lead electrocardiogram records in 100 consecutive patients of a tertiary cardiovascular care center. *Cardiology Journal, 28*(4), 543–548. https://doi.org/10.5603/cj.a2019.0001

Kurtz, C. F., & Snowden, D. J. (2003). The new dynamics of strategy: Sense-making in a complex and complicated world. *IBM Systems Journal, 42*(3), 462–483.

Larson, H. J., Jarrett, C., Eckersberger, E., Smith, D. M., & Paterson, P. (2014). Understanding vaccine hesitancy around vaccines and vaccination from a global perspective: A systematic review of published literature, 2007–2012. *Vaccine, 32*(19), 2150–2159.

Lehmann, U., & Sanders, D. (2007). Community health workers: What do we know about them? The state of the evidence on programmes, activities, costs and impact on health outcomes of using community health workers. World Health Organization. https://chwcentral.org/resources/community-health-workers-what-do-we-know-about-them-the-state-of-the-evidence-on-programmes-activities-costs-and-impact-on-health-outcomes-of-using-community-health-workers/

Mankins, J. C. (1995). *Technology Readiness Levels: A White Paper*. Washington, DC: NASA, Office of Space Access and Technology.

Medrec, M. (2024). https://medrec-m.com/

Merson, M. H., O'Malley, J., Serwadda, D., & Apisuk, C. (2008). The history and challenge of HIV prevention. *Lancet, 372*(9637), 475–488.

Palmer, R., & Zimmerman, B. (2017). Using complexity science for healthcare decision-making: A case study. *Journal of Evaluation in Clinical Practice, 23*(5), 1137–1143.

Phadke, V. K., Bednarczyk, R. A., Salmon, D. A., & Omer, S. B. (2016). Association between vaccine refusal and vaccine-preventable diseases in the United States: A review of measles and pertussis. *JAMA, 315*(11), 1149–1158.

Plsek, P. E., & Greenhalgh, T. (2001). The challenge of complexity in health care. *BMJ, 323*(7313), 625–628.

Reeves, J. J., Hollandsworth, H. M., Torriani, F. J., Taplitz, R., Abeles, S., Tai-Seale, M., Millen, M., Clay, B. J., & Longhurst, C. A. (2020). Rapid response to COVID-19: Health informatics support for outbreak management in an academic health system. *Journal of the American Medical Informatics Association, 27*(6), 853–859.

Roumeliotis, D. (2020). Diffusion of innovation: Getting past the first wave of innovators and early adopters to reach the tipping point. Unconventional Business Wisdom for the refined entrepreneurial mindset. https://theboldbusinessexpert.com/2020/11/02/diffusion-of-innovation-getting-past-the-first-wave-of-innovators-and-early-adopters-to-reach-the-tipping-point/

Shore, J. H., Schneck, C. D., Mishkind, M. C., Shore, P., & Shore, J. H. (2020). Telepsychiatry and the Coronavirus Disease 2019 Pandemic—Current and future outcomes of the rapid virtualization of psychiatric care. *JAMA Psychiatry, 77*(12), 1211–1212.

Shortell, S. M., Addicott, R., Walsh, N., & Ham, C. (2014). The NHS five year forward view: Lessons from the United States in developing new care models. *BMJ, 349*, g8317.

The Austin Common. (2013). Dell children's medical center first in the world to earn LEED for health care platinum designation, 2013, July 11. https://theaustincommon.com/dell-childrens-medical-center-first-world-earn-leed-health-care-platinum-designation/

U.S. Department of Health and Human Services. (2021). HIPAA home. https://www.hhs.gov/hipaa/index.html

van Beurden, E. K., Kia, A. M., Zask, A., Dietrich, U., & Rose, L. (2013). Making sense in a complex landscape: How the Cynefin framework from complex adaptive systems theory can inform health promotion practice. *Health Promotion International, 28*(1), 73–83.

World Health Organization (WHO). (2020). Strengthening the health systems response to COVID-19. https://www.who.int/europe/tools-and-toolkits/strengthening-the-health-system-response-to-covid-19

Wosik, J., Fudim, M., Cameron, B., Gellad, Z. F., Cho, A., Phinney, D., Curtis, S., Roman, M., Poon, E. G., Ferranti, J., Katz, J. N., & Tcheng, J. (2020). Telehealth transformation: COVID-19 and the rise of virtual care. *Journal of the American Medical Informatics Association, 27*(6), 957–962.

3 Innovation in Healthcare

Perspectives from Organizational, Societal, and Technological Dimensions

Mohit Goswami

3.1 INTRODUCTION

Service innovation in healthcare is multifaceted in that it often encompasses the development and subsequent implementation of novel approaches, technologies, know-how, and processes to improve healthcare service delivery further. Such innovations are essential for handling the difficult problems faced by healthcare systems globally, such as rising costs and the increasing need to enhance patient outcomes and experiences. Technological advancements play a key role in driving service innovation in healthcare, particularly in the developing world. For instance, increased care coordination and patient safety have been realized through the transformation of patient information storage, access, and sharing among healthcare practitioners through the usage of electronic health records (EHRs) (Länsisalmi, Kivimäki, & Aalto, 2006). Telemedicine is another technological innovation that allows for remote consultations and monitoring, thereby enhancing access to healthcare, especially in underserved areas (Bashshur et al., 2011). By monitoring vital signs, medication compliance, and lifestyle choices, wearable technologies and modern healthcare mobile apps enable people to participate actively in their treatment management, leading to improved health outcomes (Plaza et al., 2013). Moreover, service innovation in healthcare involves a shift toward patient-centered care models. This approach emphasizes the involvement of patients in decision-making processes, thus understanding their unique needs and preferences and providing tailored solutions (Bodenheimer & Sinsky, 2014). Patient-centered medical homes (PCMHs) and accountable care organizations (ACOs) are two prominent instances of service delivery models that emphasize comprehensive and coordinated treatment to meet patients' all-encompassing health requirements (Friedberg et al., 2015). Service innovation in healthcare pertains to efforts to address socioeconomic determinants of health and health inequities in addition to integrating technological breakthroughs and patient-centered methods. Extant research has shown that socioeconomic dimensions such as income, education, and access to resources impact individuals' health outcomes and healthcare utilization (Braveman, Egerter, & Williams, 2011). Therefore, innovative interventions targeting social determinants (such as community health worker programs, transportation

DOI: 10.1201/9781003513834-3

assistance, and affordable housing initiatives) are crucial for advancing health fairness and minimizing differences in healthcare outcomes and access (Gottlieb et al., 2016).

As evident from the aforementioned discussions, organizational, societal, and technological aspects become both drivers and impediments to the realization of service innovation in healthcare delivery. Therefore, this chapter intends to identify such drivers and barriers cutting across organizational, societal, and technological constructs. The rest of the chapter is arranged as follows. Section 3.2 provides the literature review related to the extant contributions. Section 3.3 enumerates drivers of service innovation in healthcare. Section 3.4 details the challenges and barriers related to service innovation in healthcare. Finally, the chapter concludes in Section 3.5 wherein conclusions are presented.

3.2 LITERATURE REVIEW

This chapter explores various nuances related to drivers and barriers emanating from organizational, societal, and technological aspects. Therefore, pertinent research literature is presented along these three dimensions.

3.2.1 Technological Innovation in Healthcare Service Delivery

Technological innovations play an important role in driving service innovation in healthcare, enabling the transformation of care delivery processes and enhancing patient outcomes. EHRs are perhaps among the most widely adopted technological innovations in healthcare, facilitating the digital storage, access, and exchange of patient information (Hillestad et al., 2005). Hillestad et al. (2005) employing a literature review approach and followed by data analysis methodologies related to electronic medical record (EMR) implementation rate indicated that technology adoption leads to significant savings, enhanced healthcare outcomes, and improved chronic disease management. Existing research indicates that EHR implementation is associated with improved healthcare coordination, mitigated medical errors, and improved patient safety (Länsisalmi et al., 2006). Länsisalmi et al. (2006) further focused on various aspects of healthcare innovation, including its definition, types, processes, and outcomes within healthcare settings. The study augmented the extant studies related to technological innovations that essentially entail the design, development, and implementation of new medical devices. Bashshur et al. (2011) further developed a taxonomy that categorized telemedicine based on various criteria including the nature of the clinical interaction, the type of technology used, and the specific medical services provided. The taxonomy further incorporated multiple facets, such as the timing of information exchange (synchronous vs. asynchronous), the purpose of the interaction (diagnostic, therapeutic, educational), and the clinical specialty involved, providing a tiered classification system. An important contribution of the study pertained to the fact that it provided technological modalities and frameworks for technological integration in healthcare services. Studies have also demonstrated the effectiveness of telemedicine in improving patient satisfaction, reducing healthcare costs, and expanding access to specialty care services (Bashshur et al., 2011). Additionally, wearable technologies and mobile-based applications have emerged as effective tools for promoting patient engagement and self-management of health conditions. With their smartphones or wearable devices, patients can monitor vital signs, track medication adherence, and access instructional resources. Current research has also indicated that the use of such interventions is associated with improved treatment compliance, better management of diseases, and enhanced patient-healthcare provider communication (Plaza et al., 2013). Plaza et al. (2013) from a technological perspective further revealed that mindfulness apps offered a range of functionalities, including guided meditations, progress tracking, reminders, and educational content. This study further highlighted the potential for integrating mindfulness apps into broader health interventions, emphasizing the need for collaboration between app developers and healthcare professionals to ensure the delivery of high-quality and evidence-based capabilities. Service innovation in healthcare also encompasses the adoption of patient-centered healthcare models that capture the needs and preferences, while additionally considering the experiences of patients. Patient-centered care underlines collaboration between patients and healthcare providers, leading to shared decision-making with a provision of personalized care plans tailored to each patient's unique circumstances (Bodenheimer & Sinsky, 2014). Rogers et al. (2024) categorized and examined three distinct types of simulated records in EMR systems, viz. fictional, confidential, and unknown patients. From a technological standpoint, the study identified several challenges such as system integration, privacy mechanisms, and error mitigation through automation.

3.2.2 Organizational Aspects in Healthcare Service Delivery

According to the extant research, patient satisfaction, treatment adherence, and health outcomes have been linked to PCMHs and ACOs (Friedberg et al., 2015). Friedberg et al. (2015) further highlighted the role PCMHs and ACOs play in innovative healthcare models that emphasize coordination, continuity, and patient engagement. These models aim to address the fragmentation and inefficiencies inherent in traditional fee-for-service healthcare delivery by promoting team-based care, care management, and health management. The study employed a difference-in-differences approach. By comparing changes over time between participating and non-participating primary care practices, the study controlled for confounding variables and isolated the effect of the intervention. The findings further suggested that the multipayer PCMH model can lead to organizational changes aimed at improving primary care delivery. Nonetheless, achieving significant improvements in patient outcomes and cost reductions may require additional time, resources, and other complementary interventions. Teigland et al. (2013) further explored medical students' attitudes toward patient safety and quality improvement education at the University of North Carolina School of Medicine. Employing an electronic survey approach, the study found that most students recognized the importance of patient safety and quality improvement. They also preferred experiential learning methods such as real-life cases and participation in quality improvement projects. From an organizational perspective, the study highlighted the need for integrating patient safety education into clinical training, thus suggesting a major shift from traditional didactic approaches to hands-on, system-based learning. This would align with student preferences and enhance institutional training frameworks.

3.2.3 Social Dimensions in Healthcare Service Delivery

In addition to technological advancements and patient-centered care models, service innovation in healthcare involves interventions targeting social dimensions of health, which significantly influence healthcare outcomes and utilization. The socioeconomic and environmental aspects that impact people's health and ability to obtain healthcare services are referred to as social determinants of health (Braveman et al., 2011). Addressing the social determinants of health remains vital to promoting health equity and reducing disparities in healthcare access and outcomes. To enhance health outcomes for marginalized and underserved communities and overcome barriers to healthcare access, a variety of treatments targeting social determinants of health have been implemented. For instance, community health worker programs engage community members to provide culturally competent care, health education, and social support to individuals with chronic conditions or complex health needs (Gottlieb et al., 2016). Research suggests that community health worker interventions are effective in enhancing health outcomes, thus reducing hospitalizations and lowering healthcare costs (Gottlieb et al., 2016). Furthermore, healthcare organizations are increasingly partnering with community-based organizations, local governments, and social agencies to address social determinants of health through collaborative initiatives. Such initiatives may include housing assistance programs, transportation support services, food insecurity interventions, and workforce development initiatives aimed at tackling the fundamental social and financial issues that lead to suboptimal health results (Gottlieb et al., 2016). Greenhalgh et al. (2017) introduced a framework to analyze factors influencing the lack of adoption (and abandonment), scaling up, and sustainability of health. By adopting systematic review and empirical case studies, the study identified barriers such as organizational culture, technological complexity, and social resistance. From a social standpoint, the findings emphasized the importance of addressing user needs, stakeholder engagement, and policy support to ensure successful technology integration in healthcare systems. Vest et al. (2019) examined the adoption of EHRs in U.S. nursing facilities, highlighting social and systemic challenges. Using a cross-sectional survey of post-acute and long-term care providers, the study identified disparities in EHR adoption rates and the barriers hindering implementation, such as costs and interoperability challenges. From a social perspective, the findings emphasized the benefits of EHRs in improving healthcare coordination, patient safety, and staff efficiency, while also addressing the digital divide and organizational resistance to technology adoption. Levaitan et al. (2021) examined the association between physicians' workload, work hours, and experience with prescription errors in the context of an acute care hospital setting. Employing data from over 1.6 million prescriptions identified by a computerized decision-support system, the findings from the study indicated that high workloads significantly increase the likelihood of prescription errors. From a social perspective, the study highlights the potential impact of physician fatigue and workload on patient safety, thereby emphasizing the need for systemic and sustainable interventions to manage shift schedules and workload distribution to deliver better healthcare outcomes.

Table 3.1 enlists some recent and key studies and highlights the research context, methodology, data collection method, key findings, and linkages (either to Organizational, Societal, and Technological or in combinations).

TABLE 3.1
Summarizing Some Recent and Key Studies

Authors	Research Context	Methodology	Data Collection Method	Key Findings	Linkage
Rogers et al. (2024)	Challenges with 'unknown' and fictional patient data in EMRs	Case-based analysis of institutional practices	Analysis of cases involving safety events and EMR practices	Fictional and unknown records can aid functionality testing but pose risks in designing clinical workflows	Technical: Issues with data integrity and integration
Campione and Liu (2024)	Perceptions of EHR usability and safety by hospital staff tenure and position	Cross-sectional survey with regression analysis	AHRQ SOPS data from 44 hospitals (8,880 staff respondents)	Staff perceptions vary by role and tenure; dissatisfaction is highest among physicians and senior staff	Organizational and technical: usability impacts satisfaction and workflow
Classen et al. (2020)	Trends in the medication safety performance of EHR systems in U.S. hospitals	Case series; descriptive analysis of safety tests	Leapfrog group's health IT safety measures test data (8,657 hospital-years)	Safety improved over time, but wide variability in performance remains	Technical: variability due to differences in EHR vendor implementations
Leviatan et al. (2021)	Impact of physicians' workload and experience on prescribing errors	Large-scale retrospective analysis using ML models	Analysis of 1,652,896 prescriptions flagged by a decision-support system	Errors correlated with workload, successive shifts, and lack of drug-specific experience; decision support reduces errors	Technical and social: role of clinical decision-support systems in mitigating errors
Vest et al. (2019)	Adoption of interoperable health IT in U.S. nursing facilities	Cross-sectional survey with regression modeling	Surveys of AMDA members; linked to secondary data sources	Innovativeness correlates with higher adoption and interoperability	Organizational and technical: focus on culture and technology integration
Greenhalgh et al. (2017)	Barriers to technology adoption, spread, and sustainability in health/ social care programs	Hermeneutic review and longitudinal case studies	Ethnographic observation, interviews, and document analysis across six programs	Complex domains rarely achieve sustainability	Organizational, social, and technical: interactions among system, technology, and users
Teigland et al. (2013)	Medical students' attitudes toward patient safety and quality improvement education	Cross-sectional electronic survey	Survey responses from medical students at a single medical school	Students value real-life examples in learning safety integration into clinical education is preferred	Social and organizational: importance of aligning curriculum with students' needs

3.3 KEY DRIVERS OF SERVICE INNOVATION IN HEALTHCARE

3.3.1 Changing Demographics and Healthcare Needs

The landscape of healthcare is continuously evolving, driven by changing demographics and shifting healthcare needs. As populations age, chronic conditions become more prevalent, and expectations for personalized, easily available, and effective medical care assurance become essential to meet these evolving demands. This section explores how changing demographics and healthcare needs serve as key drivers of service innovation in healthcare. With advancements in healthcare leading to longer life expectancies, the percentage of elderly individuals in the population is increasing globally. As individuals age, they are more likely to develop chronic conditions such as diabetes, cardiovascular diseases, and neurological disorders that require ongoing management and support (Olshansky et al., 2005). Research indicates that the prevalence of chronic conditions has been rising worldwide, thus placing significant demands on healthcare systems (Ward et al., 2014). To address the needs of an aging population with multiple chronic conditions, healthcare providers are turning to innovations to develop new care models, technologies, and interventions that enhance care coordination, improve patient outcomes, and optimize resource utilization (Friedberg et al., 2015). These models emphasize proactive, coordinated, and patient-centered care delivery that has been demonstrated to enhance health outcomes, reduce hospitalizations, and lower healthcare costs (Friedberg et al., 2015). Another key driver of service innovation in healthcare is the rising need for individualized and easily accessible medical treatment. As patients become more knowledgeable and involved when making healthcare decisions, they expect care tailored to individual needs, preferences, and circumstances. Moreover, advancements in technology have empowered patients to take a more active role in managing their health, driving demand for digital health solutions and telemedicine services (Greenhalgh et al., 2017). Extant studies suggest that patient engagement and empowerment are essential components of effective healthcare delivery and are associated with improved health outcomes and patient satisfaction (Barello et al., 2016). Service innovation in healthcare aims to leverage technology and patient-centered care models to provide personalized, accessible, and convenient healthcare services that meet the diverse needs of patients. These innovations not only significantly enhance access to care but also greatly empower patients to take an active role in managing their healthcare, which will improve health outcomes.

3.3.2 Technological Advancements and Digital Transformation

Technological advancements and digital transformation have become pivotal drivers of service innovation in healthcare, transforming the delivery of patient care and healthcare systems worldwide. This section of the chapter explores the tenets of technological advancements and digital transformation as key drivers of service innovation in healthcare. One of the foundational elements of technological advancements in healthcare is the adoption of health information technology (HIT) and EHRs. EHRs enable the digital capture, storage, and exchange of patient health information, thus replacing traditional paper-based record systems with digital ones. Research has shown that the implementation of EHRs leads to improvements in care coordination, patient safety, and healthcare quality (Hillestad et al., 2005). Furthermore, HIT encompasses a wide range of digital tools and systems that support various aspects of healthcare delivery, including clinical decision support, remote patient monitoring, etc. Such technologies enable healthcare service providers to deliver more efficient, effective, and individualized patient treatment that improves health outcomes and patient experiences (Länsisalmi et al., 2006). Remote patient monitoring and telemedicine technologies have emerged as transformative innovations in healthcare, particularly in the context of digital transformation. Additionally, technologies for remote patient monitoring allow medical professionals to monitor patients' health parameters and vital signs from a distance, thereby facilitating proactive management and early detection of health issues (Plaza et al., 2013). The widespread adoption of wearable devices and mobile health applications has further accelerated digital transformation in healthcare, empowering patients to actively engage in their health and well-being. Wearable technology allows people to track their heart rate, physical activity, sleep habits, and other health parameters. Examples of these devices are fitness trackers and smartwatches in real time (Plaza et al., 2013). Similarly, mobile health applications provide patients immediate access to health-related information, resources, and tools, thus allowing them to track medication adherence, set health goals, and receive personalized health recommendations. Research suggests that using mobile health applications and wearable technology is associated with improvements in health behaviors, medication adherence, and health outcomes (Plaza et al., 2013). Technological innovations can enable patients to participate actively in managing their health. As healthcare systems continue to evolve in response to changing patient needs and technological innovation, the role of technology in driving service innovation will remain paramount.

3.3.3 Regulatory and Policy Changes

Policy and regulatory changes play a significant role in improving healthcare delivery and driving service innovation. This section explores how regulatory and policy changes serve as key drivers of service innovation in healthcare. Regulatory agencies and policymakers often play a critical role in encouraging the adoption of technological innovations in healthcare by creating an environment that supports innovation and facilitates the implementation of new technologies. Policies that support EHR interoperability standards, for instance, EHRs and HIT systems, can facilitate the seamless and real-time exchange of patient information among healthcare providers, leading to improvements in care coordination and patient outcomes (Länsisalmi et al., 2006). Research suggests that regulatory initiatives aimed at incentivizing the adoption of telemedicine and remote patient monitoring technologies have led to increased utilization of these services, particularly in underserved or rural areas (Bashshur et al., 2011). By removing regulatory barriers and providing reimbursement incentives for telemedicine services, policymakers can stimulate innovation and expand access to care, ultimately improving patient outcomes and reducing healthcare disparities (Bashshur et al., 2011). Regulatory and policy changes can also foster collaboration and integration among healthcare stakeholders, driving service innovation through coordinated care delivery models and partnerships. By providing incentives for collaboration and rewarding value-based care delivery, policymakers can drive service innovation in healthcare and promote the adoption of innovative care models that prioritize patient-centered care, care coordination, and population health management. In some cases, regulatory and policy changes may be needed to address barriers to innovation and facilitate the adoption of new technologies and care delivery models. For example, regulatory frameworks governing data privacy and security can impact the development and implementation of options for digital health such as mobile health applications and wearable devices (Plaza et al., 2013). Research suggests that lawmakers must find a balance between ensuring patient privacy and driving innovation by implementing regulations that ensure data security while enabling the responsible use of health data for research and healthcare delivery purposes (Plaza et al., 2013). By developing clear and flexible regulatory frameworks that promote innovation while safeguarding patient rights and data privacy, policymakers can create an environment conducive to service innovation in healthcare.

3.3.4 Patient-Centered Care and Experience

Patient-centered care and experience have emerged as central components of service innovation in healthcare driving the development of innovative care models, technologies, and interventions aimed at improving patient outcomes and satisfaction. This section explores the role of patient-centered care and experience as key drivers of service innovation in healthcare. Patient-centered care emphasizes the importance of involving patients in their healthcare decisions, respecting their preferences, and addressing their concerns. Research suggests that patient-centered care is associated with improved patient outcomes, higher satisfaction with care, and increased adherence to treatment regimens (Epstein & Street Jr, 2011). As healthcare systems strive to deliver care that is more personalized, accessible, and responsive to patient needs, patient-centered care has become a driving force behind service innovation. By prioritizing the patients' perspectives and preferences, healthcare providers can develop innovative care models and interventions that better meet the needs of patients and their families (Epstein & Street Jr, 2011). Service innovation in healthcare often involves co-designing care with patients and engaging them as partners in the design, delivery, and evaluation of healthcare services. Research suggests that involving patients in the co-design process leads to the development of more patient-centered and effective care solutions (Bate & Robert, 2006). By actively and continuously seeking feedback from patients, healthcare providers can identify areas for improvement, tailor services to meet patient preferences, and co-create solutions that address patients' unique needs and circumstances (Bate & Robert, 2006). Co-design approaches have been used to develop innovative care models, digital health tools, and patient education materials that enhance patient engagement, satisfaction, and health outcomes. Consider, for instance, patient portals, mobile health applications, and virtual care platforms that empower patients to access their health information, communicate with their healthcare providers, and engage in self-management activities from the convenience of their smartphones or computers (Lupton, 2013). Research suggests that technology-enabled interventions can further improve patient engagement, satisfaction, and health outcomes by providing patients with greater control over their healthcare experience (Lupton, 2013).

3.4 CHALLENGES AND BARRIERS TO SERVICE INNOVATION WITHIN HEALTHCARE

3.4.1 Resistance to Change and Organizational Culture

While service innovation in the healthcare industry has enormous potential to improve patient outcomes and care delivery, it also faces challenges and barriers particularly related to resistance to change and organizational culture. This section examines the impact of resistance to change and organizational culture as a significant barrier to service innovation in healthcare. One prevalent problem is resistance to change encountered in healthcare organizations when implementing service innovations. Healthcare professionals may resist changes to established workflows, practices, and systems due to factors such as fear of the unknown, perceived loss of autonomy, or concerns about increased workload (Greenhalgh et al., 2017). Studies have suggested that resistance to change can hinder the adoption and implementation of innovative practices and technologies, leading to delays or failures in service innovation initiatives (Greenhalgh et al., 2004). Overcoming resistance to change requires proactive leadership, effective communication, and engagement strategies that address stakeholders' concerns, build trust, and further a culture of openness and collaboration. Organizational culture plays a significant role in shaping attitudes, behaviors, and decision-making processes within healthcare organizations, thus influencing their ability to embrace and sustain service innovation initiatives. Research suggests that organizational cultures characterized by hierarchy, rigid structures, and resistance to risk-taking may inhibit creativity, experimentation, and innovation (Scott et al., 2003). Healthcare organizations with hierarchical cultures may struggle to empower frontline staff to contribute ideas, share feedback, and participate in innovation efforts, leading to missed opportunities for service improvement (Scott et al., 2003). Additionally, those cultures that prioritize stability and conformity over innovation may be resistant to change and reluctant to adopt new practices or technologies, even when evidence suggests strong benefits (Scott et al., 2003). Addressing resistance to change and transforming organizational culture are critical steps in overcoming barriers to service innovation in healthcare. Successful innovation efforts require leadership commitment, employee engagement, and cultural change initiatives that promote a shared vision of innovation and create an environment supportive of experimentation and learning (Damschroder et al., 2009). Healthcare leaders can promote innovation by fueling a psychologically safe work environment where staff members are at ease taking chances, exchanging ideas, and questioning the embedded status quo (Edmondson, 1999). By creating opportunities for cross-functional collaboration, encouraging knowledge sharing, and rewarding innovative behavior, organizations can cultivate a culture that values creativity, continuous improvement, and service excellence (Damschroder et al., 2009).

3.4.2 Resource Constraints and Financial Pressures

In the ever-evolving landscape of healthcare services, resource constraints and financial pressures often present significant challenges and barriers to the implementation of service innovation efforts. Resource constraints, including limited funding, staffing shortages, and infrastructure limitations, pose significant challenges to healthcare organizations looking to innovate and improve service delivery. Resource constraints can impede the development, adoption, and scaling of innovative practices and technologies, thus limiting their impact and effectiveness (Greenhalgh et al., 2004). For instance, healthcare organizations may lack the necessary financial resources to invest in new technologies, staff training, or infrastructure upgrades needed to support service innovation initiatives (Greenhalgh et al., 2017). Similarly, staffing shortages and competing priorities may strain existing resources and limit the capacity of healthcare organizations to dedicate time and personnel to innovation efforts (Greenhalgh et al., 2017). Financial pressures, including budget constraints, reimbursement limitations, and rising healthcare costs, further exacerbate the challenges of implementing service innovation in healthcare. Financial considerations often drive decision-making in healthcare organizations, influencing the prioritization of innovation initiatives and the allocation of resources (Damschroder et al., 2009). Further, healthcare organizations may be hesitant to invest in innovative technologies or care delivery models if they perceive them as cost-prohibitive or if the return on investment is uncertain (Damschroder et al., 2009). Additionally, reimbursement policies and payment structures may not adequately incentivize or reward innovation, creating rather disincentives for healthcare providers to adopt new practices or technologies (Damschroder et al., 2009). Addressing resource constraints and financial pressures requires strategic planning, stakeholder engagement, and innovative financing models that support service innovation in healthcare. Collaborative partnerships, shared resources, and creative funding mechanisms can help overcome resource constraints and facilitate the implementation of innovative practices and technologies (Teigland et al., 2013). For example, healthcare organizations may collaborate with industry partners, academic institutions, or government agencies to access funding, expertise, and resources needed to support innovation initiatives (Teigland et al., 2013). Additionally, value-based payment models and alternative reimbursement structures that reward outcomes, rather than volume, can incentivize healthcare providers to invest in innovation and focus on delivering high-quality, cost-effective care (Damschroder et al., 2009).

3.4.3 Data Privacy and Security Concerns

Data privacy and security concerns represent significant challenges and barriers to the implementation of service innovation in healthcare. Healthcare organizations handle vast amounts of sensitive patient health information, including medical records, diagnostic data, and treatment histories. The protection of this data is paramount to ensuring patient privacy and confidentiality. However, concerns about data breaches, unauthorized access, and misuse of health information pose significant challenges to service innovation (Rothstein, 2010). Data breaches in healthcare can result in serious consequences, including financial losses, lasting reputational damage, and compromised patient trust (Ponemon Institute, 2021). Strict regulatory standards, including the Health Insurance Portability and Accountability Act (HIPAA) in the United States, must be followed by healthcare businesses to safeguard patient data and comply with privacy and security standards (Ponemon Institute, 2021). Data privacy and security concerns can erode patient trust and confidence in healthcare organizations and service innovation initiatives. Patients may be reluctant to share sensitive health information or participate in innovative programs if they perceive their privacy to be at risk (Prainsack & Buyx, 2013). Trust is further essential for patient engagement and participation in healthcare services as a breach of privacy can undermine trust and hinder patient-provider relationships (Prainsack & Buyx, 2013). Healthcare organizations must prioritize data privacy and security to maintain patient trust and enable engagement in service innovation initiatives. Transparent communication, informed consent processes, and robust data protection measures are essential for building patient trust and ensuring that patient privacy is respected throughout the innovation process (Prainsack & Buyx, 2013). Failure to comply with data privacy regulations can result in severe legal and financial consequences, including fines, penalties, and legal liability (Rothstein, 2010). Healthcare organizations face increased scrutiny from regulatory agencies and stakeholders, requiring them to invest in robust data privacy and security infrastructure and implement comprehensive risk management strategies to mitigate potential breaches and legal risks (Ponemon Institute, 2021). Healthcare data privacy and security issues can be mitigated by blockchain technology and artificial intelligence (AI). Because the healthcare sector deals with private patient data, the sector is particularly vulnerable to data breaches. AI improves data privacy by applying cutting-edge strategies like differential privacy and data anonymization that can enable the exchange of medical data without disclosing personally identifiable information (PII). Only authorized people can access data according to their responsibility levels and contextual requirements managed by AI-driven access control systems that can dynamically manage data permissions. Additionally, AI systems may examine enormous datasets to identify possible privacy flaws and suggest suitable fixes, thus proactively protecting patient data.

3.4.4 Interoperability and Integration Challenges

Interoperability and integration challenges pose significant barriers to the implementation of service innovation in healthcare. One of the primary challenges in healthcare is the fragmentation of health information systems that often operate in silos and use incompatible data formats and standards. Interoperability issues hinder the seamless exchange and integration of patient health information across different healthcare settings and systems (Adler-Milstein et al., 2017). Consider, for example, EHR systems from different vendors using proprietary data formats and interfaces, making it difficult to share patient information among providers, hospitals, and healthcare organizations (Adler-Milstein et al., 2017). This lack of interoperability limits the ability of healthcare providers to access comprehensive patient data, hindering care coordination and collaboration. Interoperability challenges also contribute to inefficient data exchange and communication among healthcare providers, leading to delays, errors, and redundancies in care delivery. Manual data entry, paper-based processes, and reliance on fax machines for information exchange remain common practices in healthcare, despite the availability of digital health technologies (Adler-Milstein et al., 2017). Healthcare providers may spend significant time and resources manually entering patient data into different systems or reconciling discrepancies between electronic and paper-based records (Adler-Milstein et al., 2017). This inefficiency not only impedes workflow productivity but also increases the risk of data errors and compromises patient safety. Another challenge in achieving interoperability and integration is the lack of standardized data formats, terminologies, and data governance frameworks. Variabilities in data standards and terminology mappings across healthcare systems and organizations complicate efforts to exchange and integrate health information effectively (HIMSS, 2020). Additionally, the absence of clear data governance policies and practices further exacerbates interoperability challenges, making it difficult to establish trust, accountability, and data quality assurance mechanisms (HIMSS, 2020). Addressing interoperability and integration challenges requires collaborative efforts from healthcare stakeholders, policymakers, and technology vendors. Initiatives to establish common data standards, interoperability frameworks, and data governance principles are essential for overcoming barriers to interoperability and facilitating seamless data exchange and integration (HIMSS, 2020). For instance, healthcare organizations can adopt Health Level Seven International (HL7) standards and Fast Healthcare Interoperability Resources (FHIR) specifications to enable standardized data exchange and interoperability across disparate systems (HIMSS, 2020). Additionally, policymakers can implement regulations and incentives that promote interoperability and data sharing, such as the 21st Century Cures Act in the United States, which aims to advance interoperability and empower patients with access to their health information (CMS, 2021). By facilitating smooth data transfer between various systems, AI can also significantly reduce interoperability and integration issues in the healthcare industry. By using machine learning and natural language processing (NLP) to standardize and translate various healthcare data formats, including HL7 and FHIR, AI promotes interoperability and ensures system compatibility. Additionally, by spotting trends and enhancing data consistency, AI-driven analytics streamline processes.

Table 3.2 provides a summary of the categories and subcategories for both drivers and barriers considered in the chapter.

3.5 CONCLUSIONS

This chapter underscores the multifaceted nature of service innovation in healthcare, driven by technological advancements, regulatory changes, and evolving patient expectations. The chapter also highlights that while technological innovations such as telemedicine, EHRs, and wearable health technologies offer significant benefits, their successful adoption is often hindered by organizational resistance, resource constraints, and concerns related to data privacy and interoperability. Further, three major lenses, viz. technological, social, and organizational viewpoints, are considered for assessing the innovation aspects in healthcare delivery. First, from an organizational standpoint, fostering a culture of innovation remains essential to overcome resistance and enhance adoption rates. To this end, healthcare organizations must prioritize leadership support, employee engagement,

TABLE 3.2
Categories and Subcategories for Drivers and Barriers Pertinent to Service Innovation in Healthcare

Drivers	Barriers
Changing demographic needs	**Organizational culture and resistance to change**
1. Aging population	1. Lack of awareness
2. Chronic disease burden	2. Workforce reluctance
3. Healthcare demand growth	3. Rigid structures
Technological advancements and digital transformation	**Resource constraints and financial resources**
1. Electronic health records	1. Funding storages
2. Telemedicine	2. High implementation costs
3. Wearable devices	
Regulatory and policy interventions	**Data privacy and security concerns**
1. Compliance standards	1. Cybersecurity threats
2. Incentive programs	2. Regulatory compliances
3. Healthcare reforms	3. Staffing schedules and workload
	4. Staffing issues
Patient-centered care and experience	**Interoperability and integrational issues**
1. Personalized treatment	1. System fragmentation
2. Patient engagement	2. Lack of standardization
3. Remote monitoring	

and continuous education to synchronize innovation goals for operational realities. Further, resource constraints remain a key challenge, necessitating alternative funding models and strategic Vpartnerships to drive lasting adoption. Second, from the social perspective, service innovation plays a critical role in improving health equity and access, particularly for underserved populations. Patient-centric approaches that integrate social determinants of health into service delivery can help address such disparities and lead to more inclusive healthcare models. Finally, technologically, interoperability and data security continue to pose significant barriers. Addressing these issues requires robust regulatory frameworks and industry-wide collaboration to ensure seamless information exchange without compromising patient privacy. Overall, the study suggests that an integrative approach incorporating regulatory incentives, technological advancements, and patient engagement is essential to achieve meaningful and lasting innovation in healthcare services. By tackling these barriers, healthcare stakeholders can drive impactful, patient-focused innovations that enhance service efficiency and delivery quality. Future research can consider both exploratory and confirmatory studies to further the understanding of these factors and their associated impacts. Finally, studies considering the trade-offs considering economic, social, and technological dimensions would also be valuable addition.

REFERENCES

Adler-Milstein, J., Holmgren, A. J., Kralovec, P., Worzala, C., Searcy, T., & Patel, V. (2017). Electronic health record adoption in US hospitals: The emergence of a digital "advanced use" divide. *Journal of the American Medical Informatics Association*, 24(6), 1142–1148.

Barello, S., Triberti, S., Graffigna, G., Libreri, C., Serino, S., Hibbard, J., & Riva, G. (2016). eHealth for patient engagement: A systematic review. *Frontiers in Psychology*, 6, 2013.

Bashshur, R., Shannon, G., Krupinski, E., & Grigsby, J. (2011). The taxonomy of telemedicine. *Telemedicine Journal and e-Health*, 17(6), 484–494.

Bate, P., & Robert, G. (2006). Experience-based design: From redesigning the system around the patient to co-designing services with the patient. *Quality and Safety in Health Care*, 15(5), 307–310.

Bodenheimer, T., & Sinsky, C. (2014). From triple to quadruple aim: Care of the patient requires care of the provider. *Annals of Family Medicine*, 12(6), 573–576.

Braveman, P., Egerter, S., & Williams, D. R. (2011). The social determinants of health: Coming of age. *Annual Review of Public Health*, 32, 381–398.

Campione, J., & Liu, H. (2024). Perceptions of hospital electronic health record (EHR) training, support, and patient safety by staff position and tenure," BMC Health Services Research, 24: 955. https://doi.org/10.1186/s12913-024-11322-3

Classen D.C., Holmgren A.J., Co Z., Newmark L.P., Seger D., Danforth M., & Bates D.W. National Trends in the Safety Performance of Electronic Health Record Systems From 2009 to 2018. JAMA Netw Open. 2020 May 1;3(5):e205547. doi: 10.1001/jamanetworkopen.2020.5547. PMID: 32469412; PMCID: PMC7260621.

CMS. (2021). 21st Century Cures Act: Interoperability, Information Blocking, and the ONC Health IT Certification Program. Available at https://www.federalregister.gov/documents/2020/05/01/2020-07419/21st-century-cures-act-interoperability-information-blocking-and-the-onc-health-it-certification. Last accessed 1st January 2025.

Damschroder, L. J., Aron, D. C., Keith, R. E., Kirsh, S. R., Alexander, J. A., & Lowery, J. C. (2009). Fostering implementation of health services research findings into practice: A consolidated framework for advancing implementation science. *Implementation Science*, 4, 50.

Edmondson, A. C. (1999). Psychological safety and learning behavior in work teams. *Administrative Science Quarterly*, 44(2), 350–383.

Epstein, R. M., & Street Jr, R. L. (2011). The values and value of patient-centered care. *Annals of Family Medicine*, 9(2), 100–103.

Friedberg, M. W., Schneider, E. C., Rosenthal, M. B., Volpp, K. G., & Werner, R. M. (2015). Association between participation in a multipayer medical home intervention and changes in quality, utilization, and costs of care. *JAMA*, 311(8), 815–825.

Gottlieb, L. M., Hessler, D., Long, D., Laves, E., Burns, A., R., Sweeney, P., Schudel, C., & Adler, N. E. (2016). Effects of social needs screening and in-person service navigation on child health: A randomized clinical trial. *JAMA Pediatrics,* 170(11), e162521.

Greenhalgh, T., Robert, G., Macfarlane, F., Bate, P., & Kyriakidou, O. (2004). Diffusion of innovations in service organizations: Systematic review and recommendations. *Milbank Quarterly*, 82(4), 581–629.

Greenhalgh, T., Wherton, J., Papoutsi, C., Lynch, J., Hughes, G., A'Court, C., … & Shaw, S. (2017). Beyond adoption: A new framework for theorizing and evaluating no adoption, abandonment, and challenges to the scale-up, spread, and sustainability of health and care technologies. *Journal of Medical Internet Research*, 19(11), e367.

Hillestad, R., Bigelow, J., Bower, A., Girosi, F., Meili, R., Scoville, R., & Taylor, R. (2005). Can electronic medical record systems transform health care? Potential health benefits, savings, and costs. *Health Affairs*, 24(5), 1103–1117.

HIMSS. (2020). *Interoperability and Health Information Exchange: A HIMSS Policy Call to Action*. HIMSS, Chicago, IL.

Länsisalmi, H., Kivimäki, M., & Aalto, P. (2006). Innovation in healthcare: A systematic review of recent research. *Nursing Science Quarterly*, 19(1), 66–72.
Leviatan, I., Oberman, B., Zimlichman, E., & Stein, G. Y. (2021). Associations of physicians' prescribing experience, work hours, and workload with prescription errors. *Journal of the American Medical Informatics Association,* 28(6), 1074–1080.
Lupton, D. (2013). The digitally engaged patient: Self-monitoring and self-care in the digital health era. *Social Theory & Health*, 14(3), 170–193.
Olshansky, S. J., Passaro, D. J., Hershow, R. C., Layden, J., Carnes, B. A., Brody, J., ... & Ludwig, D. S. (2005). A potential decline in life expectancy in the United States in the 21st century. *New England Journal of Medicine*, 352(11), 1138–1145.
Plaza, I., Demarzo, M. M., Herrera-Mercadal, P., & García-Campayo, J. (2013). Mindfulness-based mobile applications: Literature review and analysis of current features. *JMIR mHealth and uHealth*, 1(2), e24.
Ponemon Institute. (2021). The Cost of a Data Breach Report. Available at https://www.dataendure.com/wp-content/uploads/2021_Cost_of_a_Data_Breach_-2.pdf. Last accessed 1st January, 2025.
Prainsack, B., & Buyx, A. (2013). A solidarity-based approach to the governance of research biobanks. *Medical Law Review*, 21(1), 71–91.
Rogers, K. J., Blau, J., & Krasowski, M. D. (2024). Evaluating the utility and challenges associated with "unknown" and fictional patients in the electronic medical record. *Academic Pathology,* 11(3):100141.
Rothstein, M. A. (2010). Is deidentification sufficient to protect health privacy in research? *American Journal of Bioethics*, 10(9), 3–11.
Scott, T., Mannion, R., Davies, H., & Marshall, M. (2003). The quantitative measurement of organizational culture in health care: A review of the available instruments. *Health Services Research*, 38(3), 923–945.
Teigland, C. L., Blasiak, R. C., & Wilson, L. A. (2013). Patient safety and quality improvement education: A cross-sectional study of medical students' preferences and attitudes. *BMC Medical Education,* 13, 16.
Vest, J. R., Jung, H. Y., Wiley Jr., K., Kooreman, H., Pettit, L., & Unruh M. A. (2019). Adoption of health information technology among US nursing facilities. *Journal of the American Medical Directors Association*. doi:10.1016/j.jamda.2018.11.002.
Ward, B. W., Schiller, J. S., & Goodman, R. A. (2014). Multiple chronic conditions among US adults: A 2012 update. *Preventing Chronic Disease*, 17(11), e62.

4 Recent Initiatives in Revamping Healthcare Policies and Programmes in India

A Review of Progress and Challenges

Jiban Kumar Behera, Bhaskar Behera, and Manojit Bhattacharya

ABBREVIATIONS

ABDM	Ayushman Bharat Digital Mission
ABHA	Ayushman Bharat Health Account
AIIMS	All India Institute of Medical Sciences
AYUSH	Ayurveda, Yoga and Naturopathy, Unani, Siddha, and Homoeopathy
CBNAAT	Cartridge-Based Nucleic Acid Amplification Test
CHCs	Community Health Centres
DCGI	Drug Controller General of India
DMHP	District Mental Health Programme
eVIN	Electronic Vaccine Intelligence Network
EHR	Electronic Health Records
HPR	Health Professional Registry
HWCs	Health and Wellness Centres
IHIP	Integrated Health Information Platform
JSY	Janani Suraksha Yojana
MoHFW	Ministry of Health and Family Welfare
NCDs	Non-Communicable Diseases
NDHM	National Digital Health Mission
NHM	National Health Mission
NHP	National Health Policy
NHS	National Health Stack
NMC	National Medical Commission
NMHP	National Mental Health Programme
NRHM	National Rural Health Mission

DOI: 10.1201/9781003513834-4

NTEP	National Tuberculosis Elimination Programme
NUHM	National Urban Health Mission
ORS	Online Registration System
PGIMER	Postgraduate Institute of Medical Education and Research
PHCs	Primary Health Centres
PM-JAY	Pradhan Mantri Jan Arogya Yojana
PMSMA	Pradhan Mantri Surakshit Matritva Abhiyan
PMSSY	Pradhan Mantri Swasthya Suraksha Yojana
RNTCP	Revised National Tuberculosis Control Programme
RSBY	Rashtriya Swasthya Bima Yojana
SDGs	Sustainable Development Goals
SECC	Socio-Economic Caste Census
SHAs	State Health Agencies

4.1 INTRODUCTION

India's concerted efforts in poverty reduction have been fruitful, with the Poverty Headcount Ratio declining from 29.17% in 2013–2014 to 11.28% in 2022–2023. This means that 250 million Indians have successfully escaped multidimensional poverty (ESCAP & India, 2024). India's commitment to achieving Sustainable Development Goal (SDG) Target 1.2, which aims to halve multidimensional poverty by 2030, remains steadfast. India's healthcare sector, a dynamic force in driving economic growth and generating employment, has made significant progress in recent years (Singh, 2024). This progress is evident in the improved coverage, quality of services, and substantial investments from both government and private entities. While the public healthcare system offers essential services, it often lacks secondary and tertiary care facilities in urban areas. This gap is effectively filled by the private sector, which delivers most of these vital services in metropolitan and tier I and II cities, thereby increasing healthcare accessibility for many individuals (Gunasekaran & Harmantzis, 2007). A notable aspect of India's healthcare system is its affordability; surgical procedures are available at significantly lower rates than in the US and Western Europe, leading to a surge in medical tourism. This underscores India's healthcare achievements and instils a sense of national pride (Cancarevic, Plichtová, & Malik, 2021). Additionally, with lower expenses for clinical research, India is rapidly becoming a centre for research and development for international companies, enhancing its importance globally. Recent research shows exciting and remarkable growth in the healthcare sector, with its market value rising from US$110 billion in 2016 to an anticipated US$638 billion by 2025 (Ahmet, 2023). Looking ahead to 2024, the healthcare sector is set to thrive, playing a vital role in public health and economic progress. Encouragingly, it is predicted to create approximately 7.5 million new jobs by 2024, establishing itself as a key pillar for employment in the nation (Khare & Arora, 2023). From 431 million in 1990 to over 129 million in 2024, the number of Indians living in severe poverty has dropped dramatically, a significant milestone in our economic journey. This decline, evidence of adequate economic progress, is a testament to the impact of our collective efforts. However, the estimated poverty rate for 2023–2024, at 10%–15%, underscores the pressing need for robust social security measures to ensure access to healthcare, education, and housing (Dev, 2024).

The Indian healthcare sector is a vast and intricate system composed of various interrelated components that provide healthcare services to over 1.4 billion people. It includes public, private, and voluntary sectors and numerous healthcare delivery mechanisms, policies, and programmes (Kumar, 2023). Key components of the Indian health sector include the public healthcare system, private healthcare sector, health insurance, traditional systems of medicine, pharmaceutical and medical device industry, health infrastructure, human resources for health, health information systems, regulatory and policy framework, research and development, and health financing (Figure 4.1) (Kumar & Duggirala, 2021). India's public healthcare system, operated mainly by the government, is structured into three levels: primary, secondary, and tertiary care facilities. This systematic approach ensures comprehensive healthcare access for the whole population (Balarajan, Selvaraj, & Subramanian, 2011). Primary healthcare, structured via primary health centres (PHCs) and sub-centres (SCs), is the foundation of India's healthcare system. It focuses on preventive, promotive, and essential curative services, particularly in rural areas. Community health centres (CHCs) serve larger populations, providing more specialized care. Public health programmes, such as immunization and maternal and child health services, are mainly delivered through these centres. Secondary healthcare, which includes district hospitals and sub-district hospitals, offers more advanced medical services (Lesnik, 2004). These facilities handle referrals from PHCs and CHCs, providing specialized outpatient surgeries and inpatient care. Tertiary healthcare involves highly specialized hospitals, medical colleges, and research institutes, such as the All India Institute of Medical Sciences (AIIMS) and Postgraduate Institute of Medical Education and Research (PGIMER). These institutions offer advanced diagnostic, therapeutic, and rehabilitative services alongside cutting-edge research and training programmes (Bali, Rai, & Verma, 2021). In metropolitan areas, the private healthcare industry offers better treatment options and plays a crucial role in the Indian health system. This sector includes private hospitals, clinics, diagnostic centres, and pharmaceutical companies, offering faster and more sophisticated treatment options tailored to the needs of the middle and upper classes. Health Insurance encompasses public, private, and state-sponsored insurance plans (Nandraj, Muraleedharan, Baru, Qadeer, & Priya, 2001). The government runs health insurance programmes like Ayushman Bharat Pradhan Mantri Jan Arogya Yojana (PM-JAY), offering free health coverage to economically vulnerable families. This scheme is one of the world's most significant government-sponsored health insurance initiatives, covering over 500 million people (Naib, Kumar, Chandrashekar, Smith, & Chhabra, 2021). Several private insurance companies offer individual and group health insurance plans covering various medical expenses such as hospitalization, surgery, and maternity care. Many Indian states have launched specific health insurance programmes targeting groups like farmers, the elderly, and low-income families (Patel et al., 2015). India proudly boasts a vibrant heritage of alternative health traditions through AYUSH like Ayurveda, Yoga, Naturopathy, Unani, Siddha, and Homoeopathy offering holistic care for all. The Ministry of AYUSH oversees these systems, promoting them as complementary to modern medicine. Many Indians turn to AYUSH treatments

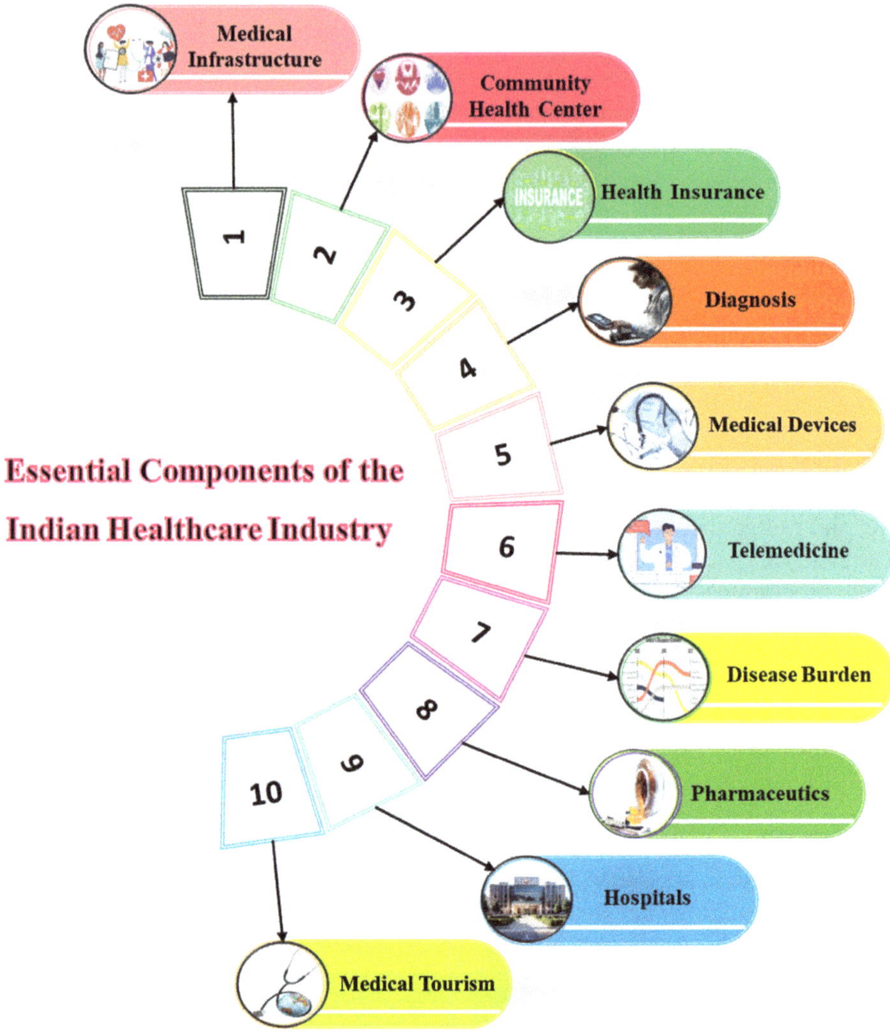

FIGURE 4.1 The key components of the Indian healthcare system are illustrated in the schematic diagram.

for chronic conditions, wellness, and preventive care (Mishra, 2020). Ongoing efforts aim to integrate AYUSH into primary healthcare while formally recognizing AYUSH practitioners to provide holistic healthcare solutions. One of the biggest generic medicine manufacturers in the world, India's pharmaceutical and medicine device sector significantly helps to meet the worldwide need for reasonably priced drugs (Greene, 2007). By offering reasonably priced medications for diseases such as TB, human immunodeficiency virus (HIV)/acquired immunodeficiency syndrome (AIDS), and malaria, the Indian pharmaceutical industry significantly helps to address world healthcare requirements (Waning, Diedrichsen, & Moon, 2010). Locally produced medical devices, including diagnostic equipment, implants, and surgical instruments, are also crucial; however, there is an increasing focus on boosting domestic manufacturing to reduce import dependency (Organization, 2012). The health infrastructure in India includes physical facilities such as hospitals, health centres, diagnostic labs, and pharmacies (Bhandari & Dutta, 2007). Significant investments are being made to enhance this infrastructure through initiatives like the Pradhan Mantri Swasthya Suraksha Yojana (PMSSY), which aims to increase the capacity of medical institutions nationwide (Kumar & Singh, 2024). Despite progress, challenges remain in ensuring equitable distribution of healthcare infrastructure, particularly in rural and remote areas. These challenges encompass inadequate funding, a shortage of skilled healthcare professionals, and the poor maintenance of existing facilities (Bajpai, 2014). India's vast workforce of healthcare professionals, including doctors, nurses, midwives, paramedics, and allied health workers, reflects the country's commitment to healthcare. While challenges such as the uneven distribution of healthcare personnel persist—especially in rural areas—the government continues to work towards addressing these issues (Sheikh & George, 2012). This exciting progress brings a wave of positive changes and initiatives. Despite the challenges faced, ongoing investments and innovations in healthcare give us hope for India's future. The chapter carefully addresses current issues and explores promising future directions for healthcare policies and programmes in the country.

4.2 INDIA'S MOST IMPORTANT HEALTHCARE POLICY AND PROGRAMMES

1. The National Health Policy (NHP) showcases the progression of its healthcare goals. Established in 1946, the Bhore Committee laid the foundation for a government-led health system that aimed to provide universal healthcare (Brimnes, 2023). Launched in 1983, the inaugural NHP prioritized universal primary healthcare, especially for underserved communities (Figure 4.2). That was accomplished by enhancing healthcare facilities in rural areas, boosting immunization initiatives, and addressing communicable diseases (Hemamalini, 2021). The policy underwent an update in 2002 to address the increasing prevalence of non-communicable diseases (NCDs) and encourage the involvement of the private sector (Figure 4.3) (Alwan et al., 2010). The aim during this period was to elevate public health expenditure to 2% of GDP and to strengthen public health infrastructure. The 2017 NHP was crafted to align with global goals such as universal health coverage and aimed to increase public health spending to 2.5% of GDP by 2025 (Table 4.1; Dehury et al., 2023). This comprehensive framework aims for universal access to quality healthcare services and aligns with the global SDGs (Lahariya, 2020). The NHP addresses critical challenges like the rising prevalence of NCDs, financial security in health, and the development of the healthcare workforce. By promoting affordable and high-quality healthcare, the policy seeks to improve health equity and ensure that all citizens, especially vulnerable populations, can access essential services without financial hardship (Nath, Shalini, & Mathur, 2021). A key focus is strengthening primary care through health and wellness centres (HWCs),

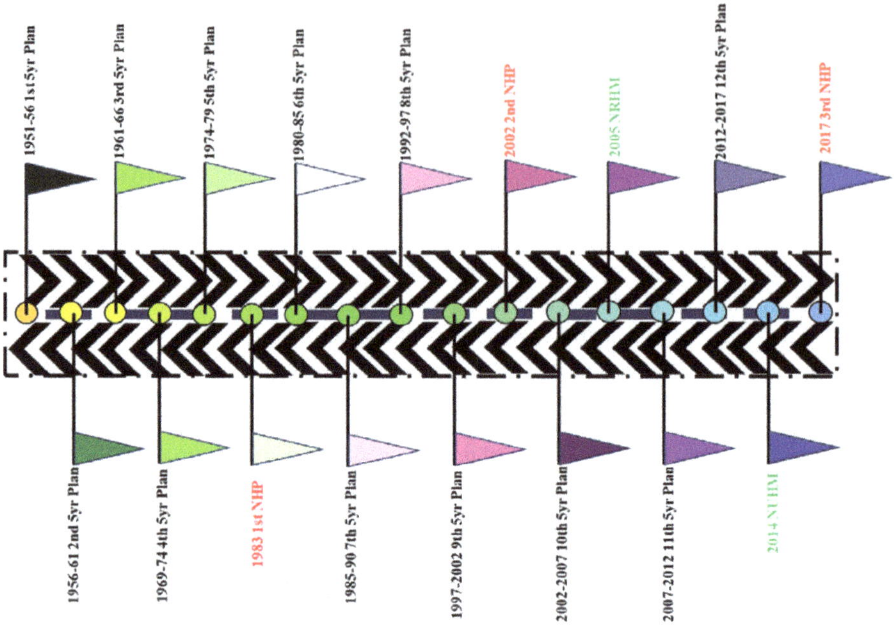

FIGURE 4.2 The graphical illustration represents a roadmap of 5-year plans, NHP, NRHM, and HUHM programmes in the Indian healthcare sector. It provides a visual overview of the key initiatives and strategies implemented over time.

which will provide comprehensive services, including mental health support and NCD management. It emphasizes improving the healthcare workforce, adopting digital technologies, and establishing regulatory frameworks for accountability in service delivery (Ghosh, 2023). NHP addresses urban health needs, setting specific health indicators for 2025, such as reducing infant and maternal mortality rates and increasing life expectancy. It aims to decrease maternal and child mortality, tackle malnutrition, integrate mental health in primary care, and combat infectious diseases like tuberculosis (TB) and malaria (Dudhraj, 2020). The NHP promotes a holistic approach to health and well-being through regular monitoring and collaboration across sectors.

2. PM-JAY is a key healthcare programme launched by the Indian government in September 2018 as part of the Ayushman Bharat scheme to support economically disadvantaged populations. It offers health insurance coverage of up to 500,000 rupees (approximately US$5,757.14) per family annually for hospitalization, benefiting over 100 million families and around 500 million individuals (Aashima & Sharma, 2024). PM-JAY covers a wide range of medical expenses, including surgeries and diagnostic services, with over 1,500 packages available. Beneficiaries can access treatment without cash or paperwork at empanelled hospitals by presenting their PM-JAY card (Saxena, Trivedi, Shroff, & Sharma, 2022). The selection of beneficiaries is based on the Socio-Economic Caste Census (SECC) 2011, with

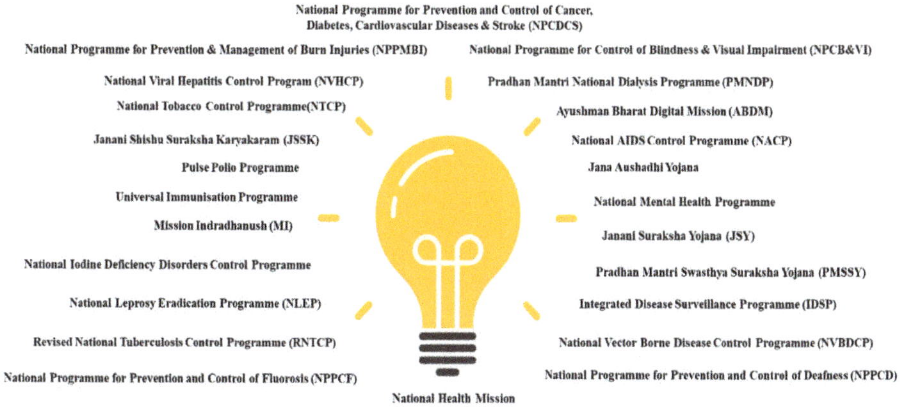

FIGURE 4.3 The diagram illustrates various policies and programmes in the Indian healthcare system that influence the overall quality of care for patients.

no restrictions on family size, age, or gender, allowing every eligible family member to access necessary services. The programme also features inter-state portability, allowing access to services nationwide. The scheme's implementation is driven by state health agencies (SHAs), which actively monitor its reach and efficacy, ensuring that the benefits genuinely reach those who need them most. The funding structure comprises 60% from the central government and 40% from state governments, promoting financial sustainability and preventive healthcare (Organization, 2018). PM-JAY has significantly enhanced healthcare access for millions, making medical care more affordable and fostering competition for quality services (Srivastava, Bertone, Basu, De Allegri, & Brenner, 2023).

3. The Rashtriya Swasthya Bima Yojana (RSBY), introduced in 2008 by the Indian government, has offered health insurance to families living below the poverty line (BPL) and other marginalized groups. By minimizing out-of-pocket costs through cashless hospital coverage of up to 30,000 rupees, RSBY has greatly enhanced healthcare access for numerous families (Karan, Yip, & Mahal, 2017). The initiative employs a unique card system that permits treatment without upfront payments. Families can acquire an RSBY card by paying a minimal annual fee of 30 rupees, allowing them to receive cashless treatment in designated hospitals, reflecting RSBY's dedication to inclusivity. Moreover, the programme has implemented inter-state portability, allowing beneficiaries to access care while relocating. Although RSBY has significantly lowered healthcare expenses, it encounters challenges related to limited coverage, fraud, and a lack of awareness. Nevertheless, the initiative has demonstrated flexibility by instituting regular audits and grievance redressal mechanisms to tackle these problems. In 2018, RSBY was merged into the PM-JAY, raising the coverage limit to 500,000 rupees per family each year and broadening its demographic. This transition builds upon RSBY's groundwork while striving for a more

TABLE 4.1
A Summary of the Implications of 5-Year Plans, NHP, NRHM, and HUHM Programmes throughout the Years, Highlighting Their Objectives and the Factors Influencing the Healthcare Sector (https://www.india.gov.in/national-health-policy-2017)

Time Period	Years	Plan	Objectives	Factors Considered
1951–1974	1951–1956	First 5-year plan	To enhance the nation's health situation. Diseases such as malaria, tuberculosis, dysentery, and diarrhoea.	Incidence of sickness, quantity of hospitals, public healthcare spending.
	1956–1961	Second 5-year plan	To manage communicable diseases such as malaria, filariasis, TB, leprosy, and sexually transmitted infections, while extending healthcare to a larger population.	Incidence of sickness, quantity of hospitals, governmental healthcare spending, private healthcare facilities.
	1961–1966	Third 5-year plan	Eradication campaign for smallpox and malaria, supplying clean drinking water to rural and urban regions. To manage filarial cholera, tuberculosis, leprosy, and other infectious illnesses.	Prevalence of sickness, quantity of hospitals, public healthcare spending, medication availability, accessibility of awareness programmes, and data on vaccination and immunization.
	1969–1974	Fourth 5-year plan	To manage and eliminate communicable illnesses while delivering curative and preventative healthcare in rural regions. To enhance the training programmes for medical and paramedical workers.	Accessibility of preventative health services, awareness initiatives, education, presence of skilled professionals, and illness prevalence.
1974–1990	1974–1979	Fifth 5-year plan	Execute the National Leprosy Control Programme. Implement the National Program for Preventing Visual Impairment. Manage filariasis strategies in rural areas. Establish a lab for simultaneous food and pharmaceutical testing.	Prevalence of illness, prevalence of mortality, and morbidity. Epidemiology of illness, accessibility of pharmaceuticals, and clinical studies.
	1983	First NHP	To provide economical basic healthcare services.	Epidemiology of diseases. Public expenditure, accessibility of pharmaceuticals, accessibility of awareness programmes, capacity for budget allocation, accessibility of financial assets.

(Continued)

TABLE 4.1 (*Continued*)
A Summary of the Implications of 5-Year Plans, NHP, NRHM, and HUHM Programmes throughout the Years, Highlighting Their Objectives and the Factors Influencing the Healthcare Sector (https://www.india.gov.in/national-health-policy-2017)

Time Period	Years	Plan	Objectives	Factors Considered
	1980–1985	Sixth 5-year plan	A national initiative for the promotion of maternity and childcare was launched, as well as the advocacy for immunization against tetanus, pertussis, diphtheria, TB, and poliomyelitis.	Incidence of illness, incidence of mortality and morbidity. Epidemiology of illness. Accessibility of financial resources, economic condition.
	1985–1990	Seventh 5-year plan	To initiate a health development initiative. Preventive and promotive dimensions, together with the organization of effective and efficient health services.	Prevalence of illness, prevalence of mortality and morbidity. Epidemiology of diseases. Accessibility of preventative healthcare services, awareness initiative.
1992–2007	1992–1997	Eighth 5-year plan	Enhancement and advancement of rural health infrastructure. Commencement of control and eradication initiatives for several communicable illnesses and vector-borne diseases, including malaria, kala-azar, and Japanese encephalitis.	Incidence of mortality and morbidity. Epidemiology of diseases. Accessibility of preventative healthcare services. Awareness initiatives.
	1997–2002	Ninth 5-year plan	The project aims to establish a district-level disease surveillance system, develop comprehensive non-communicable disease management plans, and establish emergency, disaster, accident, and trauma treatment management systems.	Technological applicability, illness epidemiology, readiness for recurrence, availability of financial resources.
	2002	Second NHP	To concentrate on the illness load of tuberculosis, malaria, visual impairment, and HIV/AIDS.	Epidemiology of illness and readiness for recurrence. Accessibility of preventative healthcare services, educational initiatives, availability of pharmaceuticals, and clinical research.

(*Continued*)

TABLE 4.1 *(Continued)*

A Summary of the Implications of 5-Year Plans, NHP, NRHM, and HUHM Programmes throughout the Years, Highlighting Their Objectives and the Factors Influencing the Healthcare Sector (https://www.india.gov.in/national-health-policy-2017)

Time Period	Years	Plan	Objectives	Factors Considered
	2002–2007	Tenth 5-year plan	The goal is to improve healthcare system efficiency, service quality, logistics, and medication use, while ensuring fair access to essential healthcare through the creation, implementation, and evaluation of healthcare finance systems.	The focus is on improving the healthcare system through preventative health services accessibility, awareness initiatives, budgetary allocation, and healthcare infrastructure, as well as addressing the epidemiology of illnesses.
	2005	NRHM	The objective is to enhance the health sector's GDP contribution from 0.9% to 2%–3% by bolstering current initiatives addressing malaria, blindness, iodine shortage, filariasis, kala-azar, tuberculosis, and leprosy.	The readiness to improve the healthcare system includes enhancing preventative health services, awareness initiatives, healthcare infrastructure, and understanding illness epidemiology, while also ensuring accessibility of financial assets.
2007–2017	2007–2012	Eleventh 5-year plan	The goal is to decrease maternal, infant, and fertility rates; reduce malnutrition; improve access to potable water; and develop a NACP-III formulation for AIDS control.	The focus is on improving the accessibility of preventative health services, educational initiatives, healthcare infrastructure, illness epidemiology, medicine availability, and clinical research.
	2012–2017	Twelfth 5-year plan	Public health services are made accessible to disabled individuals, providing specialized assistance, enhancing monitoring and assessment systems, and providing adequate training for health and rehabilitation educators.	Public health services, the supply of money, the framework of healthcare, and the spread of illness.
	2014	NUHM	To address the health requirements of the urban impoverished, particularly the residents in slums.	Healthcare infrastructure, epidemiology of diseases.
	2017	Third NHP	To enhance the secondary and tertiary healthcare facilities.	The focus is on healthcare infrastructure, disease epidemiology, financial resource availability, access to preventative health services, medicine availability, and clinical research.

inclusive healthcare framework in India, thereby improving health security for countless families (Vitsupakorn, Bharali, Yamey, & Mao, 2021).

4. The National Urban Health Mission (NUHM) was initiated in 2013 by the Indian government as a segment of the National Health Mission (NHM), aiming to tackle the healthcare issues faced by urban populations, particularly vulnerable groups such as slum residents and street vendors (Figure 4.3; Table 4.2; S. Kumar, Sharma, Sood, & Kumar, 2016). NUHM emphasizes enhancing access to quality primary healthcare services, concentrating on preventive and treatment measures while improving infrastructure in urban health facilities, including urban primary health centres (UPHCs) (Raichowdhury, Khetrapal, & Chin, 2023). Significant efforts include maternal and child health programmes, vaccination initiatives, and the management of both communicable diseases and NCDs. Urban Health and Nutrition Days (UHNDs) facilitate outreach efforts in urban slums, ensuring that every 50,000–60,000 individuals can reach a UPHC (Venkatesh, Garg, Gnanasekaran, & Pal, 2024). The involvement of Accredited Social Health Activists (ASHAs) is crucial for promoting health awareness within the community. Collaborating with campaigns like the Swachh Bharat Mission improves living conditions and health results (Raichowdhury et al., 2023). Despite the obstacles caused by swift urbanization and a workforce shortage, effective collaboration among health departments and urban development entities is vital. NUHM aims to deliver comprehensive healthcare access, setting the foundation for a healthier future for all urban dwellers in India (Venkatesh et al., 2024).
5. The Pradhan Mantri Surakshit Matritva Abhiyan (PMSMA) is a groundbreaking initiative launched by the Ministry of Health and Family Welfare (MoHFW) in 2016 to improve antenatal care (ANC) for pregnant women across India. The programme provides free, standardized ANC services to all pregnant women, focusing mainly on those in their second and third trimesters, with special attention to high-risk pregnancies to reduce maternal and infant mortality rates (Singh, Sonkaria, & Raghav, 2017). Designated as "PMSMA Day" on the ninth of each month, pregnant women are encouraged to visit government health facilities for routine check-ups and specialized care (Dandona et al., 2022). The initiative also invites private-sector doctors to volunteer their services, expanding access, especially in areas with limited healthcare resources. Participants receive a unique PMSMA maternal health card to monitor their health throughout pregnancy. Services offered include routine check-ups, blood tests, ultrasounds, immunizations, and nutritional counselling (Singh et al., 2017). PMSMA actively promotes access to quality ANC, particularly for economically disadvantaged women, through a network of health centres nationwide. Since its launch, it has effectively improved access to care and reduced the maternal mortality ratio in India, though challenges such as awareness and infrastructure in remote areas remain (Bakshi et al., 2024).
6. India's digital health initiatives are revolutionizing healthcare by enhancing accessibility and efficiency for patients. Initiatives such as the Ayushman

TABLE 4.2

An Overview of the Various Policies and Programmes Launched 2024, Funding Patterns of Schemes, Eligibility Criteria, Beneficiaries, Types of Benefits in the Indian Healthcare Sector, and the Impact of These Initiatives on Overall Public Health Outcomes (https://ihip.mohfw.gov.in/#!/programmes)

Sl No	Policy/ Programme	Launched	Funding Pattern of Scheme	Beneficiaries and Eligibility Criteria	Types of Benefits	Brief Description
1	National Health Mission (NHM)	2013	NHM is a joint venture between the central government and the state governments.	NHM aims to ensure equitable and affordable healthcare for all, with a special focus on marginalized, poor, and vulnerable populations, especially in rural and underserved areas.	NHM provides a wide range of healthcare services and benefits, with a focus on universal health coverage, equity, and affordability.	NHM is a major health initiative by the Government of India aimed at enhancing the healthcare system, especially in rural and underserved areas. It focuses on strengthening public health infrastructure, improving accessibility to services, and addressing the needs of marginalized populations.
2	Integrated Disease Surveillance Programme (IDSP)	2004	Central government and state governments and WHO	IDSP primarily benefits communities and individuals affected by infectious diseases.	IDSP enhancing disease surveillance, response mechanisms, and public health management.	IDSP is a flagship programme of the MoHFW, aimed at strengthening the disease surveillance system. It focuses on improving early detection and response to outbreaks, ensuring timely interventions to prevent further spread.
3	National Vector Borne Diseases Control Programmes (NVBDCP)	2003	Centrally sponsored scheme	Especially those living in endemic areas and high-risk regions.	NVBDCP provides a range of preventive, diagnostic, treatment, and surveillance benefits for vector-borne diseases.	NVBDCP is a central government initiative in India aimed at controlling and preventing vector-borne diseases through surveillance, control measures, and research.

(Continued)

TABLE 4.2 (*Continued*)

An Overview of the Various Policies and Programmes Launched This Year, Funding Patterns of Schemes, Eligibility Criteria, Beneficiaries, Types of Benefits in the Indian Healthcare Sector, and the Impact of These Initiatives on Overall Public Health Outcomes (https://ihip.mohfw.gov.in/#!/programmes)

Sl No	Policy/ Programme	Launched	Funding Pattern of Scheme	Beneficiaries and Eligibility Criteria	Types of Benefits	Brief Description
4	National Tuberculosis Elimination Programme (NTEP)	2020	Central government, with support from state governments, international organizations, and NGOs	NTEP is targeted towards individuals who are at risk of or affected by tuberculosis.	NTEP offers a range of services to individuals with tuberculosis to ensure early diagnosis, effective treatment, and prevention of transmission.	NTEP is a government initiative in India aiming to eradicate tuberculosis (TB) by 2025, focusing on early diagnosis, treatment, and prevention.
5	National Viral Hepatitis Control Programme (NVHCP)	2018	Central government and the state governments, with additional support from international organizations and private sector collaborations	NVHCP is designed to target individuals affected by hepatitis B and hepatitis C.	NVHCP provides a comprehensive range of services to control and manage hepatitis B and hepatitis C in India, including screening, diagnosis, treatment, and awareness.	The NVHCP is a government initiative in India aimed at controlling and preventing viral hepatitis, particularly hepatitis B and C, by improving access to screening, diagnosis, and treatment.
6	National Mental Health Programme (NMHP)	1982	Central government and state governments, along with the possibility of private sector involvement	Benefits the entire population, with a focus on individuals suffering from mental health disorders.	Services and benefits aimed at improving the mental health of the population, providing treatment, rehabilitation, and prevention of mental health conditions.	The NMHP is a government initiative in India aimed at enhancing mental health access, reducing stigma, and integrating mental health services into the primary healthcare system at district and community levels.

(*Continued*)

TABLE 4.2 (*Continued*)

An Overview of the Various Policies and Programmes Launched This Year, Funding Patterns of Schemes, Eligibility Criteria, Beneficiaries, Types of Benefits in the Indian Healthcare Sector, and the Impact of These Initiatives on Overall Public Health Outcomes (https://ihip.mohfw.gov.in/#!/programmes)

Sl No	Policy/ Programme	Launched	Funding Pattern of Scheme	Beneficiaries and Eligibility Criteria	Types of Benefits	Brief Description
7	National Programme for Health Care of the Elderly (NPHCE)	2010	Central government and state governments	Focuses on providing healthcare services to elderly citizens across India.	NPHCE provides a wide range of benefits aimed at improving the healthcare access, treatment, and well-being of elderly citizens.	The NPHCE is aimed at addressing the health issues of the elderly population, promoting active ageing, and improving their quality of life.
8	National Programme for Prevention and Control of Deafness (NPPCD)	2006	Central and state governments, PPPS sharing model	Individuals with hearing impairment or at risk of developing hearing loss. The programme focuses on both prevention and rehabilitation.	Provides a range of services and interventions aimed at preventing and managing hearing impairments.	The NPPCD, initiated by the Indian MoHFW, aims to tackle the growing issue of hearing impairment and deafness in India by preventing hearing loss, promoting early detection, and improving access to hearing aids.
9	Pradhan Mantri National Dialysis Programme (PMNDP)	2016	Central and state government, PPPS sharing model	Individuals who suffer from chronic kidney disease (CKD), particularly those in the end-stage renal disease (ESRD) phase, who require regular dialysis.	PMNDP focuses on improving access to dialysis services, ensuring quality care, and reducing the financial burden on patients who need regular dialysis.	PMNDP is a crucial health initiative by the Indian government, aimed at providing affordable and accessible dialysis services to individuals with CKD for survival.

(*Continued*)

TABLE 4.2 (*Continued*)

An Overview of the Various Policies and Programmes Launched This Year, Funding Patterns of Schemes, Eligibility Criteria, Beneficiaries, Types of Benefits in the Indian Healthcare Sector, and the Impact of These Initiatives on Overall Public Health Outcomes (https://ihip.mohfw.gov.in/#!/programmes)

Sl No	Policy/ Programme	Launched	Funding Pattern of Scheme	Beneficiaries and Eligibility Criteria	Types of Benefits	Brief Description
10	National Programme for Prevention and Control of Non-Communicable Diseases (NP-NCD)	2010	Central and state government sharing model	Individuals who (30–60 years) are at risk of or suffering from non-communicable diseases (NCDs)	Prevention and management of NCDs through various interventions.	The NP-NCD initiative, initiated by the Indian MoHFW, aims to tackle the increasing prevalence of non-communicable diseases.
11	National programme for Prevention & Management of Trauma & Burn Injuries (NPPMT&BI)	2016	Central and state government sharing model	Individuals who are affected by trauma (such as road accidents, falls, injuries from violence, etc.) or burn injuries.	Prevention of trauma and burn injuries, improved trauma and burn care, capacity building and training, infrastructure development, and rehabilitation and support.	NPPMT&BI is a crucial programme aimed at enhancing the prevention, treatment, and rehabilitation of trauma and burn victims in India.
12	National Programme for Prevention and Control of Fluorosis (NPPCF)	2008	Centre will bear 75% of the total budget and the state government will contribute 25% of the budget. In case of north eastern states it will be 90% and 10% respectively.	All people residing in areas with high fluoride content in drinking water in the districts covered so far under the programme.	Awareness about fluorosis and its effects; measures to prevent it; diagnostic facilities; management and rehabilitation of fluorosis cases.	The PPFCF was established in 2008–09 to tackle fluorosis, primarily due to high fluoride intake from drinking water.

(*Continued*)

TABLE 4.2 *(Continued)*

An Overview of the Various Policies and Programmes Launched This Year, Funding Patterns of Schemes, Eligibility Criteria, Beneficiaries, Types of Benefits in the Indian Healthcare Sector, and the Impact of These Initiatives on Overall Public Health Outcomes (https://ihip.mohfw.gov.in/#!/programmes)

Sl No	Policy/ Programme	Launched	Funding Pattern of Scheme	Beneficiaries and Eligibility Criteria	Types of Benefits	Brief Description
13	National Tobacco Control Programme (NTCP)	2007	Centrally sponsored scheme	The programme primarily targets tobacco users, vulnerable groups, and communities, particularly in regions where tobacco consumption is prevalent.	To bring about greater awareness about the harmful effects of tobacco use and about the Tobacco Control Laws. To facilitate effective implementation of the Tobacco Control Laws (COTPA 2003).	Overall policy formulation, planning, implementation, monitoring, and evaluation of the different activities envisaged under the NTCP.
14	Health Melas	2018	The centre state funding pattern will be 60:40/90:10/100%	All people	The initiative aims to boost public health awareness, motivate beneficiaries through innovative media, and provide early diagnosis screening, basic healthcare services, referrals, specialized services, and diagnostic services.	MoHFW is implementing a strategy of organizing Health Melas to provide free health education, early diagnosis, and quality care services to lakhs of people seeking essential tests and medicines.
15	Umbrella Scheme Rashtriya Arogya Nidhi (RAN)	1997	Centrally sponsored scheme	Individuals living below the poverty line	Treatment of major life-threatening diseases	The Rashtriya Arogya Nidhi is an Indian government initiative providing financial assistance to individuals below the poverty line for major life-threatening diseases.
16	Universal Immunization Programme (UIP)	1985	100% funded by the central government	All children and pregnant women.	Material and services.	UIP is one of the key interventions for protection of children from life-threatening conditions by providing vaccination.

(Continued)

TABLE 4.2 *(Continued)*

An Overview of the Various Policies and Programmes Launched This Year, Funding Patterns of Schemes, Eligibility Criteria, Beneficiaries, Types of Benefits in the Indian Healthcare Sector, and the Impact of These Initiatives on Overall Public Health Outcomes (https://ihip.mohfw.gov.in/#!/programmes)

Sl No	Policy/ Programme	Launched	Funding Pattern of Scheme	Beneficiaries and Eligibility Criteria	Types of Benefits	Brief Description
17	Pulse Polio Programme (PPP)	1995	MoHFWS, WHO, and UNICEF	Children under the age of 5 years	Health benefits, preventive measures, and community-level advantages.	The primary goal of the PPP is to eradicate polio in India by immunizing all children under the age of 5 against the poliovirus.
18	PM-Ayushman Bharat Health Infrastructure Mission (PM-ABHIM)	2021	Central and state governments	All people	The initiative focuses on enhancing healthcare infrastructure, disease surveillance, and access to healthcare in underserved areas, human resource development, promoting research and innovation.	Strengthening health infrastructure and ensuring comprehensive healthcare access at primary, secondary, and tertiary levels across rural and urban India.
19	National AIDS and STD Control Programme (NACP)	1992	Funded through a combination of government funding and support from international organizations such as the Global Fund, World Bank, and UNAIDS	The NACP primarily targets people at high risk of HIV/AIDS and sexually transmitted infections (STIs), as well as individuals living with HIV/AIDS.	NACP provides a wide range of benefits to people living with HIV/AIDS, high-risk populations, and the general public. The benefits focus on prevention, treatment, and care.	The National Action Plan for Prevention of HIV/AIDS and Sexually Transmitted Diseases (STDs) is a government initiative in India aimed at reducing HIV infections, improving the quality of life for those living with HIV/AIDS, and reducing the impact of STDs.

(Continued)

TABLE 4.2 (*Continued*)

An Overview of the Various Policies and Programmes Launched This Year, Funding Patterns of Schemes, Eligibility Criteria, Beneficiaries, Types of Benefits in the Indian Healthcare Sector, and the Impact of These Initiatives on Overall Public Health Outcomes (https://ihip.mohfw.gov.in/#!/programmes)

Sl No	Policy/ Programme	Launched	Funding Pattern of Scheme	Beneficiaries and Eligibility Criteria	Types of Benefits	Brief Description
20	National Sickle Cell Anaemia Elimination Mission (NSCAEM)	2021	Central government, and the implementation involves active collaboration with state governments, local health departments, and tribal welfare organizations	The NSCAEM focuses on the tribal population, which is particularly affected by sickle cell anaemia, but the mission also benefits the general population at risk of the condition.	The NSCAEM offers various types of benefits to those affected by sickle cell anaemia and aims to prevent its spread through early detection and genetic counselling.	The Indian government has launched NSCAEM, a mission to eradicate sickle cell anaemia, focusing on the tribal population, through screening, awareness, and treatment, aiming to improve health outcomes.
21	National Urban Health Mission (NUHM)	2013	Central government and the state/UT governments	The NUHM primarily targets the urban poor, vulnerable groups, and migrants in cities and towns across India.	The NUHM offers a range of services and benefits aimed at improving healthcare access and outcomes for urban poor and vulnerable populations in urban settings.	The NUHM programme, launched by the Indian government, aims to improve healthcare access and services in urban areas, particularly those with high concentrations of economically and socially disadvantaged groups, particularly the poor, migrants, and slum dwellers.
22	National Tele Mental Health Programme (NTMHP)	2022	Central and state government, private sector, and NGOs	NTMHP primarily targets individuals facing mental health issues who require timely intervention, but who may have limited access to healthcare services due to geographic, financial, or social barriers.	NTMHP offers a wide range of benefits to ensure comprehensive and timely mental healthcare across the country.	The NTMHP is a government initiative in India aimed at addressing mental health issues by improving mental healthcare services through telemedicine and digital technologies, for all citizens.

(Continued)

TABLE 4.2 (*Continued*)

An Overview of the Various Policies and Programmes Launched This Year, Funding Patterns of Schemes, Eligibility Criteria, Beneficiaries, Types of Benefits in the Indian Healthcare Sector, and the Impact of These Initiatives on Overall Public Health Outcomes (https://ihip.mohfw.gov.in/#!/programmes)

Sl No	Policy/ Programme	Launched	Funding Pattern of Scheme	Beneficiaries and Eligibility Criteria	Types of Benefits	Brief Description
23	Pradhan Mantri Swasthya Suraksha Yojana (PMSSY)	2003	Central and state government, private sector, and NGOs	All people	Improved healthcare access, upgraded medical education, healthcare infrastructure improvement, improved healthcare delivery, promotion of research and innovation, boost to local economy.	PMSSY is a government initiative aimed at enhancing healthcare infrastructure, ensuring quality services, and modernizing facilities in underdeveloped and remote areas of India, thereby reducing urban-rural disparity.
24	Ayushman Bharat Digital Mission (ABDM)	2021	Centrally sponsored scheme	All people	Health ID, electronic health records (EHRs), telemedicine services, improved access to healthcare, real-time health data, interoperability across healthcare systems, empowered citizens, reduction in fraud and errors.	The Indian government has launched ABDM, a digital health initiative aimed at transforming healthcare delivery through digital technologies, making it more accessible, efficient, and affordable. This is part of the Ayushman Bharat scheme, a flagship programme for universal health coverage and financial protection.

(*Continued*)

TABLE 4.2 *(Continued)*

An Overview of the Various Policies and Programmes Launched This Year, Funding Patterns of Schemes, Eligibility Criteria, Beneficiaries, Types of Benefits in the Indian Healthcare Sector, and the Impact of These Initiatives on Overall Public Health Outcomes (https://ihip.mohfw.gov.in/#!/programmes)

Sl No	Policy/ Programme	Launched	Funding Pattern of Scheme	Beneficiaries and Eligibility Criteria	Types of Benefits	Brief Description
25	Nikshay Poshan Yojana	2018	Centrally sponsored scheme	All TB patients	Nutritional support, improved treatment adherence, reduced treatment failure, reduction in mortality and morbidity, empowerment of health workers.	Nikshay Poshan Yojana under NTEP to provide nutritional support to tuberculosis (TB) patients in India. It aims to improve their overall health and support the treatment.
26	Janani Suraksha Yojana (JSY)	2005	Central government and the state governments.	The scheme is primarily targeted at pregnant women belonging to the BPL category, although general category women may also be eligible for financial support.	Cash incentive for pregnant women, incentives for healthcare providers, improved maternal and neonatal health.	The JSY is a national scheme under the Ministry of Health and Family Welfare, aimed at reducing maternal and neonatal mortality by promoting institutional deliveries and improving access to maternal healthcare services.
27	National Iodine Deficiency Disorders Control Programmes (NIDDCP)	1992	Centrally sponsored scheme	All people	Universal salt iodization, quality control, and public awareness.	The NIDDCP is a health initiative under the MoHFW, aimed at eliminating iodine deficiency disorders by ensuring all citizens, especially in areas with prevalent iodine deficiency, consume sufficient iodine.

(Continued)

TABLE 4.2 (*Continued*)

An Overview of the Various Policies and Programmes Launched This Year, Funding Patterns of Schemes, Eligibility Criteria, Beneficiaries, Types of Benefits in the Indian Healthcare Sector, and the Impact of These Initiatives on Overall Public Health Outcomes (https://ihip.mohfw.gov.in/#!/programmes)

Sl No	Policy/ Programme	Launched	Funding Pattern of Scheme	Beneficiaries and Eligibility Criteria	Types of Benefits	Brief Description
28	National Programme for Prevention and Control of Cancer, Diabetes, Cardiovascular Disease and Stroke (NPCDCS)	2010	Central government and state governments	General population of India, with a focus on high-risk groups	Prevention, early detection, treatment, and health promotion.	The NPCDCS reduces the burden of non-communicable diseases (NCDs), including cancer, diabetes, cardiovascular diseases, and stroke, which are leading causes of morbidity and mortality.
29	National Programme for Control of Blindness and Visual Impairment (NPCB&VI)	1976	Central government and state governments	All age groups	Focusing on screening, early detection, affordable treatment, and rehabilitation services, the programme aims to reduce the burden of visual impairment and ensure that all individuals are benefited.	The NPCB&VI is a government initiative aimed at preventing blindness and improving visual health by focusing on prevention, treatment, and rehabilitation of individuals with visual impairments, particularly cataracts.
30	National Oral Health Programme (NOHP)	2014	Central government and state governments	The programme targets the entire population, especially those with limited access to oral health services in rural, remote, and underserved areas.	Oral health awareness, free or subsidized treatment, oral health screening, fluoride supplements, rehabilitation and support.	The NOHP is launched by the Ministry of Health and Family Welfare to tackle the increasing oral health issues in the country, focusing on promoting oral hygiene, preventing dental caries, gum diseases, and oral cancers, and improving overall oral health awareness.

(*Continued*)

TABLE 4.2 *(Continued)*

An Overview of the Various Policies and Programmes Launched This Year, Funding Patterns of Schemes, Eligibility Criteria, Beneficiaries, Types of Benefits in the Indian Healthcare Sector, and the Impact of These Initiatives on Overall Public Health Outcomes (https://ihip.mohfw.gov.in/#!/programmes)

Sl No	Policy/ Programme	Launched	Funding Pattern of Scheme	Beneficiaries and Eligibility Criteria	Types of Benefits	Brief Description
31	National Organ Transplant Programme (NOTP)	2013	Centrally sponsored scheme	Patients in need of organ transplants, organ donors.	The programme emphasizes awareness, capacity building, and the ethical and legal aspects of organ donation, making it a comprehensive and vital healthcare initiative for the nation.	The NOTP is a health initiative by the Indian government, under the Ministry of Health and Family Welfare, aimed at enhancing organ transplant access and addressing the country's organ shortage by establishing a coordinated system, promoting awareness, and establishing infrastructure.
32	National Leprosy Eradication Programme (NLEP)	2000	Centrally sponsored scheme	People who have been diagnosed with leprosy benefit from free treatment and support for disability prevention.	Free medical treatment, community awareness, and rehabilitation.	NLEP is an Indian government initiative aiming to eradicate leprosy, a chronic infectious disease affecting skin, peripheral nerves, respiratory tract, and eyes, through early detection, treatment, and prevention.
33	National Health Policy (NHP)	2017	Centrally sponsored scheme	General population of India.	Financial protection, access to health services, preventive healthcare, health education, improved mental health, and improvement in health infrastructure.	The NHP of India 2017 aims to ensure universal health coverage, equity, accessibility, and affordability for all citizens, with a focus on vulnerable and marginalized populations. It aims to improve healthcare quality, ensure affordability, and promote preventive care, aligning with the Sustainable Development Goals, particularly SDG 3.

Bharat Digital Mission (ABDM), telemedicine, and mHealth applications utilize technology to close healthcare gaps and improve patient outcomes (Figure 4.3; Table 4.2; Sharma, Rohatgi, Jain, & Singh, 2023). Notable features include the health ID, which holds medical records, and the Health Facility Registry (HFR), which provides healthcare options. The Health Professional Registry (HPR) links citizens with verified healthcare providers, while Personal Health Records (PHR) allows individuals to take control of their health information. These advancements foster improved collaboration among healthcare professionals and enable more tailored services nationwide (Kesavadev, Krishnan, & Mohan, 2021). eSanjeevani Telemedicine Services, introduced by MoHFW, is a leading initiative that facilitates virtual consultations to minimize the necessity for physical hospital visits, particularly in remote regions (Dastidar, Jani, Suri, & Nagaraja, 2024). It consists of two models: eSanjeevani OPD, which enables patients to connect with doctors from their homes, and eSanjeevani Ayushman Bharat—Health and Wellness Centre (AB-HWC), which connects PHCs with specialists for doctor-to-doctor consultations (Dastidar et al., 2024; Kaladharan, Dhanya, Drisya, & Raj, 2023). This service improves healthcare accessibility, decreases patient travel, and lessens the load on medical facilities. Furthermore, the eHospital and Online Registration System (ORS) created by the National Informatics Centre enhances hospital management by unifying patient registration, appointment scheduling, and billing, improving service delivery and patient experience (Sharma, Aggarwal, Arora, & Bahuguna, 2022). The CoWIN (COVID Vaccine Intelligence Network) platform became an essential digital resource during the COVID-19 pandemic, facilitating the registration, distribution, and monitoring of vaccinations throughout India (Arjun, Singh, & Parida, 2023). Its functionalities, such as simple registration, appointment booking, digital vaccination certificates, and real-time tracking, significantly improved the nation's vaccination initiatives. In addition to CoWIN, India rolled out various mHealth applications to enhance health results (Inampudi & Gaurav, 2024). The Aarogya Setu app offered contact tracing, local COVID-19 case tracking, symptom self-evaluation, and access to urgent health services (Gupta, Bedi, Goyal, Wadhera, & Verma, 2020). mDiabetes provides timely guidance on managing diabetes, while Kilkari delivers voice messages to expectant mothers and new parents, supplying advice on maternal and child health (Small et al., 2024). The Integrated Health Information Platform (IHIP) is a real-time disease surveillance mechanism that enhances disease reporting and encourages data-informed decision-making. Moreover, the Revised National Tuberculosis Control Programme (RNTCP) has developed Nikshay, a digital platform for managing TB cases, which includes real-time patient monitoring, treatment oversight, and incentives to encourage patient engagement and adherence to treatment. Nikshay has dramatically enhanced the detection of cases and the treatment management for TB patients, improving the reporting and tracking of TB across various states (Rajoria, Maula, Vyas, Ray, & Nischal, 2024). The Electronic Vaccine

Intelligence Network (eVIN) streamlines the distribution of vaccines and cold chain management in India, ensuring adequate storage and transportation of vaccines (Gurnani et al., 2020). Its key features include real-time vaccine supply monitoring, supporting routine immunizations and initiatives such as COVID-19 vaccinations. Another project, the National Health Stack (NHS), seeks to establish a robust healthcare delivery framework, standardizing data sharing and ensuring interoperability. Components of the NHS consist of health IDs and Electronic Health Records (EHR), promoting a cohesive health system and improving healthcare accessibility and efficiency for all citizens (Malhotra, Kotwal, & Basu, 2019).

7. In 2013 the Indian government launched the NHM which seeks to enhance the public health system and provide fair, reasonably priced, high-quality treatment for every member of society (Figure 4.3; Table 4.2; A. Ghosh & Ghosh, 2020). Combining the National Rural Health Mission (NRHM) with the NUHM, the NHM emphasizes underprivileged groups in the rural and metropolitan setting (Nagarajan, Paul, Yadav, & Gupta, 2015). The main goals are lower infant mortality, better mother health, and managing communicative and non-communicative disorders. Programmes like Janani Suraksha Yojana (JSY) and Janani Shishu Suraksha Karyakram (JSSK) are crucial in these initiatives (Krishnamoorthy, 2024). The NHM also supports projects like HWCs, ASHAs, and Rashtriya Bal Swasthya Karyakram (RBSK) to provide complete healthcare and stresses community involvement via Village Health, Sanitation and Nutrition Committees (VHSNCs) (Choudhary & Singh, 2018). India has seen significant progress under the NHM with expanded vaccination efforts, improved healthcare infrastructure, and a focus on enhancing service delivery (Bhardwaj, 2023). However, challenges remain, including needing more healthcare professionals and addressing ongoing quality issues in public hospitals. The NHM's commitment to vulnerable populations aims to foster healthier communities nationwide (Chauhan, Dumka, Hannah, Ahmed, & Kotwal, 2022; Golechha, Bohra, Rana, & Panchamia, 2025).
8. Initiated on December 25, 2014, Mission Indradhanush is a key immunization initiative by the Government of India aimed at boosting vaccination rates among children who are either unvaccinated or only partially vaccinated, as well as pregnant women (Figure 4.3; Table 4.2; Singh, 2018). The main objective is to provide complete immunization for children under the age of two and expectant mothers, especially in underserved regions like urban slums, tribal areas, and among nomadic groups (Thakur, Awasthi, Taneja, & Janardhanan, 2020). The programme administers vaccines for 12 diseases, which include TB, polio, diphtheria, hepatitis B, and measles (Bhadoria, Mishra, Singh, & Kishore, 2019). Initially concentrated on 201 high-priority districts with immunization rates lower than 50% from 2014 to 2017, the initiative was expanded with the launch of the Intensified Mission Indradhanush (IMI) in October 2017, focusing on districts with the least coverage (Chatterjee et al., 2021). IMI 2.0 was introduced in December 2019, aiming for complete immunization in selected areas (Thakur et al., 2020).

Mission Indradhanush 3.0, launched in February 2021, centred on vaccinating individuals overlooked during the COVID-19 pandemic (Tawde, Quazi, Gaidhane, & Choudhari, 2024). With customized micro-plans for each district and cooperation among various ministries and organizations, the mission has successfully immunized more than 37.64 million children and 9.46 million pregnant women by the time of IMI 2.0. Despite facing several challenges, Mission Indradhanush continues influencing public health significantly and aspires to universal vaccination.

9. The National Mental Health Programme (NMHP), initiated by the Government of India in 1982, seeks to tackle mental health issues nationwide, focusing on at-risk and marginalized groups. Its goals encompass the early identification, diagnosis, and treatment of mental health disorders (Figure 4.3; Table 4.2; Roy & Rasheed, 2015). A significant element is the incorporation of mental health services within PHCs to ensure accessibility in remote regions and to enhance human resource development. Additionally, to counteract mental health stigma, the programme highlights the importance of public education and awareness initiatives (Wig & Murthy, 2015). The District Mental Health Programme (DMHP), launched in 1996, improves mental health services at the district level, connecting them with primary healthcare (Kirpekar, Faye, Bhave, Gawande, & Tadke, 2024). In 2020, the KIRAN Helpline was established, marking a vital initiative that offers round-the-clock support during the COVID-19 pandemic in various languages, providing comfort and assistance to those in distress (Parmar, Rina, & Padhy, 2020). This initiative underscores the commitment of the NMHP to provide support even in the most challenging times. Organizations like the National Institute of Mental Health and Neurosciences (NIMHANS) are crucial in training professionals and influencing policies (Kalaivanan et al., 2020). Despite advancements, ongoing challenges like stigma, a lack of trained professionals, and insufficient funding remain, especially in rural regions. The Mental Healthcare Act of 2017 is a notable achievement, highlighting the entitlement to mental health services and confirming that everyone should have access to these essential services. Increasing investment in mental health infrastructure and expanding training opportunities for professionals is vital to addressing the growing mental health issues in India (Duffy & Kelly, 2019). Fortifying the DMHP to integrate mental health with primary care is essential to enhance overall service accessibility.
10. The National Programme for Prevention and Control of Cancer, Diabetes, Cardiovascular Diseases, and Stroke (NPCDCS) was launched by the Government of India in 2010 to address the rising public health challenges posed by NCDs (Figure 4.3; Table 4.2; Venugopal, Richa, Singh, Gautam, & Jahnavi, 2023). This comprehensive initiative empowers communities to adopt healthier lifestyles by promoting awareness and positive changes, such as reducing tobacco and alcohol consumption, encouraging nutritious diets, and increasing physical activity (Venugopal et al., 2023). A key aspect of NPCDCS is early diagnosis and management of NCDs,

enhancing primary healthcare facilities for timely detection and treatment at the community level. It also prioritizes capacity building for healthcare professionals through comprehensive training on screening and management (Krishnan, Gupta, Nongkynrih, & Thakur, 2011). The programme emphasizes health promotion and behaviour change communication (BCC) opportunistic screening for diabetes, hypertension, and various cancers at health centres, particularly for those aged 30 and above. Population-based screening is implemented in high-priority districts to expand early detection efforts. Additionally, NPCDCS provides compassionate palliative care for individuals facing severe complications from NCDs. With a robust surveillance system, NPCDCS monitors NCD prevalence and risk factors, conducting regular district-level surveys to track progress (Earnest & Gnanadurai, 2022). The programme is making significant strides in early detection, routine screenings, and awareness initiatives to reduce the incidence and mortality rates associated with NCDs, particularly strokes and heart diseases. Collaborative efforts with other health initiatives ensure holistic healthcare services are delivered effectively at the district level, providing a comprehensive approach to public health.

11. The National Tuberculosis Elimination Programme (NTEP), previously known as the RNTCP, is India's primary effort to combat TB (Burugina Nagaraja et al., 2021). Established in 1997, the NTEP implemented the Directly Observed Treatment, Short-course (DOTS) approach to improve TB management (Zaman, 2021). Its rebranding in 2020 introduced an ambitious objective of eradicating TB by 2025, five years earlier than the target set by the World Health Organization (WHO; Figure 4.3; Table 4.2; Sharath et al., 2024). NTEP prioritizes early diagnosis and treatment to provide timely, high-quality care to every patient, including those who have drug-resistant TB. The programme stresses universal access to TB care, particularly for rural and underserved populations. It relies on modern diagnostic technologies such as CBNAAT and GeneXpert (Sarkar, 2018), which ensure precise early identification and treatment of multidrug-resistant (MDR-TB) and extensively drug-resistant TB (XDR-TB), instilling confidence in the programme's approach (Chowdhury, Ahmad, Sinha, Dutta, & Haque, 2023). Support programmes like Nikshay Mitra and the Nikshay Poshan Yojana offer nutritional and psychosocial support, which helps enhance treatment compliance (Yadav, 2024). Although the DOTS strategy has achieved over 85% success in managing new TB cases, issues such as social stigma and the complexities of treating MDR-TB and XDR-TB continue to pose challenges (Law, 2019). NTEP is dedicated to eliminating TB by 2025 through the early identification of cases and enhanced treatment methods. Future initiatives include adopting digital monitoring technologies, forming partnerships with the private sector, launching community awareness campaigns, and consistently investing in innovative research related to diagnostics and vaccines.
12. Initiated by the Indian government in 1995, the Pulse Polio Immunization Program aims to eliminate poliomyelitis through extensive immunization,

supporting the global initiative led by the WHO (Shigh, Suresh, Kumar, & Singh, 1997). Its primary goal is to halt poliovirus transmission by administering the Oral Polio Vaccine (OPV) to children under five during National and Sub-National Immunization Days, held twice a year, typically in January and February. The programme relies on the unwavering commitment of healthcare workers who ensure that children in remote areas receive their polio drops (Gomber, Taneja, & Mohan, 1996). Surveillance measures, such as monitoring acute flaccid paralysis (AFP) and analysing sewage samples, help identify potential polio cases (Biru et al., 2024). India was declared polio-free by the WHO on March 27, 2014, following the last reported case in 2011 (Figure 4.3; Table 4.2; Bahl et al., 2014). However, challenges like vaccine hesitancy in underserved regions persist, necessitating targeted awareness campaigns and innovative outreach strategies. With the addition of the inactivated polio vaccine (IPV) to the Universal Immunization Programme (UIP), India continues to prioritize community health and maintain high vaccination rates. The collaboration with organizations like the WHO, Rotary International, and UNICEF is a testament to the programme's sustainability and its ability to prevent imported cases (Carvalho & Weckx, 2006).

13. The Government of India launched a programme called the Integrated Child Development Services (ICDS) in 1975, which is vital for supporting young children, expectant and nursing mothers, and adolescent girls. Recognized as a leading early childhood development initiative, ICDS focuses on addressing malnutrition and infant mortality while advancing maternal and child health (Gupta, Gupta, & Nongkynrih, 2013). Recent campaigns like Poshan Abhiyaan aim to enhance service quality by empowering Anganwadi workers. Anganwadi centres (AWCs) play a crucial role by providing hot meals and take-home food to combat malnutrition and offering immunization services in collaboration with the Ministry of Health (Vir, 2023). They conduct regular health check-ups, prenatal and postnatal care, and monitor children's growth. Early childhood education is also provided for children aged 3–6, promoting cognitive and social development through play. Nutrition and Health Education (NHED) initiatives empower mothers with information on nutrition and hygiene (Vir, 2017). Despite the programme's successes in improving health outcomes and raising awareness in rural areas, challenges remain, including varying service quality, inadequate infrastructure, and better coordination with other health programmes. Launched in 2018, POSHAN Abhiyaan aims to improve nutritional outcomes and reduce stunting and undernutrition through technology and better coordination. Efforts to upgrade AWCs and enhance service delivery are ongoing, with initiatives like Saksham Anganwadi and Poshan 2.0 promoting a comprehensive nutrition and early childhood care approach (Paul, Singh, & Palit, 2018).
14. The JSY programme, established in 2005 by the MoHFW as part of the NHM, aims to improve maternal and neonatal health by encouraging safe institutional deliveries, particularly for economically disadvantaged women in rural settings (Figure 4.3; Table 4.2; Rai & Singh, 2012). JSY

offers financial support to pregnant women, motivating them to give birth in medical facilities and increasing access to skilled birth attendants. Women 19 years or older from below-poverty line (BPL) families can receive assistance for their first two live births, with varying monetary incentives based on whether they live in low-performing or high-performing states (Gupta et al., 2012). ASHA workers are essential in linking women to healthcare services providing help with ANC, transportation, and postnatal assistance. Although the initiative has led to a rise in institutional births in India, issues such as awareness, infrastructure, and quality of care continue to pose challenges (Lim et al., 2010). Furthermore, focusing on postnatal care is vital for safeguarding mothers' and newborns' health. Collaborative efforts are necessary to address these obstacles and improve maternal health outcomes (Das, Rao, & Hagopian, 2011).

15. The Deendayal Antyodaya Yojana-National Urban Livelihoods Mission (DAY-NULM) is a comprehensive initiative, launched by India in 2013, to combat urban poverty (Kamble, 2024). It empowers the urban poor by promoting self-employment and skilled job opportunities through the establishment of self-help groups (SHGs) and the provision of training, support, and affordable financial resources. This initiative is a lifeline for marginalized communities, especially women, as it enhances their access to economic opportunities and promotes gender equality (Kumar, 2022). DAY-NULM is a multifaceted programme with several interrelated components: the Social Mobilization and Institutional Development (SMID) organizes urban poor households into SHGs; the Employment through Skill Training and Placement (EST&P) enhances the employability of youth and migrant workers; and the Self-Employment Programme (SEP) provides financial aid for starting small enterprises (Raghunathan, Trivedi, Gupta, Chakraborty, & Mankad, 2024). It also aims to bring street vendors into the formal economy by providing them with legal locations, training, and social security benefits as supported by the Street Vendors Act (2014). The initiative also includes the Shelters for Urban Homeless (SUH) programme, which offers vital services such as sanitation and healthcare (Ghosh, Goel, & Ojha, 2020). The programme is executed at state and municipal levels by State Urban Livelihoods Missions (SULMs) and Urban Local Bodies (ULBs) in partnership with NGOs and community organizations (Panday, 2020). Despite challenges such as limited financial resources and the need for improved outcome monitoring, DAY-NULM is a testament to the effectiveness of a comprehensive approach in empowering millions of impoverished families and improving livelihoods through technology and sustainable practices.
16. The National Digital Health Mission (NDHM), launched by the Government of India in 2020, represents a joint initiative to establish a digital health ecosystem connecting patients, healthcare providers, hospitals, and insurance companies (Chakravarthi, 2024). Overseen by the MoHFW, it aims to improve the accessibility, efficiency, and transparency of healthcare services. Important elements include the health ID, which serves as a unique identifier for citizens' health information, and the PHR, designed for secure information

sharing (Gudi, Lakiang, Pattanshetty, Sarbadhikari, & John, 2021). The mission includes the Healthcare Professionals Registry, HFR, Ayushman Bharat Health Account (ABHA), eHospital, eSanjeevani for telemedicine services, and DigiDoctor for locating certified doctors (Bhardwaj, 2023). NDHM streamlines healthcare service delivery, decreases wait times, and enhances treatment results, particularly in rural regions. Nevertheless, challenges such as digital literacy, concerns regarding data privacy, and insufficient infrastructure in rural areas remain. With more than 100 million registrations for ABHA, the mission seeks to incorporate private sector solutions and enhance healthcare access, especially for low-income families, through programmes like Ayushman Bharat PM-JAY (Raj, Dananjayan, & Agarwal, 2023).

4.3 ESSENTIAL COMPONENTS OF THE INDIAN HEALTHCARE INDUSTRY

An important framework that guarantees all Indian residents access to high-quality medical care is the country's healthcare system. This system includes various services, such as preventative care, chronic disease management, and emergency medical services (Kumar & Duggirala, 2021). Nonetheless, obstacles such as geographical differences and resource constraints persistently affect the overall efficacy and accessibility of healthcare services nationwide.

1. Healthcare Infrastructure: At its core is the Public Healthcare System, which encompasses government hospitals, clinics, and health centres across different levels (Burns, 2014). Primary healthcare is delivered through SCs, PHCs, and CHCs, emphasizing essential services. District hospitals provide secondary care, while tertiary healthcare institutions offer specialized services. The Private Healthcare System complements this by providing hospitals and clinics with more advanced treatments (Figure 4.1; Dey et al., 2013).
2. Human Resources for Health (HRH): India boasts a diverse array of healthcare professionals, including specialists and community health workers, who play a vital role, particularly in rural regions. The expansion of medical education is leading to an increase in healthcare professionals (Figure 4.1; Rao, Rao, Kumar, Chatterjee, & Sundararaman, 2011).
3. Health Insurance and Financing: Programmes like Ayushman Bharat PM-JAY promote health equity by offering insurance coverage to economically disadvantaged groups. Despite existing challenges, such as out-of-pocket expenses, the market for private insurance is expanding, presenting various options (Figure 4.1; A. S. Kumar et al., 2011).
4. Public Health Programmes: The government implements national health initiatives to address diseases like TB, malaria, and HIV, along with vaccination drives to enhance public health (Figure 4.1; Abinash Singh & Vellakkal, 2021).
5. Pharmaceuticals and Medical Devices: India plays a significant role in the pharmaceutical industry, manufacturing affordable generic medications

and vaccines. The medical devices sector is also expanding to meet local and international demands (Figure 4.1; P. Paul, 2022).

6. Digital Health and Technology: Technological advancements, such as telemedicine and mobile health applications, are enhancing access to healthcare. The NDHM seeks to improve healthcare efficiency via unique health IDs and integrated digital health records (Figure 4.1; Bagga, Singh, & Hood, 2024).
7. Public Health Surveillance and Research: The NHM aims to bolster health infrastructure and adapt to public health challenges through targeted surveillance and research initiatives (Prasad, Mithilesh, & Rao, 2010).
8. Regulatory and Governing Bodies: The MoHFW supervises India's health policy. The National Medical Commission (NMC) oversees the supervision of medical education and the licensure of doctors. The Drug Controller General of India (DCGI) guarantees the safety and efficacy of pharmaceuticals and medical equipment. The National Accreditation Board for Hospitals and Healthcare Providers (NABH) accredits healthcare facilities to maintain quality standards (Figure 4.1; A. S. Bali & Ramesh, 2021).
9. Traditional Medicine Systems: India accepts alternative medicine, particularly AYUSH. The Ministry of AYUSH vigorously advocates for these important practices and is committed to incorporating AYUSH professionals into the national healthcare system (Figure 4.1; Srikantha, Bhat, Singh, & Singh, 2015).
10. Health Communication and Awareness: Public health initiatives aim to enhance sanitation, vaccination, nutrition, and NCD awareness. BCC programmes encourage healthy behaviours related to hygiene, family planning, and preventive measures (Figure 4.1; Jadhav, 2024).

4.4 CRUCIAL CHALLENGES FACING THE INDIAN HEALTHCARE INDUSTRY

The Indian healthcare industry is poised for a substantial overhaul, offering remarkable chances to elevate the quality, accessibility, and fairness of healthcare services for numerous individuals. This transformation promises to improve the country's public health and overall wellness significantly.

1. **Gaps in Healthcare Infrastructure**: There is a notable divide between healthcare facilities in rural and urban areas. Prompt measures are necessary to guarantee all communities access to quality healthcare (Figure 4.4; Agrawal, 2015).
2. **Shortage of Healthcare Workforce**: India is experiencing a deficiency of doctors, nurses, and allied health professionals, particularly in rural regions. Supporting initiatives that help retain healthcare personnel in these areas can assist in rectifying this imbalance (Figure 4.4; Sinha & Sigamani, 2016).
3. **Accessibility to Healthcare Services**: Geographic obstacles impede access to healthcare options. Investments in transportation and emergency medical services are critical to ensuring prompt care for all individuals (Figure 4.4; Balarajan et al., 2011).

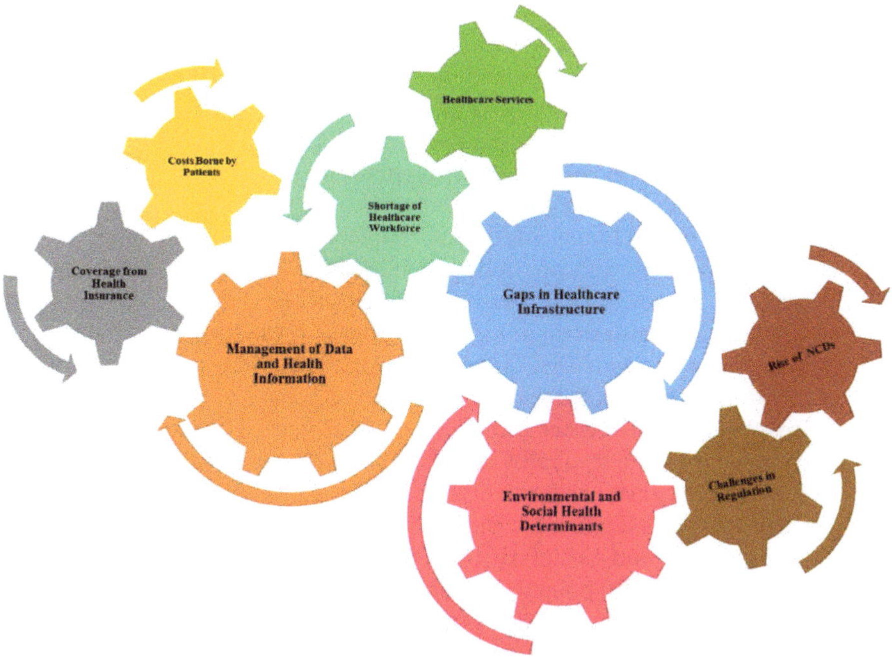

FIGURE 4.4 A schematic diagram highlights the significant challenges confronting the Indian healthcare sector. Addressing these issues is vital for enhancing the quality and accessibility of healthcare services throughout the nation.

4. **Healthcare Costs Borne by Patients**: Despite initiatives such as Ayushman Bharat (PM-JAY), many still face significant medical expenses. Advocating for comprehensive health insurance solutions can help alleviate this financial strain (Figure 4.4; A. S. Kumar et al., 2011).
5. **Coverage from Health Insurance**: While government programmes are a positive step, many remain uninsured. Promoting universal health coverage has the potential to significantly reduce the uninsured population, fostering a more equitable healthcare system (Figure 4.4; Binny & Gupta, 2017).
6. **Rise of NCDs**: The increasing prevalence of NCDs, such as diabetes and hypertension, necessitates a stronger emphasis on preventive healthcare and education about healthy lifestyles to manage these diseases effectively (Figure 4.4; Barik & Arokiasamy, 2016).
7. **Concerns of Infectious Diseases**: The threat of infectious diseases continues to be pressing, especially accentuated by the COVID-19 pandemic. Enhancing public health initiatives and disease surveillance is essential for future preparedness (Figure 4.4; Quinn & Kumar, 2014).
8. **Financing for Health Systems**: Public healthcare expenditure is low at around 1.2% of GDP. Increasing investment can improve facilities and the compensation of healthcare professionals, leading to a more sustainable health system for coming generations (Figure 4.4; Kadarpeta, Anand, & Achungura, 2024).

9. **Quality of Healthcare Services**: The quality of healthcare significantly varies between public and private providers. Private institutions frequently excel with cutting-edge technology, while public facilities face staff shortages. Tackling medical errors and improving patient care quality is crucial for delivering outstanding healthcare (Figure 4.4; Gopal, 2019).
10. **Management of Data and Health Information**: Initiatives like the ABDM are advancing digital health, but there are still challenges in data collection and utilization. Enhancing accuracy, interoperability, and data privacy can revolutionize healthcare delivery and lead to better decision-making (Figure 4.4; Pandey, Roy, Bhawsar, & Mishra, 2010).
11. **Challenges in Regulation**: Frameworks such as the Central Drugs Standard Control Organisation (CDSCO) maintain high standards for pharmaceuticals and medical devices, yet problems such as counterfeit drugs and slow approval processes present difficulties. The Clinical Establishments Act intends to standardize quality across healthcare facilities in India, and strengthening regulations for healthcare professionals is vital to uphold high practice standards (Figure 4.4; Bhattacharya et al., 2015).
12. **Environmental and Social Health Determinants**: Environmental challenges, including air pollution, unsafe drinking water, and poor waste management, greatly influence public health. Collaborative efforts and investment in healthcare infrastructure are crucial to creating healthier settings (Figure 4.4; Sengupta, 2016).
13. **Disparities in Health Equity**: Significant health inequities are prevalent, influenced by socio-economic status, geography, gender, and caste. Vulnerable populations often face hurdles in accessing healthcare, particularly in urban-rural dynamics. By fostering inclusivity and ensuring healthcare accessibility for everyone, we can work towards a more equitable society (Figure 4.4; Sherlin & Karunanidhi, 2024).

4.5 PROSPECTIVE COURSE OF ACTION AND OPPORTUNITIES

The Indian healthcare sector is experiencing rapid changes driven by demographic shifts, technological advances, and government reforms to improve health equity. While these changes offer opportunities, they pose challenges, such as the need for better infrastructure and enhanced workforce skills (Ramani & Mavalankar, 2006). Digital health solutions, such as telemedicine, are poised to help bridge the gap between urban and rural areas, especially in rural regions. Advancements in artificial intelligence (AI) are improving diagnostic capabilities, and wearable technology enables remote monitoring of chronic illnesses (Bhat, 2015). The government's emphasis on enhancing health infrastructure, notably through HWCs, presents investment prospects. Smart hospitals that employ integrated technology can enhance patient experiences while lowering costs (Haleem, Javaid, Singh, & Suman, 2022). Public-private partnerships (PPPs) are vital in increasing access to quality healthcare, particularly in underserved communities. India's pharmaceutical industry, recognized for its generic medicines, shows significant growth potential in vaccines and biotechnology, bolstered by government initiatives in gene therapy and precision medicine (Thomas, 2008). The Ayushman Bharat scheme is set to further stimulate healthcare demand by offering insurance coverage to more than 500 million individuals while increasing health awareness, likely boosting private insurance enrolment (Lahariya, 2018). However, challenges persist, particularly the lack of healthcare professionals, especially in rural areas, highlighting the need for more medical and nursing educational institutions. The country's strong appeal for medical tourism and advancements in AI and robotics create additional opportunities. The NDHM, with its potential to establish a digital health ecosystem and improve access and accountability, offers a promising future for digital healthcare in India (Agarwal, 2023). Finally, India's dynamic startup landscape concentrates on healthcare innovations, offering growth potential in telemedicine, diagnostics, and digital therapeutics (Bhatia, Vasaikar, & Wali, 2018). Merging traditional Indian medical practices like Ayurveda with modern healthcare can deliver comprehensive treatment alternatives and broaden access to global markets (Patwardhan & Partwardhan, 2005).

4.6 CONCLUSION

The recent initiatives to transform healthcare policies and programmes in India reflect a strong dedication to achieving universal health coverage and enhancing the overall health system. Programmes such as Ayushman Bharat, the NDHM, and significant investments in health infrastructure are steering the country towards improved accessibility, affordability, and quality in healthcare. Nonetheless, addressing rural-urban disparities, strengthening the healthcare workforce, and ensuring financial sustainability are crucial for the long-term effectiveness of these reforms. India's path towards a more resilient healthcare system is encouraging, but ongoing efforts and innovation are vital to effectively addressing the healthcare needs of its varied population. Despite notable challenges in implementation, the recent emphasis on healthcare reform showcases an ambitious pledge to achieve universal health coverage. The Ayushman Bharat initiative, especially PM-JAY, significantly extends health insurance to millions of vulnerable families. The success of these initiatives depends on tackling core challenges such as insufficient healthcare infrastructure, a lack of healthcare professionals, and disparities in access between urban and rural areas. The COVID-19 pandemic has highlighted India's healthcare system's weaknesses and strengths, leading to digital health infrastructure reforms through efforts like the NDHM. Furthermore, the emphasis on preventive healthcare through HWCs and incorporating traditional medicine via AYUSH reflect a comprehensive approach to healthcare delivery. Going forward, the effectiveness of these reforms will depend on ongoing political commitment, increased healthcare expenditure (below 2% of GDP), stronger public-private collaborations, and a focus on healthcare workforce development. Policymakers, healthcare practitioners, and stakeholders interested in India's healthcare landscape have important roles in this endeavour. The accurate measure of success will be whether these reforms, with our engaged participation, can effectively lower out-of-pocket expenses and ensure that quality healthcare reaches the most vulnerable populations in India, particularly in rural and remote regions.

REFERENCES

Aashima, & Sharma, R. (2024). A systematic review of the world's largest government sponsored health insurance scheme for 500 million beneficiaries in India: Pradhan Mantri Jan Arogya Yojana. *Applied Health Economics and Health Policy*, 22(1), 17–32.

Agarwal, L. (2023). Building a resilient digital health ecosystem in India. In: *Accelerating Global Health*, p. 82. ISBN:978-81-963864-8-1. https://www.undp.org/sites/g/files/zskgke326/files/2023-09/orf-path_health-n1.pdf.

Agrawal, P. (2015). *Infrastructure in India: Challenges and the Way Ahead*, Institute of Economic Growth, University of Delhi Enclave. https://www.iegindia.org/upload/publication/Workpap/wp350.pdf.

Ahmet, E. (2023). Risk analysis and assessment of artificial intelligence usage in healthcare. *Arel Üniversitesi Sağlık Bilimleri Dergisi*, 7(2), 110–129.

Alwan, A., MacLean, D. R., Riley, L. M., d'Espaignet, E. T., Mathers, C. D., Stevens, G. A., & Bettcher, D. (2010). Monitoring and surveillance of chronic non-communicable diseases: Progress and capacity in high-burden countries. *The Lancet*, 376(9755), 1861–1868.

Arjun, M., Singh, A. K., & Parida, S. P. (2023). CoWIN: The future of universal immunization program in India. *Indian Journal of Community Medicine*, 48(4), 514–517.

Bagga, G., Singh, H., & Hood, M. M. (2024). Revolutionizing Indian healthcare: The impact of digital health, AI, telemedicine, and data security. *IOSR Journal of Business and M*anagement, 26(9), 30–34.

Bahl, S., Kumar, R., Menabde, N., Thapa, A., McFarland, J., Swezy, V., … Wassilak, S. (2014). Polio-free certification and lessons learned—South-East Asia region, March 2014. *MMWR Morbidity and Mortality Weekly Report*, 63(42), 941–946.

Bajpai, V. (2014). The challenges confronting public hospitals in India, their origins, and possible solutions. *Advances in Public Health*, 2014(1), 898502.

Bakshi, R. K., Kumar, N., Sharma, S., Singh, K. J., Chakma, J. K., & Singh, R. (2024). Advancing maternal health: India's recent initiatives. *Journal of the Epidemiology Foundation of India*, 2(4), 163–181.

Balarajan, Y., Selvaraj, S., & Subramanian, S. (2011). Health care and equity in India. *The Lancet*, 377(9764), 505–515.

Bali, A. S., & Ramesh, M. (2021). Governing healthcare in India: A policy capacity perspective. *International Review of Administrative Sciences*, 87(2), 275–293.

Bali, R. K., Rai, S., & Verma, D. K. (2021). Tertiary healthcare institutions and maxillofacial surgery: A case for reform. *Journal of Maxillofacial and Oral Surgery*, 20, 337–339. doi:10.1007/s12663-021-01616-y.

Barik, D., & Arokiasamy, P. (2016). Rising health expenditure due to non-communicable diseases in India: An outlook. *Frontiers in Public Health*, 4, 268.

Bhadoria, A. S., Mishra, S., Singh, M., & Kishore, S. (2019). National immunization programme–mission Indradhanush programme: Newer approaches and interventions. *The Indian Journal of Pediatrics*, 86, 633–638.

Bhandari, L., & Dutta, S. (2007). Health infrastructure in rural India. *India Infrastructure Report*, 2007, 265–285.

Bhardwaj, N. D. (2023). Challenges in healthcare in India. In: *Administration in India: Challenges and Innovations*, Routledge, London, pp. 52–69. ISBN:978-1-032-55975-9, doi:10.4324/9781003433187.

Bhat, T. (2015). International trade in health care services: Prospects and challenges for India. *India Quarterly*, 71(3), 239–254.

Bhatia, P., Vasaikar, S., & Wali, A. (2018). A landscape of nanomedicine innovations in India. *Nanotechnology Reviews*, 7(2), 131–148.

Bhattacharya, S., Sharma, V., Dubey, R., Bhasin, T., Bhattacharya, D., Mulukutla, R. D., … Aysola, U. (2015). Some key issues and challenges facing India: Perspectives on policies and action. *Vikalpa*, 40(2), 209–241.

Binny, M. G., & Gupta, M. (2017). Health insurance in India–opportunities and challenges. *International Journal of Latest Technology, Engineering, Management and Applied Sciences (IJLTEMAS)*, 6(8), 36–43.

Biru, G., Gemechu, H., Gebremeskel, E., Daba, H., Dese, K., Wakjira, E., … Murad, H. (2024). Community-based surveillance of acute flaccid paralysis: A review on detection and reporting strategy, 1–34. doi:10.2139/ssrn.4939522.

Brimnes, N. (2023). Rallying around the magic wand: Visions of social medicine, public health and disease control in India 1946–1957. *Health and Development*, 2, 175.

Burns, L. R. (2014). India's healthcare industry: A system perspective. In: Burns, L. R. (Ed.), *India's Healthcare Industry: Innovation in Delivery, Financing, and Manufacturing*, Cambridge University Press, Cambridge, pp. 3–37.

Burugina Nagaraja, S., Thekkur, P., Satyanarayana, S., Tharyan, P., Sagili, K. D., Tonsing, J., … Sachdeva, K. S. (2021). Active case finding for tuberculosis in India: A syntheses of activities and outcomes reported by the national tuberculosis elimination programme. *Tropical Medicine and Infectious Disease*, 6(4), 206.

Cancarevic, I., Plichtová, L., & Malik, B. H. (2021). Healthcare systems around the world. In: *International Medical Graduates in the United States: A Complete Guide to Challenges and Solutions*, pp. 45–79. doi:10.1007/978-3-030-62249-7.

Carvalho, L. H. F., & Weckx, L. Y. (2006). Universal use of inactivated polio vaccine. *Jornal de Pediatria*, 82, s75–s82.

Chakravarthi, I. (2024). *Digital Health and the National Digital Health Mission–Leveraging "Universal Health Care" for Technology and Capital?* pp. 1–19. https://rupe-india.org/aspects-no-81-82/digital-health-and-the-national-digital-health-mission/.

Chatterjee, S., Das, P., Pinheiro, A., Haldar, P., Ray, A., Brenzel, L., & Resch, S. (2021). The incremental cost of improving immunization coverage in India through the Intensified Mission Indradhanush programme. *Health Policy and Planning*, 36(8), 1316–1324.

Chauhan, V., Dumka, N., Hannah, E., Ahmed, T., & Kotwal, A. (2022). Recent initiatives for transforming healthcare in India: A political economy of health framework analysis. *Journal of Global Health Economics and Policy*, 2, e2022002, doi:10.52872/001c.34300.

Choudhary, R., & Singh, M. M. (2018). Exploring key issues and challenges in tribes healthcare programmes. *Tribal Healers of India*, 102–104.

Chowdhury, K., Ahmad, R., Sinha, S., Dutta, S., & Haque, M. (2023). Multidrug-resistant TB (MDR-TB) and extensively drug-resistant TB (XDR-TB) among children: Where we stand now. *Cureus*, 15(2), e35154. doi:10.7759/cureus.35154.

Dandona, R., Majumder, M., Akbar, M., Bhattacharya, D., Nanda, P., Kumar, G. A., & Dandona, L. (2022). Assessment of quality of antenatal care services in public sector facilities in India. *BMJ Open*, 12(12), e065200.

Das, A., Rao, D., & Hagopian, A. (2011). India's Janani Suraksha Yojana: Further review needed. *The Lancet*, 377(9762), 295–296.

Dastidar, B. G., Jani, A. R., Suri, S., & Nagaraja, V. H. (2024). Reimagining India's national telemedicine service to improve access to care. *The Lancet Regional Health-Southeast Asia*, 30, 100480, doi:10.1016/j.lansea.2024.100480.

Dehury, R. K., Dehury, P., Sripathi, N., Acharyulu, G., Behera, M. R., & Neeragatti, S. (2023). Health sector development in India: An account from Bhore Committee 1946 to National Health Policy 2017. *Journal of Development Policy and Practice*, 8(2), 209–242.

Dev, S. M. (2024). Regional dimensions in India: Economic growth, inclusive and sustainable development. *Journal of Quantitative Economics*, 22(2), 245–296.

Dey, B., Mitra, A., Prakash, K., Basu, A., Ray, S., & Mitra, A. (2013). Gaps in health infrastructure in Indian scenario: A review. *Indo Global Journal of Pharmaceutical Sciences*, 3(2), 156–166.

Dudhraj, V. (2020). National health policy 2017: Can it release health-related burden of diseases towards achieving health-related sustainable development goals? *International Journal of Creative Research Thoughts*, 8(8), 675–687.

Duffy, R. M., & Kelly, B. D. (2019). India's mental healthcare act, 2017: Content, context, controversy. *International Journal of Law and Psychiatry*, 62, 169–178.

Earnest, D., & Gnanadurai, A. (2022). Exploring the concept of good death among the terminally ill patients. *Indian Journal of Continuing Nursing Education*, 23(2), 179–183.

ESCAP, U., & India, I. (2024). *Landscape Study of Inclusive Business in Agrifood Systems in India*. https://repository.unescap.org/handle/20.500.12870/7415.

Ghosh, A., & Ghosh, R. (2020). Maternal health care in India: A reflection of 10 years of national health mission on the Indian maternal health scenario. *Sexual & Reproductive Healthcare*, 25, 100530.

Ghosh, P., Goel, G., & Ojha, M. (2020). Homeless shelters in urban India: Life sans dignity. *International Journal of Housing Markets and Analysis*, 13(1), 4–18.

Ghosh, S. M. (2023). National health mission and the status of public healthcare in Indian States. *Social Change*, 53(4), 562–574.

Golechha, M., Bohra, T., Rana, R., & Panchamia, J. (2025). Impact of India's flagship national health mission on governance, human resources for health, and the health system: A scoping review. *World Medical & Health Policy*, 1–25, https://onlinelibrary.wiley.com/doi/epdf/10.1002/wmh3.636.

Gomber, S., Taneja, D., & Mohan, K. (1996). Awareness of pulse polio immunisation. *The Indian Journal of Pediatrics*, 63, 99–103.

Gopal, K. M. (2019). Strategies for ensuring quality health care in India: Experiences from the field. *Indian Journal of Community Medicine*, 44(1), 1–3.

Greene, W. (2007). *The Emergence of India's Pharmaceutical Industry and Implications for the US Generic Drug Market*, US International Trade Commission, Office of Economics Washington DC, pp. 1–41. https://www.usitc.gov/publications/332/EC200705A.pdf.

Gudi, N., Lakiang, T., Pattanshetty, S., Sarbadhikari, S. N., & John, O. (2021). Challenges and prospects in India's digital health journey. *Indian Journal of Public Health*, 65(2), 209–212.

Gunasekaran, V., & Harmantzis, F. C. (2007). Emerging wireless technologies for developing countries. *Technology in Society*, 29(1), 23–42.

Gupta, A., Gupta, S., & Nongkynrih, B. (2013). Integrated child development services (ICDS) scheme: A journey of 37 years. *Indian Journal of Community Health*, 25(1), 77–81.

Gupta, R., Bedi, M., Goyal, P., Wadhera, S., & Verma, V. (2020). Analysis of COVID-19 tracking tool in India: Case study of Aarogya Setu mobile application. *Digital Government: Research and Practice*, 1(4), 1–8.

Gupta, S. K., Pal, D. K., Tiwari, R., Garg, R., Shrivastava, A. K., Sarawagi, R., … Lahariya, C. (2012). Impact of Janani Suraksha Yojana on institutional delivery rate and maternal morbidity and mortality: An observational study in India. *Journal of Health, Population, and Nutrition*, 30(4), 464.

Gurnani, V., Singh, P., Haldar, P., Aggarwal, M. K., Agrahari, K., Kashyap, S., … Nandi, P. (2020). Programmatic assessment of electronic vaccine intelligence network (eVIN). *PLoS One*, 15(11), e0241369.

Haleem, A., Javaid, M., Singh, R. P., & Suman, R. (2022). Medical 4.0 technologies for healthcare: Features, capabilities, and applications. *Internet of Things and Cyber-Physical Systems*, 2, 12–30.

Hemamalini, M. (2021). Health planning and policies and problems. In: *Community Health Nursing: Framework for Practice*, Vol. 28, S. Gangadharan, M. Hemamalini (Eds.), Delhi, India. Elsevier.

Inampudi, S., & Gaurav, A. K. (2024). Integrated approaches of technology applications for COVID vaccination: Administrative successes of CoWIN program in India. In: *Perspectives and Practices of Public Administration in South Asia: Post-Pandemic Recovery and Sustainable Development Agenda*, pp. 39–60. doi:10.1007/978-3-031-49841-1_3.

Jadhav, S. (2024) Health and health care communication in India 4. *Journal of Shivaji University (Humanities and Social Sciences)*, 368, 4199.

Kadarpeta, R. S. R., Anand, J. S., & Achungura, G. (2024). Strengthening public financing of primary healthcare in India: A perspective. *Health Services Insights*, 17, 11786329241249289.

Kaladharan, S., Dhanya, M., Drisya, R., & Raj, M. B. (2023). Intention to use eSanjeevani-OPD app: An empirical investigation using health belief model. In: *Paper Presented at the 2023 Advanced Computing and Communication Technologies for High Performance Applications (ACCTHPA)*, pp. 1–6. doi:10.1109/ACCTHPA57160.2023.10083374.

Kalaivanan, R. C., Basavaraju, V., Sadh, K., Rahul, P., Nagabhushana, S. H., Manjunatha, N., … Math, S. B. (2020). Implementing national mental health program: Local leaders' perspectives and lessons for national action. *Asian Journal of Psychiatry*, 53, 102233.

Kamble, S. A. (2024). The Antyodaya philosophy: Government plan to rural development and rural livelihood security. *Aksharasurya*, 4(06), 119–127.

Karan, A., Yip, W., & Mahal, A. (2017). Extending health insurance to the poor in India: An impact evaluation of Rashtriya Swasthya Bima Yojana on out of pocket spending for healthcare. *Social Science & Medicine*, 181, 83–92.

Kesavadev, J., Krishnan, G., & Mohan, V. (2021). Digital health and diabetes: Experience from India. *Therapeutic Advances in Endocrinology and Metabolism*, 12, 20420188211054676.

Khare, M., & Arora, S. (2023). Skills for sustainable employability: Strategies in India. In: *Sustainable and Dynamic Graduate Employability*, pp. 95–117. Routledge, London.

Kirpekar, V., Faye, A., Bhave, S., Gawande, S., & Tadke, R. (2024). District mental health program: Then and now. *Indian Journal of Psychiatry*, 66(7), 603–613.

Krishnamoorthy, A. (2024). Did the Government achieve its aim by implementing the Janani Shishu Suraksha Karyakaram program in India? pp. 1–22. SSRN https://papers.ssrn.com/sol3/papers.cfm?abstract_id=4911766.

Krishnan, A., Gupta, V., Nongkynrih, B., & Thakur, J. (2011). How to effectively monitor and evaluate NCD programmes in India. *Indian Journal of Community Medicine*, 36(Suppl1), S57–S62.

Kumar, A. (2023). The transformation of the Indian healthcare system. *Cureus*, 15(5), e39079. doi:10.7759/cureus.39079.

Kumar, A. S., Chen, L. C., Choudhury, M., Ganju, S., Mahajan, V., Sinha, A., & Sen, A. (2011). Financing health care for all: Challenges and opportunities. *The Lancet*, 377(9766), 668–679.

Kumar, N., & Singh, B. (2024). Pradhan Mantri Swasthaya Suraksha Nidhi, Vol. 2, pp. 11–20. Community Welfare Schemes in Vikas-Sheel Bharat.

Kumar, P. (2022). An analysis of some poverty alleviation and employment generation programmes in India. *Ideal Research Review*, 72(1), 1–7.

Kumar, R., & Duggirala, A. (2021). Health insurance as a healthcare financing mechanism in India: Key strategic insights and a business model perspective. *Vikalpa*, 46(2), 112–128.

Kumar, S., Sharma, A., Sood, A., & Kumar, S. (2016). Urban health in India: Policies, practices and current challenges. *Journal of Health Management*, 18(3), 489–498.

Lahariya, C. (2018). 'Ayushman Bharat' program and universal health coverage in India. *Indian Pediatrics*, 55(6), 495–506.

Lahariya, C. (2020). Health & wellness centers to strengthen primary health care in India: Concept, progress and ways forward. *The Indian Journal of Pediatrics*, 87(11), 916–929.

Law, S. (2019). *Exploring TB Patient Journeys and the Emergence of MDR-TB in India and South Africa: A Multi-Methods Study*, McGill University, Canada, pp. 1–24. https://www.proquest.com/openview/8a56e22505d44033b8d5e2a74483ee7e/1?pq-origsite=gscholar&cbl=44156.

Lesnik, J. (2004). Community health centers: Health care as it could be. *JL & Health*, 19, 1.

Lim, S. S., Dandona, L., Hoisington, J. A., James, S. L., Hogan, M. C., & Gakidou, E. (2010). India's Janani Suraksha Yojana, a conditional cash transfer programme to increase births in health facilities: An impact evaluation. *The Lancet*, 375(9730), 2009–2023.

Malhotra, C., Kotwal, V., & Basu, A. (2019). Designing national health stack for public health:

Role of ICT-based knowledge management system. In: *Paper Presented at the 2019 ITU Kaleidoscope: ICT for Health: Networks, Standards and Innovation (ITU K)*, pp. 1–8. doi:10.23919/ITUK48006.2019.8996135.

Mishra, K. (2020). *The Indic Quotient: Reclaiming Heritage through Cultural* Enterprise, Bloomsbury Publishing, Delhi, p. 1. https://www.bloomsbury.com/in/indic-quotient-9789389391909/.

Nagarajan, S., Paul, V. K., Yadav, N., & Gupta, S. (2015). The national rural health mission in India: Its impact on maternal, neonatal, and infant mortality. *Paper Presented at the Seminars in Fetal and Neonatal Medicine*, 20(5), 315–320. doi:10.1016/j.siny.2015.06.003.

Naib, P., Kumar, P., Chandrashekar, S., Smith, O., & Chhabra, S. (2021). Trends in cardiac care utilization under Ayushman Bharat Pradhan Mantri Jan Arogya Yojana, India. *Annals of Clinical Cardiology*, 3(2), 63–68.

Nandraj, S., Muraleedharan, V., Baru, R., Qadeer, I., & Priya, R. (2001). *Private Health Sector in India*, Centre for Enquiry into Health and Allied Themes/Indian Institute of Technology/Jawaharlal Nehru University, Mumbai, Madras, Delhi, India, pp. 1–170. https://www.researchgate.net/profile/Vr-Muraleedharan/publication/283559565_Private_health_sector_in_India_CEHAT/links/5712635408ae39beb87a43e2/Private-health-sector-in-India-CEHAT.pdf.

Nath, A., Shalini, M. A., & Mathur, P. (2021). Health systems challenges and opportunities in tackling non-communicable diseases in rural areas of India. *National Medical Journal of India*, 34(1), 29.

Panday, P. K. (2020). Global best practices of urban slum development. In: *The Face of Urbanization and Urban Poverty in Bangladesh: Explaining the Slum Development Initiatives in the light of Global Experiences*, pp. 87–119.

Pandey, A., Roy, N., Bhawsar, R., & Mishra, R. M. (2010). Health information system in India: Issues of data availability and quality. *Demography India*, 39(1), 111–128.

Parmar, A., Rina, K., & Padhy, S. K. (2020). COVID-19 pandemic and people who use opioids in India: Opportunities and evolutions. *Indian Journal of Psychological Medicine*, 42(6), 566–568.

Patel, V., Parikh, R., Nandraj, S., Balasubramaniam, P., Narayan, K., Paul, V. K.,… Reddy, K. S. (2015). Assuring health coverage for all in India. *The Lancet*, 386(10011), 2422–2435.

Patwardhan, B., & Partwardhan, A. (2005). Traditional medicine: Modern approach for affordable global health, World Health Organization, Switzerland, pp. 1–172.

Paul, P. (2022). Medical device and equipment sector in India: Towards sophisticated digital healthcare systems: An overview. In: Dutta, G. (Ed.), Next-Generation Nanobiosensor Devices for Point-of-Care Diagnostics, pp. 211–225.

Paul, V. K., Singh, A., & Palit, S. (2018). POSHAN Abhiyaan: Making nutrition a Jan Andolan. *Proceedings of the Indian National Science Academy*, 84(4), 835–841.

Prasad, M. N., Mithilesh, M., & Rao, G. R. (2010). Public health surveillance in India–challenges and opportunities. *Indian Emergency Journal*, 5, 21–26.

Quinn, S. C., & Kumar, S. (2014). Health inequalities and infectious disease epidemics: A challenge for global health security. *Biosecurity and Bioterrorism: Biodefense Strategy, Practice, and Science*, 12(5), 263–273.

Raghunathan, N., Trivedi, P., Gupta, R., Chakraborty, S., & Mankad, S. (2024). Transformative impact of the national livelihood missions on livelihoods of women. *State of India's Livelihoods*, 49, 63–83.

Rai, R. K., & Singh, P. K. (2012). Janani Suraksha Yojana. *WHO South-East Asia Journal of Public Health*, 1(4), 362–368.

Raichowdhury, S., Khetrapal, S., & Chin, B. (2023). Core interventions contributing to the effectiveness of the National Urban Health Mission in India. *Journal of Global Health*, 13, 03009. doi:10.7189/jogh.13.03009.

Raj, G. M., Dananjayan, S., & Agarwal, N. (2023). Inception of the Indian digital health mission: Connecting… the… dots. *Health Care Science*, 2(5), 345–351.

Rajoria, C., Maula, M. T., Vyas, S., Ray, A., & Nischal, N. (2024). Paving a way for "TB Mukt Bharat": A snapshot of India's TB elimination program. *Indographics*, 3(2), 27–32.

Ramani, K., & Mavalankar, D. (2006). Health system in India: Opportunities and challenges for improvements. *Journal of Health Organization and Management*, 20(6), 560–572.

Rao, M., Rao, K. D., Kumar, A. S., Chatterjee, M., & Sundararaman, T. (2011). Human resources for health in India. *The Lancet*, 377(9765), 587–598.

Roy, S., & Rasheed, N. (2015). The national mental health programme of India. *International Journal of Current Medical and Applied Sciences*, 7, 7–15.

Sarkar, S. (2018). Recent development in the molecular diagnosis of tuberculosis. *Bengal Physician Journal*, 5(2), 10–15.

Saxena, A., Trivedi, M., Shroff, Z. C., & Sharma, M. (2022). Improving hospital-based processes for effective implementation of Government funded health insurance schemes: Evidence from early implementation of PM-JAY in India. *BMC Health Services Research*, 22, 1–13.

Sengupta, K. (2016). *Determinants of Health Status in* India, Springer, New York, pp. 1–172, doi:10.1007/978-81-322-2535-5.

Sharath, B., Menon, S., Balakrishnan, R., Hombaiah, C., Reddy, R. H., & Anil, S. (2024). Healthcare providers' perspectives on tuberculosis control in a district of Southern India–insights from 2022 sub-national TB free certification. *Clinical Epidemiology and Global Health*, 101655, 1–71, doi:10.1016/j.cegh.2024.101655.

Sharma, N., Aggarwal, A. K., Arora, P., & Bahuguna, P. (2022). Association of waiting time and satisfaction level of patients with online registration system in a tertiary level medical institute outpatient department (OPD). *Health Policy and Technology*, 11(4), 100687.

Sharma, R., Rohatgi, A., Jain, S., & Singh, D. (2023). The Ayushman Bharat digital mission (ABDM): Making of India's digital health story. *CSI Transactions on ICT*, 11(1), 3–9.

Sheikh, K., & George, A. (2012). *Health Providers in India: On the Frontlines of Change*, Routledge, India, pp. 1–40. ISBN:978-0-415-57977-3.

Sherlin, S., & Karunanidhi, K. (2024). Community health workers in India: Bridging the gap in healthcare access and equity. In: Oruganti, S. K., Karras, D. A., Thakur, S. S., Nagpal, K., Gupta, S. K. (Eds.), *Case Studies on Holistic Medical Interventions*, pp. 506–510.

Shigh, B., Suresh, K., Kumar, S., & Singh, P. (1997). Pulse polio immunization in Delhi—1995–96: A survey. *Indian Journal of Pediatrics*, 64, 57–64.

Singh, A. (2018). Mission Indradhanush (MI) and intensified mission Indradhanush (imi): The immunization programmes in India–a brief review. *Gut Gastroenterology*, 1, 1–2.

Singh, A., & Vellakkal, S. (2021). Impact of public health programs on maternal and child health services and health outcomes in India: A systematic review. *Social Science & Medicine*, 274, 113795.

Singh, M., Sonkaria, L., & Raghav, P. (2017). Pradhan Mantri Surakshit Matritva Abhiyan (PMSMA): New initiative to deliver quality maternal health care in India. *MOJ Womens Health*, 4(2), 00081.

Singh, U. K. (2024). Implementation of sustainable development goals in India: Progress and challenges. *Regional Dimensions of Human Development in India and South Africa: Through Sustainable Development Goals*, pp. 39–91.

Sinha, P., & Sigamani, P. (2016). Key challenges of human resources for health in India. *Global Journal of Medicine and Public Health*, 5(4), 1–10.

Small, Z., Thompson, S. E., Sharma, A., Majumdar, S., Thout, S. R., Praveen, D., & Hirst, J. E. (2024). Mobile health (mHealth) interventions for health promotion during the perinatal period in India: A scoping review. *Frontiers in Global Women's Health*, 5, 1427285.

Srikantha, N., Bhat, S., Singh, A., & Singh, R. (2015). Healthcare seeking attitude and utilization of traditional medicine in India-an overview. *World Journal of Pharmaceutical Science and Research*, 4(7), 722–738.

Srivastava, S., Bertone, M. P., Basu, S., De Allegri, M., & Brenner, S. (2023). Implementation of PM-JAY in India: A qualitative study exploring the role of competency, organizational and leadership drivers shaping early roll-out of publicly funded health insurance in three Indian states. *Health Research Policy and Systems*, 21(1), 65.

Tawde, P. P., Quazi, Z., Gaidhane, A., & Choudhari, S. G. (2024). Developments and trends of immunization in India: A narrative review. *Cureus*, 16(8), e66547.

Thakur, R., Awasthi, A. A., Taneja, N., & Janardhanan, R. (2020). The evaluation of immunization coverage under mission Indradhanush: A review. *International Journal of Community Medicine and Public Health*, 7(12), 5229.

Thomas, J. J. (2008). *Innovation in India and China: Challenges and Prospects in Pharmaceuticals and Biotechnology*, Madras School of Economics, pp. 1–28. https://eaber.org/wp-content/uploads/2011/05/MSE_Thomas_2008.pdf.

Venkatesh, U., Garg, S., Gnanasekaran, S., & Pal, G. K. (2024). The National Urban Health Mission (NUHM): Impact, challenges, and future directions for urban health care. *Journal of the Epidemiology Foundation of India*, 2(4), 152–162.

Venugopal, V., Richa, R., Singh, D., Gautam, A., & Jahnavi, G. (2023). National programme for prevention and control of cancer, diabetes, cardiovascular diseases, and stroke: A scoping review in the context of hypertension prevention and control in India. *Indian Journal of Public Health*, 67(Suppl 1), S50–S57.

Vir, S. C. (2023). *Poshan Abhiyaan and Poshan 2.0: Experiences and Plan of Actions Child, Adolescent and Woman Nutrition in India*, Routledge, London, pp. 729–773.

Vir, S. C. (2017). Re-examining and re-positioning India's nutrition programme for accelerating improvements in maternal and child nutrition. Observer Research Foundation, pp. 1–28.

Vitsupakorn, S., Bharali, I., Yamey, G., & Mao, W. (2021). *Early Experiences of Pradhan Mantri Jan Arogya Yojana (PM JAY) in India: A Narrative Review*, pp. 1–32, https://ssrn.com/abstract=3797792.

Waning, B., Diedrichsen, E., & Moon, S. (2010). A lifeline to treatment: The role of Indian generic manufacturers in supplying antiretroviral medicines to developing countries. *Journal of the International AIDS Society*, 13, 1–9.

Wig, N. N., & Murthy, S. R. (2015). The birth of national mental health program for India. *Indian journal of Psychiatry*, 57(3), 315–319.

World Health Organization. (2012). *Local Production and Technology Transfer to Increase Access to Medical Devices: Addressing the Barriers and Challenges in Low-and Middle-Income Countries*, pp. 1–154. https://iris.who.int/bitstream/handle/10665/336774/9789241504546-eng.pdf.

World Health Organization. (2018). *A Vision for Primary Health Care in the 21st Century: Towards Universal Health Coverage and the Sustainable Development Goals*, World Health Organization, pp. 1–64. https://iris.who.int/bitstream/handle/10665/328065/WHO-HIS-SDS-2018.15-eng.pdf.

Yadav, S. (2024). Nikshay Mitra: A remarkable initiative in efforts against tuberculosis. *Cureus*, 16(6), e62615.

Zaman, F. A. (2021). Journey of tuberculosis control in India: From then till now. *Journal of Comprehensive Health*, 9(1), 5–10.

5 Examining the Inclusivity of India's National Urban Transport Policy for Senior Citizens

Shashikant Nishant Sharma and Kavita Dehalwar

5.1 INTRODUCTION

Most countries in the world have a large number of senior citizen population, which can be attributed to the fact that there are declining fertility rates and rising life expectancies due to improvements in medical facilities (Musselwhite, 2022). The increasing number of senior citizen population in India is a significant demographic trend with wide-ranging social, economic, and healthcare implications. This demographic shift is characterized by a growing proportion of elderly individuals (typically defined as those aged 60 and above) within the total population (Badji et al., 2021). The pace of expansion or improvement of public transportation in India is languid compared to the growth of its demand (Lunani et al., 2022). Advances in healthcare, nutrition, and medical technology have contributed to higher life expectancy, resulting in a larger proportion of the population living into old age. Falling birth rates over the years have led to a reduced number of young people in the population pyramid, contributing to the overall senior citizens of the population. Access to better healthcare and medical facilities has led to lower mortality rates and improved quality of life for older individuals, leading to longer lifespans (Galvin et al., 2021). As senior citizen population places greater demand on healthcare services, including hospitals, clinics, long-term care facilities, and public transport, government policies need to address the unique needs and challenges faced by older adults, including healthcare access, social security, and legal protection. The increasing senior citizen population in India is a multifaceted phenomenon with both challenges and opportunities (Addanki & Venkataraman, 2017). Addressing the needs of this demographic group requires comprehensive policies, social support systems, and a proactive approach to healthcare, economic planning, and urban development.

The National Urban Transport Policy (NUTP) in India was introduced in 2006 to promote sustainable and efficient urban transport systems across the country. While the policy does not explicitly focus on the senior citizen population, it does address several aspects that are relevant to their needs (Ministry of Housing and Urban Affairs, 2006). Here's a document analysis of the NUTP concerning the senior citizen population based on the revised NUTP 2014 (MOHUA, 2016). The NUTP

DOI: 10.1201/9781003513834-5

recognizes the importance of providing accessible transport options for all citizens, including senior citizens. It emphasizes the need to develop infrastructure that enables easy access to public transport, such as ramps, elevators, and priority seating for older people and disabled individuals. The policy promotes the development of efficient and affordable public transport systems as a means to address the mobility needs of all citizens. It highlights the need to improve the quality and coverage of public transport, including buses, metro systems, and paratransit services, to make them more accessible and senior-friendly (Lodhi et al., 2024). The NUTP emphasizes the creation of pedestrian-friendly infrastructure to ensure safe and convenient mobility for all residents, including older adults (Bala & Kumar, 2023). It encourages the development of wide and well-maintained footpaths, pedestrian crossings, and traffic calming measures to enhance the walking experience and promote active senior citizens. The policy acknowledges the vulnerability of older adults to traffic fatalities and emphasizes the importance of road safety. It calls for the implementation of measures to reduce traffic congestion, improve road design, and enhance traffic management systems, ultimately ensuring safer mobility for seniors (Kuriakose & Bhattacharjee, 2021). Recent developments in urban transportation services are rapidly transforming the way people make their trips (Raj et al., 2023).

The NUTP emphasizes the integration of different modes of transport, including public transport, non-motorized transport, and paratransit services (Dawda et al., 2021). This integration aims to provide seamless connectivity, reduce travel time, and enhance accessibility, benefiting all citizens, including older adults (Sharma, Kumar, et al., 2024). The policy recognizes the importance of promoting non-motorized modes of transport, such as walking and cycling, for short-distance travel. For senior citizens, these modes of transport can provide health benefits for seniors and create age-friendly urban environments. The NUTP encourages the use of technology and innovation in urban transport planning and management (Charaniya, 2018). This includes the development of intelligent transportation systems (ITS), mobile applications, and online platforms that can provide real-time information about transport services and accessibility features, thus aiding older adults in navigating the transport system more effectively.

It's important to note that while the NUTP sets out guidelines and objectives for urban transport planning in India, the implementation of these measures can vary across different cities and states. Local governments and urban planning authorities play a crucial role in translating the policy's provisions into practical solutions that cater to the specific needs of the senior citizen population in their respective areas. The mobility and accessibility expectations of seniors in the senior citizen population have been increasing due to the expansion of the public transport system in many metropolitan cities of India (Alsnih & Hensher, 2003). The improvement of the pedestrian amenities is necessary to attract more passengers (Dube et al., 2023).

In this research, we have tried to find answers to the two pertinent research questions based on the principles of the NUTP of India 2014 which was revised based on the comments and suggestions from different committees. We have tried to find answers to the following research questions:

- How does the NUTP of India address the mobility needs of the senior citizen population?
- What provisions does the NUTP of India have in place to ensure accessibility and convenience for the senior citizen population?

5.2 METHODOLOGY

This research chapter utilizes a document analysis approach (Bowen, 2009) to examine the NUTP (2014) of India and its provisions regarding the needs of the senior citizen population. Document analysis is a research method that involves the systematic examination and interpretation of written or textual sources to gain insights into a particular subject methodology, as shown in the flowchart in Figure 5.1.

Data Collection: The primary data sources for this research include official documents related to the NUTP, such as policy documents, guidelines, reports, and publications from relevant government agencies and urban planning authorities. These documents were accessed through online databases, official websites, and government portals as shown in Table 5.1. Secondary data sources, such as scholarly articles, research chapters, and reports, were also consulted to provide additional context and analysis.

A comprehensive search was conducted using specific keywords NUTP or NUTP India or NUTP and senior citizens population. The selected documents were screened based on their relevance to the research objective, ensuring they contained information about the policy's impact on the mobility and transportation needs of the senior citizen population. The research relies on the availability and quality of the selected documents. The accuracy and comprehensiveness of the analysis are contingent

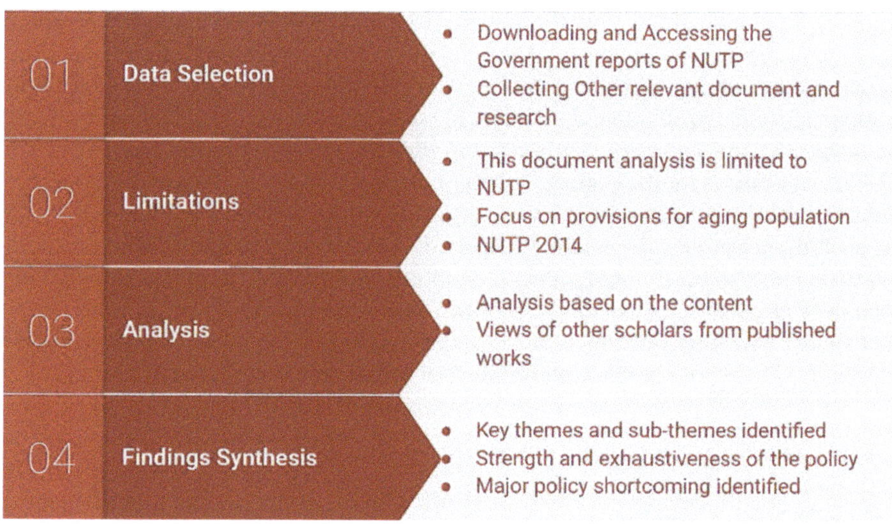

FIGURE 5.1 Document analysis adopted by the authors (conceptualized based on the research question).

TABLE 5.1
List of Documents Referred for This Research

Sl. No.	Policies and Documents	Year of Publication	Authority
1	National Urban Transport Policy	2006	Govt. of India
2	National Urban Transport Policy	2014	Govt. of India
3	Delhi Master Plan 2021	2007	Govt. of India
4	Toolkit for Comprehensive Mobility Plan	2014	Ministry of Housing and Urban Affairs, Govt. of India
5	Accessible India Campaign (Sugamya Bharat Abhiyan)	2016	Govt. of India
6	Smart Cities Mission	2015	Ministry of Urban Development, Govt. of India
7	Public Transport and Mobility Guidelines for All	2016	Ministry of Urban Development, Govt. of India

upon the transparency and thoroughness of the policy documents. Additionally, as the research is based on existing documents listed in Table 5.1, it does not provide insights into the implementation and impact of the policy on the ground. Future research could incorporate interviews, surveys, or case studies to complement the findings from document analysis. The analysis involved a systematic review and interpretation of the selected documents. The information was categorized and organized thematically to identify key provisions and recommendations within the NUTP concerning the senior citizen population. This involved examining sections related to accessibility, public transport, pedestrian infrastructure, traffic safety, integration, non-motorized transport, and technology and innovation. The findings from the document analysis were synthesized to provide an overview and analysis of the NUTP's provisions for the senior citizen population. The key themes and sub-themes identified during the analysis were discussed, highlighting how the policy addresses the specific needs of older adults in terms of accessibility, safety, public transport, pedestrian infrastructure, integration, non-motorized transport, and technology. This document analysis serves as a valuable research methodology in examining policy documents, enabling a comprehensive understanding of the NUTP's provisions for the senior citizen population in the context of urban transport planning in India.

5.3 FINDINGS AND DISCUSSION

Regular public transportation users, particularly those from low- and middle-income backgrounds, often share apprehensions regarding safety, security, and overall comfort during their journeys. Addressing these concerns involves several measures such as monitoring the speed of public transportation, enhancing accessibility at stations, installing surveillance systems and panic buttons, enabling GPS tracking, and refining mechanisms for reporting instances of harassment or theft. By implementing these strategies, the perception of safety and security among public transportation commuters can be significantly enhanced, thereby improving their overall commuting experience (Jayakumar & Maji, 2023). The document analysis of the NUTP of India provides valuable insights into how the policy addresses the specific needs of the senior citizen population in terms of mobility and transportation. The analysis reveals several provisions and recommendations within the NUTP that aim to cater to the requirements of older adults. The following analysis and discussion highlight key themes and findings from the document analysis.

5.3.1 Accessibility

The NUTP lays down a comprehensive framework for addressing various aspects of urban transport planning and development in the country. One crucial aspect highlighted by the policy is the significance of accessibility for all citizens, with particular attention given to the needs of senior citizens (Verma et al., 2021). Recognizing the demographic shift and the challenges faced by older adults in accessing public transport, the NUTP emphasizes the development of infrastructure that caters to their specific requirements. To ensure easy access to public transport for senior citizens, the NUTP recommends the incorporation of various features in transport infrastructure. Ramps are one such feature that allow wheelchair users and individuals with mobility issues to access public transportation facilities more easily. By installing ramps at bus stops, metro stations, and other transport hubs, older adults can comfortably board and alight from vehicles, promoting independence and enhancing their overall mobility. Elevators are another essential component of inclusive infrastructure highlighted by the NUTP (Saxena, 2022). Installing elevators at transit stations, particularly in multi-level facilities, enables older adults to move between different levels effortlessly (Sharma & Dehalwar, 2025). This eliminates the physical strain of climbing stairs, making it more convenient for seniors to access various modes of transportation and navigate through complex urban transport networks. The Comprehensive Mobility Plan (CMP) prioritizes the development of an efficient, accessible, and well-connected public transportation system that accommodates the mobility needs of older adults. This might include low-floor buses, priority seating, and designated spaces for mobility aids like wheelchairs and walkers (MOHUA, 2016). Accessibility of healthcare is especially important for older people (Choi et al., 2019). Likewise, accessible community centres, parks, and public spaces that provide opportunities for social interaction and recreational activities are also extremely important for older people (Temelová & Dvořáková, 2012).

Accessibility is a key focus of the NUTP, aiming to make public transport more inclusive for older adults. The policy emphasizes the provision of accessible boarding and alighting facilities in buses, metro systems, and other modes of public transportation (Kar et al., 2022). This includes the installation of ramps, lifts, or low-floor buses to facilitate easy entry and exit for individuals with mobility challenges. The NUTP also encourages the development of user-friendly ticketing systems, information displays, and signage that are easily understandable and accessible to senior citizens. These measures help older adults navigate public transport networks independently, fostering their mobility and overall well-being (Lambat et al., 2022). The NUTP recognizes that senior citizens may require priority seating due to mobility limitations or health conditions. As such, the policy advocates for the provision of designated priority seating areas in public transport vehicles. These seats are easily identifiable and are reserved for older adults, ensuring that they have a comfortable and accessible place to sit during their journeys. The NUTP encourages awareness campaigns and training programmes for both transport staff and passengers to promote understanding and respect for priority seating, thereby creating a culture of inclusivity and support for senior citizens (Abass, 2023). Priority seating is a crucial provision emphasized by the NUTP to address the specific needs of senior citizens. Even the city administration is focusing on policies for improving public transport access through intermedia public transport (Kar et al., 2022). Designating priority seating areas in buses, trains, and other public transport vehicles ensures that older adults have access to seats that are easily accessible and comfortable. These designated seats serve as a visible reminder to other passengers to offer their seats to older individuals, promoting a culture of respect and consideration within public transportation. Creating age-friendly urban environments includes provisions for accessible public transportation, pedestrian-friendly streets, ramps, and sidewalks. The plan may incorporate designs that make it easier for elderly individuals to navigate the city safely and comfortably (Govt. of India, 2007).

Furthermore, the NUTP encourages the development of integrated transport systems that cater to the diverse needs of older adults. This includes seamless integration between different modes of transport, such as buses, trains, and non-motorized transport, to provide convenient and efficient travel options (Abdel Wahed Ahmed & Abd El Monem, 2020). By integrating various modes of transport, seniors can choose the most suitable option based on their mobility requirements, reducing travel time and enhancing their overall experience. In addition to physical infrastructure, the NUTP also emphasizes the importance of sensitizing transport personnel and creating awareness among the general public about the needs of senior citizens. Training programmes can be implemented to educate transport staff on providing assistance and support to older passengers. Awareness campaigns can be conducted to encourage passengers to be more considerate and accommodating towards seniors, fostering a supportive and inclusive transport environment. By incorporating these provisions, as outlined by the NUTP, India can develop transportation systems that prioritize the accessibility needs of senior citizens. This approach not only improves the mobility and quality of life for older adults but also contributes to building a more inclusive society where everyone can participate actively in urban life. The NUTP serves as a guiding framework to ensure that urban transport planning and development in India align with the principles of inclusivity and equitable access for all citizens, including the elderly.

5.3.2 Public Transport

The NUTP policy emphasizes the enhancement of comfort, safety, and accessibility features in various modes of public transportation, including buses, metro systems, and paratransit services. Tiwari et al. (2018) talk about the need for service level benchmarking for public transport in India as it has been found that many of the cities in India don't have proper public transport systems (Tiwari et al., 2018). This really shows the low level of the implementation of the NUTP 2014 in many cities in India. This should be noted in future policy revisions so that there is a proper system of service level benchmarking of public transport so that a more improved version of the public transport can be developed which will help in better catering to the needs of the senior citizen population of India.

One of the key objectives of the NUTP is to ensure that senior citizens can travel comfortably. To achieve this, the policy encourages the installation of features that enhance the overall comfort of public transport vehicles. This includes improved seating arrangements, cushioning, and suspension systems that reduce vibrations and jolts during travel. By upgrading the seating and interior design, public transport becomes more conducive to the needs of older adults, allowing them to travel with ease and in relative comfort. The Delhi Metro provides a good public transport system to the users and older people find it easy to travel in the metro as all metro stations have lift and escalator facilities for the older people (Kuriakose & Bhattacharjee, 2021). The bus rapid transit (BRT) system is facing a lot of challenges in its implementation as there is not enough right of way of the road which can be used for the dedicated BRT corridor. That there is missing infrastructure for physically challenged people and older people and they find it difficult to cross the road where the bus stop is planned at the centre of the road (i.e., median of the road). Safety is another critical aspect addressed by the NUTP concerning older adults.

Huge financial resources are needed for the successful implementation of the metro rail projects (Yang et al., 2020). While it is found that metro rail services are more sympathetic to older people, it is found increasingly difficult to develop metro rails in all million-plus cities in India. By emphasizing the improvement of public transport systems to meet the needs of older adults, the NUTP seeks to create a more age-friendly and inclusive urban environment. Through enhanced comfort, safety, and accessibility features in buses, metro systems, and paratransit services, senior citizens can enjoy more convenient and independent travel experiences within urban areas. The NUTP serves as a guiding policy framework to ensure that public transport planning and development in India align with the principles of inclusivity, equity, and dignity for older adults.

5.3.3 Pedestrian Infrastructure

The NUTP acknowledges the significance of pedestrian infrastructure in ensuring safe and convenient mobility for older adults. The policy recognizes that many seniors rely on walking as their primary mode of transportation, and therefore emphasizes the development of pedestrian-friendly environments that cater to their specific needs. One of the key provisions highlighted by the NUTP is the development of wide and well-maintained footpaths. These footpaths provide dedicated space for pedestrians, including older adults, to walk comfortably and safely along urban roads. Wide footpaths allow for easier manoeuvring, particularly for individuals with mobility aids such as walking frames or wheelchairs. The NUTP recommends the implementation of appropriate surface materials, such as non-slip tiles or tactile paving, to ensure that footpaths are accessible to seniors with varying physical abilities (Patel & Dave, 2016).

There is a lack of proper parking policy in many cities in India which makes it problematic for pedestrian users (Parmar et al., 2023). Most of the pedestrian users who are children, school-going youths, women, older people, and physically challenged people face parking as a problem when drivers park their vehicles on the footpaths. The NUTP also emphasizes the importance of pedestrian crossings that prioritize the safety of older adults. The policy recommends the installation of zebra crossings, signalized pedestrian crossings, and other forms of safe crossing facilities at strategic locations. Clear signage, audible signals, and extended crossing times can be incorporated to assist older pedestrians in safely navigating busy intersections. By ensuring safe crossing opportunities, the NUTP promotes independent mobility for senior citizens to remain active and engaged in their communities (Joshi & Joseph, 2015). Furthermore, the NUTP advocates for the implementation of traffic calming measures to enhance pedestrian safety. Slowing down vehicle speeds in residential areas, near schools, and in areas with high pedestrian activity is crucial to protect older adults who may have slower reflexes or reduced mobility. Traffic calming measures such as speed humps, raised pedestrian crossings, and narrower lanes help create a safer environment for seniors to navigate urban spaces.

The development of age-friendly urban environments through pedestrian infrastructure aligns with the concept of active senior citizens. By providing well-designed footpaths, pedestrian crossings, and traffic calming measures, the NUTP promotes physical activity and encourages older adults to walk as a mode of transport (Saxena, 2022). Regular physical activity has numerous health benefits and contributes to the overall well-being of seniors. The availability of safe and convenient pedestrian infrastructure helps older adults maintain their independence, social connections, and access to essential services within their communities. In addition to infrastructure development, the NUTP also emphasizes the importance of comprehensive urban planning that takes into account the needs of older adults. This includes creating mixed-use neighbourhoods that incorporate a variety of amenities, such as parks, healthcare facilities, and retail centres, within walking distance. By designing cities and towns that are walkable and accessible, the NUTP supports active senior citizens and ensures that older adults can participate fully in community life (Gough et al., 2021). The NUTP recognizes the significance of pedestrian infrastructure in promoting safe and convenient mobility for older adults. By developing wide footpaths, pedestrian crossings, and implementing traffic calming measures, the policy creates age-friendly urban environments that facilitate walking and active senior citizens. These provisions cater to the mobility needs of older adults, ensuring their continued engagement and quality of life within urban areas. The CMP emphasize infrastructure improvements such as well-maintained sidewalks, ramps, pedestrian crossings, and kerb cuts to ensure that older residents can navigate the city safely and comfortably (Govt. of India, 2014). The CMP promotes age-friendly urban design principles, such as bench seating at transit stops, shade and shelter options, and rest areas along pedestrian pathways.

5.3.4 Traffic Safety

The NUTP recognizes the vulnerability of older adults to fatalities and injuries in urban areas. The policy places significant emphasis on road safety measures in urban transport planning, aiming to create safer environments for senior citizens to navigate and reduce the risks associated with their mobility. The CMP could prioritize road safety measures, including traffic calming measures, improved lighting at crossings, and awareness campaigns, to enhance the safety of elderly pedestrians and drivers (Govt. of India, 2014). The policy promotes the implementation of safety measures in public transport systems to protect senior citizens during their journeys. This includes ensuring well-maintained vehicles with functional safety features such as seat belts, handrails, and non-slip flooring. Adequate lighting and clear signage are also emphasized to enhance visibility and reduce the risk of traffic crashes. By prioritizing safety considerations, the NUTP aims to instil confidence in senior citizens while using public transport, enabling them to travel with peace of mind. Sometimes lack of low-floor buses may be a hindrance for older people and physically challenged people (Waghmare, 2024).

The NUTP acknowledges that older adults may face unique challenges when it comes to road safety. Factors such as reduced mobility, diminished sensory abilities, and slower reaction times can make them more susceptible to road crashes (Sharma et al., 2024). To address these concerns, the policy advocates for the implementation of traffic management systems that prioritize the safety of older people. One of the key provisions of the NUTP is the development of well-maintained roads (Tiwari & Jain, 2012). The policy recognizes the importance of good road conditions in ensuring safe mobility for older adults. Well-paved roads with proper signage and markings reduce the risk of slips, trips, and falls. Regular maintenance of roads, including repairs of potholes and removal of obstacles, ensures a smoother and safer journey for senior citizens.

The NUTP also encourages the installation of appropriate traffic control devices to enhance road safety for older adults. This includes the implementation of traffic signals, pedestrian crossings, and signage at strategic locations, particularly in areas with high senior pedestrian activity. Well-designed and visible road signs provide clear instructions to drivers and pedestrians, reducing confusion and potential conflicts. By improving visibility and communication on the roads, the NUTP aims to create safer conditions for older adults to navigate urban areas. In addition, the NUTP promotes the integration of technology and ITS to enhance road safety for older people (Verma et al., 2021). This can include the use of traffic surveillance cameras, vehicle detection systems, and adaptive traffic signal control to improve the flow of traffic and minimize the risk of fatalities. ITS can also provide real-time information to older pedestrians, such as crossing times at signalized intersections, helping them make informed decisions and navigate safely.

Education and awareness campaigns are another essential aspect of the NUTP's provisions for road safety among older adults. The policy emphasizes the need to educate both older individuals and the general public about road safety practices. Older adults can benefit from educational programmes that focus on safe road crossing techniques, understanding traffic signals, and being aware of potential hazards

(Bivina & Parida, 2020). The NUTP also encourages awareness campaigns that promote mutual respect and consideration between different road users, fostering a culture of safe and inclusive mobility for all. Furthermore, the NUTP highlights the importance of community engagement and involvement in road safety initiatives. Local authorities, community organizations, and senior citizens' groups can collaborate to identify specific road safety challenges older adults face in their neighbourhoods and develop targeted solutions. This participatory approach ensures that the concerns and needs of older adults are taken into account when implementing road safety measures. By implementing these provisions, as outlined in the NUTP, India can create safer environments for older adults to navigate in urban areas (Priya Uteng & Turner, 2019). By prioritizing road safety measures, including well-maintained roads, traffic management systems, and education campaigns, the NUTP aims to reduce the risks associated with urban mobility for senior citizens. These provisions contribute to creating inclusive and age-friendly cities, where older adults can move around safely, maintain their independence, and actively participate in community life.

5.3.5 Integration and Multi-Modal Transport

The NUTP of India, established in 2014, recognizes the importance of integrating different modes of transport to enhance mobility options for all citizens, including older adults. The policy emphasizes the integration of public transport, non-motorized transport, and paratransit services to create a comprehensive and seamless urban transport network (Ghosh & Kalra, 2016). By promoting the integration of different modes of transport, the NUTP aims to provide flexibility and convenience to senior citizens. Older adults may have varying mobility needs and preferences, and by offering a range of transport options, they can choose the mode that best suits their requirements. Some seniors may prefer the comfort and accessibility of public transport, while others may opt for non-motorized options such as walking or cycling. Paratransit services, designed specifically for individuals with mobility challenges, can cater to the needs of older adults who require specialized transportation. There is a need for the energization of travel modes and institutional integration to solve the issues of multi-modal transit (Hidalgo et al., 2013).

The integration of public transport plays a significant role in the NUTP's provisions for older adults. The policy emphasizes the need to develop an efficient and interconnected public transport system that includes buses, trams, trains, and metro networks. Integration can be achieved through measures such as coordinated schedules, integrated ticketing systems, and seamless transfers between different modes of transport. This integration ensures that senior citizens can easily access and navigate the public transport network, reducing travel time and increasing convenience. There is a need for adopting comprehensive indicators based on sustainable transport which will help in avoiding the fragmented implementation of the policy (Jain, 2019). Non-motorized transport, such as walking and cycling, is another important component of the NUTP's multi-modal approach. The policy recognizes that many older adults prefer walking as a mode of transport for shorter trips, and cycling can also be a viable option for those who are physically fit. To support non-motorized transport, the NUTP advocates for the development of pedestrian and cycling infrastructure, including well-maintained footpaths, dedicated cycling lanes, and safe crossing facilities. This infrastructure encourages active modes of transport, promotes physical activity among seniors, and provides additional options for them to travel within urban areas.

Paratransit services are essential in meeting the specific needs of older adults with mobility challenges. The NUTP emphasizes the importance of integrating paratransit services into the overall urban transport system to ensure that seniors with disabilities or limited mobility have access to reliable and convenient transportation. Paratransit vehicles, such as accessible vans or mini-buses, can be equipped with features like ramps or lifts to facilitate easy boarding and alighting. By integrating paratransit services with the broader transport network, the NUTP aims to provide a comprehensive and inclusive range of options for older adults. Ramachandraiah (2012) raises the question of equitable road spaces for different modes of transport so that all users can use it effectively, which is another cause of concern due to the rising number of private vehicles (Ramachandraiah, 2012). The integration of different modes of transport in line with the NUTP not only benefits older adults but also has broader advantages for urban transport systems. It reduces congestion, promotes sustainable transportation, and improves overall connectivity within cities. By offering a variety of transport options and facilitating seamless connections, the NUTP contributes to creating age-friendly cities that prioritize the needs of senior citizens and enable them to maintain their independence and active lifestyles (Adlakha et al., 2020). The NUTP's emphasis on multi-modal integration recognizes the diverse mobility needs of older adults and aims to provide flexible and convenient transport options. By integrating public transport, non-motorized transport, and paratransit services, the policy enables older adults to choose the mode of transport that best suits their requirements. This multi-modal approach promotes connectivity, reduces travel time, and enhances the overall mobility experience for seniors within urban areas.

5.3.6 Non-Motorized Transport

The NUTP of India, established in 2014, places significant emphasis on promoting non-motorized modes of transport, such as walking and cycling, for short-distance travel (Islam et al., 2023). The policy recognizes that these modes of transport have multiple benefits for older adults, contributing to their overall health, well-being, and quality of life. The NUTP acknowledges that walking and cycling are low-impact physical activities that can help older adults maintain their mobility, strength, and cardiovascular health. Regular physical activity, even short walks or leisurely cycling, can improve balance, coordination, and muscle strength, reducing the risk of falls and related injuries. By actively promoting walking and cycling, the NUTP aims to encourage seniors to engage in regular physical activity, leading to improved health outcomes and enhanced overall well-being (Islam et al., 2023).

To support and encourage walking and cycling among older adults, the NUTP highlights the need for infrastructure that facilitates these modes of transport. This includes the development of dedicated pathways, footpaths, and sidewalks that are well-maintained, accessible, and free from obstacles. Wide footpaths with non-slip surfaces provide safe and comfortable spaces for seniors to walk while cycling lanes and tracks offer designated areas for cyclists, separate from motorized traffic. The policy also emphasizes the need for appropriate signage and clear markings to guide pedestrians and cyclists and ensure their safety (Sadhu et al., 2014). In addition to dedicated infrastructure, the NUTP recognizes the importance of creating a connected network of walking and cycling paths. This involves developing pedestrian-friendly neighbourhoods, where essential amenities such as schools, shops, and healthcare facilities are within walking or cycling distance. By designing compact and mixed-use urban areas, the policy promotes the concept of age-friendly communities, where older adults can easily access the services they require without relying solely on motorized transport.

The NUTP also encourages the implementation of initiatives to raise awareness about the benefits of walking and cycling among older adults (Khurana et al., 2020). This can include educational programmes, campaigns, and community events that promote active modes of transport and highlight the importance of physical activity for seniors. By fostering a culture of walking and cycling, the policy seeks to create a supportive environment that motivates older adults to choose these modes of transport and integrate them into their daily routines. Furthermore, the NUTP recognizes that the promotion of non-motorized modes of transport is beneficial not only for older adults but also for the broader community and the environment. Increased walking and cycling can contribute to reduced congestion, improved air quality, and a more sustainable urban transport system. By prioritizing infrastructure and policies that support walking and cycling, the NUTP aligns with the principles of sustainable development and addresses the environmental and health challenges associated with motorized transport. The NUTP's recognition of the importance of promoting non-motorized modes of transport, such as walking and cycling, for short-distance travel, has significant benefits for older adults (Agarwal et al., 2017). By encouraging senior citizens to physical activity, improving health outcomes, and fostering age-friendly communities, the policy enhances the well-being and quality of life of seniors. The development of infrastructure that supports walking and cycling, along with awareness campaigns, contributes to creating inclusive and sustainable urban environments that prioritize the needs of older adults.

5.3.7 Technology and Innovation

NUTP recognizes the importance of technology and innovation in enhancing urban transport services for older adults. The policy emphasizes the role of ITS, mobile applications, and online platforms in providing real-time information and improving accessibility features for seniors. One of the key provisions of NUTP is the integration of ITS into the urban transport network (Telang et al., 2021). ITS utilize advanced technologies such as sensors, cameras, and communication networks to collect and analyse real-time data about traffic conditions, vehicle movement, and passenger flows. For older adults, ITS can provide valuable information about public transport schedules, delays, and alternative routes. This allows seniors to plan their journeys more efficiently, reducing waiting times and minimizing inconveniences.

Mobile applications and online platforms also play a crucial role in enhancing urban transport services for older adults. The NUTP encourages the development of user-friendly mobile apps that provide comprehensive information about public transport options, routes, schedules, and fares. These apps can be customized to include accessibility features such as wheelchair-friendly routes, priority seating availability, and real-time updates about crowded buses or trains. By accessing such information on their smartphones, older adults can make informed decisions and choose the most suitable transport options based on their specific needs. Online platforms can further support older adults by providing centralized information and resources related to urban transport. Dedicated websites or portals can offer a range of services, including trip-planning tools, accessibility guidelines, and feedback mechanisms. These platforms can also serve as a means of communication between seniors and transport authorities, enabling them to voice their concerns, provide suggestions, and seek assistance regarding transport services. New technologies, especially smartphone-based mobility services, are extremely elderly unfriendly and may severely exacerbate transport-related social exclusion.

The NUTP also emphasizes the importance of integrating technology with existing infrastructure to improve accessibility features for older adults (Saxena, 2022). For example, digital signage at bus stops or train stations can display real-time information about arrival and departure times, allowing seniors to plan their journeys more effectively. Furthermore, the use of contactless smart cards or mobile payment systems can simplify the fare payment process, eliminating the need for physical tickets and reducing the barriers faced by older adults. By leveraging technology and innovation, the NUTP aims to empower older adults to navigate the urban transport system more effectively. Access to real-time information, trip-planning tools, and improved accessibility features through ITS, mobile apps, and online platforms enable older adults to make informed decisions and travel with greater ease and confidence. These technological advancements contribute to creating an inclusive and user-friendly transport environment for seniors, enhancing their independence, mobility, and overall experience within urban areas. The NUTP recognizes the significance of technology and innovation in enhancing urban transport services for older adults (Chhabra et al., 2021). By integrating ITS, mobile applications, and online platforms, the policy provides real-time information, trip-planning tools, and improved accessibility features. These technological advancements empower older adults to make informed decisions, navigate the transport system more effectively, and enhance their overall experience within urban areas.

While the NUTP demonstrates a commitment to addressing the needs of the senior citizen population, the effectiveness of these provisions in practice may vary across different cities and states in India. Local governments and urban planning authorities play a crucial role in implementing and enforcing the policy measures to create age-friendly urban transport systems. The document analysis reveals that the NUTP incorporates various provisions and recommendations to cater to the needs of the senior citizen population. By emphasizing accessibility, improving public transport, enhancing pedestrian infrastructure, ensuring traffic safety, promoting integrated and multi-modal transport, and leveraging technology and innovation, the policy aims to create urban transport systems. Age-friendly urban planning seeks to prevent isolation and promote social engagement among the elderly. This might involve integrating community centres, cultural facilities, and spaces for leisure activities into the urban fabric (Govt. of India, 2007). The master plan addresses concerns related to the safety of the elderly population, including well-lit streets, crime prevention measures, and emergency response systems, ensuring that public infrastructure, such as public buildings, transportation hubs, and public facilities, are designed with the needs of older individuals in mind. This could involve incorporating features like ramps, handrails, and seating areas. Involving older residents in the planning process to understand their specific needs, preferences, and challenges could include conducting surveys, focus groups, and consultations (Govt. of India, 2007). It's important to note that the effectiveness of a master plan in addressing the needs of senior citizens depends on its implementation, enforcement, and ongoing evaluation. As the demographic landscape continues to evolve, urban planners need to adapt their strategies to ensure that cities remain inclusive, accessible, and supportive of all age groups (Govt. of India, 2007).

The Accessible India Campaign, also known as the Sugamya Bharat Abhiyan, is an initiative launched by the Government of India to create a barrier-free and inclusive environment for persons with disabilities. While the primary focus of the campaign is on improving accessibility for people with disabilities, many of the measures taken under this initiative can also benefit the elderly population (Aguiar & Macário, 2017).

5.3.8 Inconsistencies between Different Documents

From Table 5.2, we can find that there are inconsistencies among the policies. While the NUTP emphasizes the need for sustainable and inclusive urban transport systems, it might lack specific provisions addressing the unique mobility challenges of the senior citizen population (Saxena, 2022). The policies could benefit from more explicit inclusion of age-friendly design and accessibility features in public transport. The master plan should ideally incorporate measures to enhance the accessibility, safety, and convenience of public transportation for older residents. The Master Plan of Delhi is inconsistent towards the level of availability of housing, accessibility to public transport, and quality of the built environment in all three Master Plans of Delhi 1962, 2001, and 2021 (Shrivastava & Singh, 2021). Without the specific content of the toolkit, it's challenging to identify any inconsistencies. However, if the toolkit does not comprehensively address the needs of the senior citizen population in mobility planning, it could be considered inconsistent with the goal of inclusivity (Jain, 2019).

The campaign's primary focus is on accessibility for persons with disabilities. While it indirectly benefits the senior citizen population, there could be a potential inconsistency in not explicitly addressing the broader needs of the senior citizen population in public transport. While the Smart Cities Mission aims to develop smart and sustainable cities, there might be a gap in addressing the specific mobility needs of the senior citizen population. It could benefit from incorporating age-friendly transportation features and services (Prasad & Alizadeh, 2020). While these guidelines emphasize inclusive mobility, they might not extensively cover the needs of the senior citizen

TABLE 5.2
Various Policies and Inconsistencies among Them

Policy Name	Year	Key Focus/Description
National Urban Transport Policy	2006 and 2014	Emphasizes the need for sustainable and inclusive urban transport systems, but lacks specific provisions addressing the unique mobility challenges of the senior citizen population. Could benefit from more explicit inclusion of age-friendly design and accessibility features in public transport.
Delhi Master Plan 2021	2021	Ideally incorporates measures to enhance the accessibility, safety, and convenience of public transportation for older residents. Inconsistent towards the level of availability of housing, accessibility to public transport, and quality of the built environment in all three Master Plans of Delhi 1962, 2001, and 2021.
Toolkit for Comprehensive Mobility Plan	2014	Without the specific content of the toolkit, it's challenging to identify any inconsistencies. However, if the toolkit does not comprehensively address the needs of the senior citizen population in mobility planning, it could be considered inconsistent with the goal of inclusivity.
Accessible India Campaign (Sugamya Bharat Abhiyan)	2016	The campaign's primary focus is on accessibility for persons with disabilities. While it indirectly benefits the senior citizen population, there could be a potential inconsistency in not explicitly addressing the broader needs of the senior citizen population in public transport.
Smart Cities Mission	2015	While the Smart Cities Mission aims to develop smart and sustainable cities, there might be a gap in addressing the specific mobility needs of the senior citizen population. It could benefit from incorporating age-friendly transportation features and services.
Public Transport and Mobility Guidelines for All	2016	While these guidelines emphasize inclusive mobility, they might not extensively cover the needs of the senior citizen population. There could be an inconsistency if the guidelines do not comprehensively address accessibility and comfort for older adults.

population. There could be an inconsistency if the guidelines do not comprehensively address accessibility and comfort for older adults (Mahapatra et al., 2021). The document does not use explicit language and provisions that address the needs of the senior citizen population in public transport, considering accessibility, safety, comfort, and social inclusion. The is a lack of provision to incorporate age-friendly design principles into public transportation infrastructure, including vehicles, stations, and stops.

5.4 CONCLUSIONS

The document analysis of the NUTP of India provides valuable insights into how the policy addresses the needs of the senior citizen population in terms of mobility and transportation. The NUTP recognizes the vulnerability of older adults to fatalities and injuries in urban areas. It highlights the importance of road safety measures, such as traffic management systems and well-maintained roads, to mitigate risks for senior citizens. The policy promotes the integration of different modes of transport, including public transport, non-motorized transport, and paratransit services, to provide seamless connectivity and reduce travel time for older adults. The NUTP policy document serves as the torchbearer for aligning transport-related development in urban areas. In order to enhance the mobility of all groups of people, there is a lack of dedicated provision for facilities like low-floor buses plying between locations like health facilities and residential areas more frequently as compared to other routes. While the NUTP demonstrates a commitment to addressing the needs of the senior citizen population, the implementation and effectiveness of these provisions may vary across different cities and states in India. Local governments and urban planning authorities play a crucial role in translating the policy into practical solutions that cater to the specific needs of older adults in their respective areas. The document analysis of the NUTP highlights the efforts made to address the needs of the senior citizen population in urban transport planning in India.

5.4.1 Policy Recommendations

To ensure that India's NUTP effectively addresses the mobility needs of senior citizens, future policies must focus on inclusive, accessible, and senior-friendly transport systems. The following recommendations provide a roadmap for making urban transport more inclusive and convenient for older adults:

1. **Improved Physical Accessibility**: Public transport infrastructure should incorporate universally accessible designs, including ramps, elevators, tactile pathways, and priority seating. Bus stops, metro stations, and railway platforms must be designed to accommodate individuals with mobility challenges. Additionally, low-floor buses should be introduced widely to facilitate easier boarding and deboarding.
2. **Audio-visual Announcement Systems**: Real-time, multi-sensory communication is essential for senior citizens, particularly those with hearing or visual impairments. Public transport vehicles and stations should be equipped with clear audio and visual announcement systems that provide real-time updates about routes, stops, and delays.

3. **Subsidized Travel and Optimized Scheduling**: To promote greater mobility among senior citizens, policies should introduce subsidized fares or free transport services during non-peak hours. Additionally, scheduling should be optimized to ensure frequent and reliable services during times that are most beneficial for older adults, avoiding rush hours and long waiting times.
4. **Training Programmes for Transport Staff**: Public transport personnel, including drivers, conductors, and station attendants, should be trained to assist senior citizens and differently abled passengers. Sensitization programmes should focus on handling emergencies, offering appropriate guidance, and fostering an inclusive transport culture.
5. **Integration of Smart Technology**: Senior-friendly technology solutions such as mobile applications with simplified interfaces, emergency alert systems, and digital ticketing should be introduced to enhance convenience. These tools should be designed with accessibility features, including voice navigation and larger font sizes for ease of use.
6. **Strengthening Public Participation and Feedback Mechanisms**: Engaging senior citizens in policy planning and implementation through focus groups, community consultations, and regular feedback mechanisms will ensure that their needs are effectively addressed. Establishing dedicated helplines and grievance redressal mechanisms for transport-related concerns will further enhance inclusivity.
7. **Last-Mile Connectivity and Safe Transit Environments**: Senior citizens often face challenges in accessing transport hubs. Therefore, policies should promote better last-mile connectivity through accessible footpaths, electric shuttles, and paratransit services. Additionally, improved lighting, security measures, and resting areas at transit points will create safer and more comfortable environments for elderly passengers.

By incorporating these recommendations, the NUTP can significantly enhance its inclusivity, ensuring that senior citizens have a reliable, safe, and comfortable public transport experience that fosters independent and active living.

REFERENCES

Abass, A. S. (2023). Prioritised seating arrangement on public transport: A focus on the disadvantaged group. *Transport Policy*, *131*, 32–44. https://doi.org/10.1016/j.tranpol.2022.12.003

Abdel Wahed Ahmed, M. M., & Abd El Monem, N. (2020). Sustainable and green transportation for better quality of life case study greater Cairo—Egypt. *HBRC Journal*, *16*(1), 17–37. https://doi.org/10.1080/16874048.2020.1719340

Addanki, S. C., & Venkataraman, H. (2017). Greening the economy: A review of urban sustainability measures for developing new cities. *Sustainable Cities and Society*, *32*, 1–8. https://doi.org/10.1016/j.scs.2017.03.009

Adlakha, D., Krishna, M., Woolrych, R., & Ellis, G. (2020). Neighbourhood supports for active ageing in urban India. *Psychology and Developing Societies*, *32*(2), 254–277. https://doi.org/10.1177/0971333620937497

Agarwal, P. K., Gurjar, J., & Gupta, V. (2017). Evaluation of socio-economic impact of city bus services in developing countries. *Transportation Research Procedia*, *25*, 4589–4605. https://doi.org/10.1016/j.trpro.2017.05.379

Aguiar, B., & Macário, R. (2017). The need for an Elderly centred mobility policy. *Transportation Research Procedia*, *25*, 4355–4369. https://doi.org/10.1016/j.trpro.2017.05.309

Alsnih, R., & Hensher, D. A. (2003). The mobility and accessibility expectations of seniors in an aging population. *Transportation Research Part A: Policy and Practice*, *37*(10), 903–916. https://doi.org/10.1016/S0965-8564(03)00073-9

Badji, S., Badland, H., Rachele, J. N., & Petrie, D. (2021). Public transport availability and healthcare use for Australian adults aged 18–60 years, with and without disabilities. *Journal of Transport & Health*, *20*, 101001. https://doi.org/10.1016/j.jth.2020.101001

Bala, A. K., & Kumar, A. (2023). Way forward with best practices in transportation systems. 060005. https://doi.org/10.1063/5.0154009

Bivina, G. R., & Parida, M. (2020). Prioritizing pedestrian needs using a multi-criteria decision approach for a sustainable built environment in the Indian context. *Environment, Development and Sustainability*, *22*(5), 4929–4950. https://doi.org/10.1007/s10668-019-00381-w

Bowen, G. A. (2009). Document analysis as a qualitative research method. *Qualitative Research Journal*, *9*(2), 27–40. https://doi.org/10.3316/QRJ0902027

Charaniya, S. (2018). A state-level framework for integrated land use and transport. In M. Sethi & J. A. Puppim De Oliveira (Eds.), *Mainstreaming Climate Co-Benefits in Indian Cities* (pp. 285–302). Springer, Singapore. https://doi.org/10.1007/978-981-10-5816-5_12

Chhabra, D., Chowdhury, A., & Chowdhury, J. (2021). Examining sustainability of heritage on wheels: The case of autorickshaws in Delhi (India). *Journal of Heritage Tourism*, *16*(3), 349–362. https://doi.org/10.1080/1743873X.2020.1788567

Choi, M., Schuster, A. M., & Schoenberg, N. E. (2019). Solutions to the challenge of meeting rural transportation needs: Middle-aged and older adults' perspectives. *Journal of Gerontological Social Work*, *62*(4), 415–431. https://doi.org/10.1080/01634372.2019.1575133

Dawda, N. H., Joshi, G. J., & Arkatkar, S. S. (2021). Synthesizing the evolution of multimodal transportation planning milestones in Indian cities. *Procedia Computer Science*, *184*, 484–491. https://doi.org/10.1016/j.procs.2021.03.061

Dube, S., Kumar, N., Bhatia, O. P., & Narulkar, S. (2023). Study on the elements affecting the pedestrian movements around the bus stations of Indore BRT. *Transportation in Developing Economies*, *9*(1), 9. https://doi.org/10.1007/s40890-023-00180-z

Galvin, A. E., Friedman, D. B., & Hébert, J. R. (2021). Focus on disability-free life expectancy: Implications for health-related quality of life. *Quality of Life Research*, *30*(8), 2187–2195. https://doi.org/10.1007/s11136-021-02809-1

Ghosh, A., & Kalra, K. (2016). Institutional and financial strengthening of intermediate public transport services in Indian cities. *Transportation Research Procedia*, *14*, 263–272. https://doi.org/10.1016/j.trpro.2016.05.063

Gough, C., Lewis, L. K., Barr, C., Maeder, A., & George, S. (2021). Community participation of community dwelling older adults: A cross-sectional study. *BMC Public Health*, *21*(1), 612. https://doi.org/10.1186/s12889-021-10592-4

Govt. of India. (2007). Master plan for 2021. Delhi Development Authority. https://dda.gov.in/master-plan-2021

Govt. of India. (2014). Toolkit for comprehensive mobility plan. Ministry of Urban Development. https://mohua.gov.in/upload/uploadfiles/files/CMP%20Report%20Revised.pdf

Hidalgo, D., Pai, M., Carrigan, A., & Bhatt, A. (2013). Toward people's cities through land use and transport integration: A review of India's national urban investment program. *Transportation Research Record: Journal of the Transportation Research Board*, *2394*(1), 10–18. https://doi.org/10.3141/2394-02

Islam, Z., Abdel-Aty, M., Goswamy, A., Abdelraouf, A., & Zheng, O. (2023). Effect of signal timing on vehicles' near misses at intersections. *Scientific Reports*, *13*(1). https://doi.org/10.1038/s41598-023-36106-3

Jain, D. (2019). Application of indicators in transport planning: Insight from India. In S. S. Muthu (Ed.), *Development and Quantification of Sustainability Indicators* (pp. 65–90). Springer, Singapore. https://doi.org/10.1007/978-981-13-2556-4_3

Jayakumar, M., & Maji, A. (2023). Decision tree analyses of safety and comfort perceptions for public transportation in Kalyan-Dombivli region of Maharashtra. *Transportation in Developing Economies*, *9*(2), 14. https://doi.org/10.1007/s40890-023-00184-9

Joshi, R., & Joseph, Y. (2015). Invisible cyclists and disappearing cycles. *Transfers*, *5*(3), 23–40. https://doi.org/10.3167/TRANS.2015.050303

Kar, M., Sadhukhan, S., & Parida, M. (2022). Assessing commuters' perceptions towards improvement of intermediate public transport as access modes to metro stations. *Transport Policy*, *129*, 140–155. https://doi.org/10.1016/j.tranpol.2022.10.011

Khurana, A., Kumar, V. V. R., & Sidhpuria, M. (2020). A study on the adoption of electric vehicles in India: The mediating role of attitude. *Vision: The Journal of Business Perspective*, *24*(1), 23–34. https://doi.org/10.1177/0972262919875548

Kuriakose, P. N., & Bhattacharjee, J. (2021). India's public transport systems: The role of metro rail. In S. Mitra, S. Bandyopadhyay, S. Roy, & T. Ponce Dentinho (Eds.), *Railway Transportation in South Asia* (pp. 131–152). Springer. https://doi.org/10.1007/978-3-030-76878-2_8

Lambat, N., Kapse, V., & Sabnani, C. (2022). Public transport (MRTS) and the need of choice mechanism: A case of the Indian public transport. *Current Science*, *122*(8), 888. https://doi.org/10.18520/cs/v122/i8/888-899

Lodhi, A. S., Jaiswal, A., & Sharma, S. N. (2024). Assessing bus users satisfaction using discrete choice models: A case of Bhopal. *Innovative Infrastructure Solutions*, *9*(11), 437. https://doi.org/10.1007/s41062-024-01652-w

Lunani, K., Vasudevan, V., & Kumar, V. (2022). People's preferences for improvements in public transportation systems: An experience from India. *Transportation in Developing Economies*, *8*(2), 24. https://doi.org/10.1007/s40890-022-00155-6

Mahapatra, G. D., Mori, S., & Nomura, R. (2021). Universal mobility in old core cities of India: People's perception. *Sustainability*, *13*(8), 4391. https://doi.org/10.3390/su13084391

MOHUA. (2016). National Urban Transport Policy [Policy Document]. Ministry of Housing and Urban Affairs. https://www.mohua.gov.in/upload/uploadfiles/files/TransportPolicy(2).pdf

Musselwhite, C. (2022). A research agenda on transport and health and public buses: More research on the buses please! *Journal of Transport & Health*, *24*, 101355. https://doi.org/10.1016/j.jth.2022.101355

Parmar, J., Saiyed, G., & Dave, S. (2023). Analysis of taste heterogeneity in commuters' travel decisions using joint parking—and mode—choice model: A case from urban India. *Transportation Research Part A: Policy and Practice*, *170*, 103610. https://doi.org/10.1016/j.tra.2023.103610

Patel, M., & Dave, S. (2016). Modeling the response to paid on street parking policy for two wheelers and four wheelers on busy urban streets of CBD area: A case study of Surat city. *Transportation Research Procedia*, *17*, 576–585. https://doi.org/10.1016/j.trpro.2016.11.112

Prasad, D., & Alizadeh, T. (2020). What makes Indian cities smart? A policy analysis of smart cities mission. *Telematics and Informatics*, *55*, 101466. https://doi.org/10.1016/j.tele.2020.101466

Priya Uteng, T., & Turner, J. (2019). Addressing the linkages between gender and transport in low- and middle-income countries. *Sustainability*, *11*(17), 4555. https://doi.org/10.3390/su11174555

Raj, P., Bhaduri, E., Moeckel, R., & Goswami, A. K. (2023). Analyzing user behavior in selection of ride-hailing services for urban travel in developing countries. *Transportation in Developing Economies*, *9*(1), 1. https://doi.org/10.1007/s40890-022-00172-5

Ramachandraiah, C. (2012). A superficial picture. *Economic and Political Weekly*, *47*(19), 35–37.

Sadhu, S. L. N. S., Tiwari, G., & Jain, H. (2014). Impact of cycle rickshaw trolley (CRT) as non-motorised freight transport in Delhi. *Transport Policy*, *35*, 64–70. https://doi.org/10.1016/j.tranpol.2014.05.015

Saxena, A. (2022). Is street design and infrastructure perceived differently by persons of different ages, genders, and hierarchy of street? *Innovative Infrastructure Solutions*, *7*(4), 278. https://doi.org/10.1007/s41062-022-00880-2

Sharma, S. N., & Dehalwar, K. (2025). Assessing the transit-oriented development (TOD) and travel behavior of the residents in developing countries—case of Delhi. *Journal of Urban Planning and Development*. https://doi.org/10.1061/JUPDDM.UPENG-5468

Sharma, S. N., Kumar, A., & Dehalwar, K. (2024). The precursors of transit-oriented development. *Economic and Political Weekly*, *59*(14), 16–20. https://doi.org/10.5281/ZENODO.10939448

Sharma, S. N., Singh, D., & Dehalwar, K. (2024). Surrogate safety analysis—leveraging advanced technologies for safer roads. *Suranaree Journal of Science and Technology*, *31*(4), 010320(1–14). https://doi.org/10.55766/sujst-2024-04-e03837

Shrivastava, S., & Singh, D. P. (2021). Assessment of urban quality of life in built environment: A case of Delhi. In U. Iyer-Raniga (Ed.), *Sustainability in the Built Environment in the 21st Century: Lessons Learned from India and the Region* (pp. 169–183). Springer. https://doi.org/10.1007/978-3-030-61891-9_11

Telang, S., Chel, A., Nemade, A., & Kaushik, G. (2021). Intelligent transport system for a smart city. In S. C. Tamane, N. Dey, & A.-E. Hassanien (Eds.), *Security and Privacy Applications for Smart City Development* (Vol. 308, pp. 171–187). Springer. https://doi.org/10.1007/978-3-030-53149-2_9

Temelová, J., & Dvořáková, N. (2012). Residential satisfaction of elderly in the city centre: The case of revitalizing neighbourhoods in Prague. *Cities*, *29*(5), 310–317. https://doi.org/10.1016/j.cities.2011.11.015

Tiwari, G., & Jain, D. (2012). Accessibility and safety indicators for all road users: Case study Delhi BRT. *Journal of Transport Geography*, *22*, 87–95. https://doi.org/10.1016/j.jtrangeo.2011.11.020

Tiwari, R., Puntambekar, K., & Parida, P. (2018). Redefining the service level benchmarking for public transport system in India. In: *International Conference on Transportation and Development 2018*, pp. 229–237. https://doi.org/10.1061/9780784481547.022

Verma, A., Harsha, V., & Subramanian, G. H. (2021). Evolution of urban transportation policies in India: A review and analysis. *Transportation in Developing Economies*, *7*(2), 25. https://doi.org/10.1007/s40890-021-00136-1

Waghmare, M. (2024). Democratic participation and smart city citizenship in emerging economies: Case of smart cities in India. *Cities*, *148*, 104910. https://doi.org/10.1016/j.cities.2024.104910

Yang, J., Zhu, L., Duan, Y., Zhou, J., & Ma, H. (2020). Developing metro-based accessibility: Three aspects of China's Rail+Property practice. *Transportation Research Part D: Transport and Environment*, *81*, 102288. https://doi.org/10.1016/j.trd.2020.102288

6 Increasing Burden of Non-Communicable Disease on Health Systems in Aging Populations and Possible Approaches to Lessen the Burden

Berrak Itır Aylı

6.1 THE RISE OF NON-COMMUNICABLE DISEASES

Non-communicable diseases (NCDs), also known as chronic diseases, are the number one cause for death and disability worldwide. They are long-term illnesses that are not contagious between individuals. They include a range of serious health issues, the main ones being cardiovascular diseases (CVDs), cancers, chronic respiratory diseases (CRDs), diabetes, and mental health issues. NCDs are often of prolonged duration and slow progression, often requiring long-term management and treatment. They are rarely completely curable and thus require medical care going throughout a person's lifetime [1].

According to the World Health Organization (WHO), as of 2023, NCDs are responsible for approximately 74% of all global deaths, translating to around 41 million deaths annually. Of these 41 million deaths, more than 15 million occur among people under 70. Alarmingly, 77% of NCD deaths occur in low- and middle-income countries (LMICs), and among people under the age of 70, this percentage rises to 85% [2]. It is estimated that 80% of NCD-related deaths are preventable. In addition, three out of four years lived with a disability can be attributed to NCDs [3].

Throughout the past few decades, there has been a notable increase in the prevalence of NCDs. For example, a 2018 WHO study found that 80% of deaths in the Western Pacific Region are attributable to NCDs [4]. In Brazil, Latin America's largest country, in 2019, 1 million and 26,000 deaths were due to NCDs, representing 75.0% of all deaths. It is estimated that most of these deaths occurred prematurely in individuals between the ages of 25 and 65 [5].

DOI: 10.1201/9781003513834-6

According to global data from 2016, high-income countries (HICs) in regions like Asia-Pacific, Western Europe, Australasia, and Canada had the lowest rates of mortality due to NCDs, whereas LMICs, particularly in sub-Saharan Africa, faced significantly higher risks of NCD-related deaths. Women in 164 (88%) and men in 165 (89%) of 186 countries and territories had a higher probability of dying before 70 years of age from an NCD than from communicable, maternal, perinatal, and nutritional conditions combined. This disparity was especially apparent among men in Central Asia and Eastern Europe [6].

Numerous interrelated reasons, including changes in the population, differences in socioeconomic status, and changes in lifestyle brought about by urbanization and globalization, are responsible for both this inequality and this increase. It is anticipated that as populations age, the burden of NCDs will rise, increasing morbidity, disability, and mortality among older adults. Individuals in LMICs will be more affected by this compared to their counterparts in HICs.

6.2 RISK FACTORS FOR NCD

Multifactorial risk factors frequently contribute to the development of NCDs. Tobacco use, physical inactivity, excessive alcohol intake, and poor diets are important behavioral factors. These lifestyle decisions may contribute to the development of chronic illnesses, including diabetes, obesity, and hypertension, which are markers for more serious health problems [7].

Tobacco use is one of the leading avoidable causes of death worldwide, accounting for over eight million deaths annually [8]. Cigarette smoking causes approximately one of every five deaths in the United States each year, causing over 480,000 deaths; 41,000 of these deaths are attributed to secondhand smoking [9,10]. Over the course of the 20th century, it is estimated that over 100 million people suffered premature deaths because of smoking, of whom over 70% were in HICs [11]. It is estimated that close to 400 million people will die from smoking between 2010 and 2050, and over the course of the 21st century, the number of deaths caused by smoking will reach one billion people. At least half will die before the age of 69 [12].

Physical inactivity is another major risk factor for NCDs. Over 9% of all deaths globally can be attributed to physical inactivity [13]. A study in the United States estimated that inactive persons would gain 1.3–3.7 life years from age 50 by becoming active [14,15]. Another study showed that among East Asians, life expectancy from age 30 was 2.6–4.2 years longer for the active compared to the inactive [16]. In a study conducted by Lee et al., it was estimated that physical inactivity is responsible for 6% of the burden of disease from coronary heart disease, 7% of type 2 diabetes, and 10% each for breast cancer and colon cancer [13]. The cost of physical inactivity is not only measured in life years lost, but also in economic terms; it is estimated that the total cost of physical inactivity globally would be approximately INT$520 billion over an 11-year period (2020–30) [17].

Diet is another one of the modifiable behavioral risk factors that contributes to NCDs. In 2017, a study conducted across 195 countries determined that 11 million deaths and 255 million disability-adjusted life-years (DALYs) could be attributed to dietary risk factors. High intake of sodium, low intake of whole grains, and low intake of fruits and vegetables were found to be the leading dietary risk factors for deaths and DALYs globally [18]. In another study carried out in Ethiopia, dietary factors were responsible for 60,402 deaths, which accounted for almost a quarter (23.0%) of all NCD deaths [19]. Similarly, a study conducted in Australia found dietary factors were responsible for 23% of all NCD deaths, while 42.3% of cardiovascular deaths were attributed to dietary risk factors [20].

Alcohol consumption is another of the behavioral risk factors in the WHO's Global Action Plan for the Prevention and Control of NCDs [21,22]. The annual global burden of alcohol-attributable NCDs is high, with more than 1.8 million deaths and 52 million years of life lost due to premature mortality (YLLs) and close to 29 million years of life lost due to disability (YLDs) [23,24]. Alcohol consumption has been linked to eight different cancers with variable attribution rates, in addition to being linked with liver disease and cardiovascular outcomes, including hypertension, hemorrhagic stroke, and atrial fibrillation [25].

In addition to behavioral risk factors, socioeconomic determinants like income level, education, and access to healthcare facilities also contribute to high NCD rates. There is compelling evidence that people with low socioeconomic status are more likely to be unhealthy, and therefore this group also has the highest prevalence of NCDs [26]. However, socioeconomic status or education does not always correlate with risky behaviors. For instance, unhealthy eating habits and inadequate levels of physical activity have long been known to be significant risk factors for NCDs. Yet, in a study conducted among medical students in India, it was found that 63% had low levels of physical activity, 85% had inadequate fruit and vegetable intake, and 24% consumed extra salt during meals [27]. In research carried out in Nepal, smoking rates were 38% higher among men of middle-income status compared to men of low-income status, while higher educational status reduced the prevalence of insufficient fruit and vegetable consumption [28].

In another study conducted in Algeria, although people with higher education levels showed decreased levels of tobacco use and inadequate fruit/vegetable (FV) consumption, increased levels of inadequate physical activity were also observed [29].

Although the factors listed above are the main risk factors for NCDs, there are a number of others. In Table 6.1, NCD categories and risk factors are summarized. Some of these factors, like smoking and dietary habits, are modifiable; however, some of them, like family history and genetics, are not.

Another aspect of NCDs is multimorbidity, which refers to one person suffering from several chronic diseases. More and more people around the world are now suffering from more than one chronic illness, particularly in the older population. In a study conducted by Calkins and colleagues in 1999, it was seen that while almost 75% of the elderly (aged 65 and over) have at least one chronic illness, about 50% have at least two [30]. This complex constellation of diseases complicates treatment protocols, impacts quality of life, and leads to higher costs and heightened mortality. According to Banthin and colleagues, about 14% of people aged 65 and over require assistance with bathing, dressing, preparing meals, or shopping [31].

6.3 KEY TYPES OF NCDs

NCDs are a leading cause of death and disability worldwide, with the primary types being CVDs, cancer, CRDs, diabetes, and mental health disorders. In addition to these major categories, other significant types include obesity, dental and oral

TABLE 6.1
NCD Categories

NCD Category	Risk Factors
Cardiovascular diseases	• High blood pressure (hypertension) • High cholesterol levels • Smoking • Physical inactivity • Poor diet (high in saturated fats, sugar, and salt) and obesity • Diabetes • Family history of heart disease
Cancer	• High-calorie diet (processed foods, sugary beverages) • Sedentary lifestyle • Genetics • Psychological factors (stress, depression) • Socioeconomic status • Exposure to carcinogenic substances
Diabetes	• Overweight and obesity • Physical inactivity • Poor diet (high in refined sugars and fats) • Family history of diabetes • Age (risk increases with age)
Chronic respiratory diseases	• Tobacco smoke (active and passive) • Air pollution (indoor and outdoor) • Occupational dust and chemicals • Respiratory infections (especially in childhood) • Physical inactivity
Mental health disorders	• Diabetes • High blood pressure • Obesity • Smoking • Family history of kidney disease • Age

diseases, chronic kidney disease, hypertension, metabolic syndrome, cerebrovascular disease, and cognitive impairment [2]. The NCD classification is illustrated in Figure 6.1.

1. CVD, including heart attacks and strokes, has been the leading cause of mortality worldwide for the last 20 years. In 2008, 48% of all NCD deaths—17 million in total—were due to CVD [32]. Recent numbers show that 33% of all global deaths can be attributed to CVDs. Alarmingly, the cases of CVDs nearly doubled from 1990 to 2019; the identified number of CVD cases in 1990 was 271 million, while in 2019, this number increased to 550 million, with deaths rising from 12.1 to 18.6 million [33]. Much like cancers, a great number of deaths caused by CVD are avoidable. In 2016, the burden of CVD caused by alcohol was 593,000 deaths (3.3% of all CVD

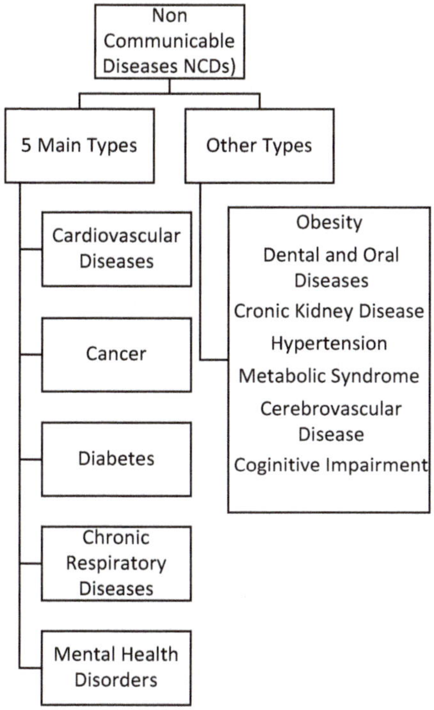

FIGURE 6.1 NCD types.

deaths) and 13 million DALYs [34]. According to a study about avoidable mortality in the European Union, between 1995 and 2020, 11.4 million deaths from CVDs in Europe were avoidable, meaning that 213.1 million potential life years lost could have been saved [35].

2. Cancer is a predominant cause of mortality associated with chronic diseases globally, resulting in around ten million fatalities per year. Two million new cancer cases are diagnosed each year in the United States alone [36], whereas globally, 20 million diagnoses of cancer were made in 2022. About one in every five people are diagnosed with cancer during their lifetime, and approximately one in nine men and one in 12 women die from their diagnosis [37,38]. According to International Agency for Research on Cancer (IARC)'s Global Cancer Observatory, lung cancer is the most common cancer worldwide. In 2022, 2.5 million new cases were diagnosed; this accounted for 12.4% of all new cancer cases [37]. The second most common cancer type was identified as breast cancer among women, with 2.3 million new cases (11.6% of all cases). The third most common cancer type was colorectal cancer, with 1.9 million cases, accounting for 9.6% of all new cancer patients [39].

   The most fatal type of cancer was identified as lung cancer, killing almost 1.8 million people in a year—18.7% of all cancer deaths. This was followed by colorectal cancer (900,000 deaths), liver cancer (760,000 deaths), breast cancer (670,000 deaths), and stomach cancer (660,000 deaths) [40]. It should be noted that many cases of lung cancer and fatalities caused by lung cancer could have been avoided if tobacco use was prevented. Similarly, many colorectal and stomach cancers could have been non-fatal if they had been identified early through proper screening programs [41].

3. Diabetes is a metabolic disease characterized by hyperglycemia, defined as the pancreas being unable to produce the insulin necessary for survival. It is among the most prevalent diseases worldwide. Type 2 diabetes, which accounts for 95% of cases, is a leading cause of CVD, blindness (diabetic retinopathy), kidney failure (diabetic nephropathy), and lower limb amputations (related to diabetic neuropathy) [42]. Out of every 10 people alive, one lives with diabetes. Diabetes is currently affecting 537 million adults, with this number expected to rise to 643 million by 2030 and 784 million by 2045.

   In addition to the 537 million cases identified in 2021, 541 million additional people live with impaired glucose tolerance, placing them at significant risk for developing type 2 diabetes. A large part of the people diagnosed with diabetes live in LMICs, where access to medication and care presents a significant global health challenge. Although it has been a century since the discovery of insulin, it is still estimated that close to 50% of individuals with diabetes lack a consistent supply of the insulin necessary for their survival. Studies show that 86% of people with a type 2 diabetes diagnosis in Africa are unable to access insulin, while in LMICs worldwide, this percentage is 63%. In HICs, 97.2% of adults with type 2 diabetes are believed to have access to insulin [43].

   Deaths from diabetes have risen by 70% since the beginning of the 21st century, with 6.7 million people losing their lives in 2021 because of diabetes and its complications. It is estimated that three million premature deaths occur because of diabetes, with type 2 diabetes causing a decrease in life expectancy of between five and ten years [44]. Diabetes-related healthcare costs account for 11.5% of all healthcare costs worldwide, with a cost of €176 billion in Europe alone in 2021 [45].

4. CRDs are long-term conditions affecting the airways and lungs, greatly contributing to global DALYs lost. CRDs are classified as chronic obstructive pulmonary disease (COPD), asthma, lung cancer, and occupational lung diseases. These diseases affect between 550 million and one billion people and result in about 4.2 million deaths per year, accounting for approximately 7% of all fatalities worldwide. According to studies, lung cancer accounts for an additional 1.4 million deaths (approximately 2.4% of global mortality) [46].

   Among children under five, lung diseases (including asthma and pneumonia) are one of the most significant causes of death, with asthma affecting 14% of all children worldwide. Between 1990 and 2017, the global prevalence of CRDs increased by 40%. Although many CRDs are readily preventable or treatable with cost-effective interventions, these conditions receive less attention than other NCDs. COPD—which includes emphysema and chronic bronchitis—is a preventable and treatable disease, with 300 million cases globally, or about 4% of the population. It was the third leading cause of death in 2017, resulting in 3.2 million deaths [47].

Although cigarette smoking remains the number one risk factor for COPD, it is notable that more than 90% of COPD-related deaths in people under age 70 occur in LMICs, due to underdiagnosis and restricted access to care. COPD also poses a considerable economic burden, costing the European Union €48.4 billion annually [48].

Another frequent CRD is asthma, which has been diagnosed in an estimated 262 million persons worldwide, although that number has been reported to be as high as 350 million. The disease is one of the most prevalent chronic illnesses among children and led to approximately 500,000 deaths in 2019 [49].

5. Mental health disorders include, but are not limited to, depression, anxiety, and dementia. It must be noted that mental health disorders do not limit their effects to a person's mental well-being but also serve as a significant risk factor for other NCDs. Conditions like depression and anxiety play a crucial role in physical health deterioration, as they are associated with behaviors such as increased alcohol and tobacco use, poor diet, and reduced physical activity. In addition, physiological mechanisms, such as abnormalities in the stress response system, further intensify the link between mental illness and physical NCDs [50]. Mental health disorders also complicate the treatment of other NCDs; patients with a mental health disorder are more likely to be noncompliant to treatments, making the need for coordinated prevention strategies more critical [51]. Despite their profound effect on health, mental health issues are often underrepresented in mortality studies like the Global Burden of Disease, where the final cause of death is usually recorded as the physical condition, not the underlying mental illness. Nonetheless, the long-established burden of mental disorders, particularly when measured by years lived with disability, highlights the significant role mental health plays in global health.

6.4 DEMOGRAPHIC SHIFT: THE AGING POPULATION AND ITS IMPLICATIONS

Globally, in the last 50 years, there have been significant developments in healthcare services, the accessibility of health services, the effectiveness of the services provided, pharmaceutical technologies, and several other social and economic developments that have caused human life expectancy to reach levels that seemed impossible at the beginning of the 20th century, when life expectancy was only 32 years [52]. By 2021, this number had more than doubled, reaching 71 years. The proportion of older individuals in society is expected to grow; while only one in every 11 people in the world was older than 65 in 2021, estimations suggest that by 2050, one in every six people will be in this group.

This increase, of course, occurred in varying amounts across different parts of the world. Unfortunately, many countries lack the capacity to deal with the longer human life expectancy, which is characterized by a higher prevalence of NCDs, higher disability rates, increased dependency, and reduced ability to work [53]. As human life continues to extend, more and more countries are expected to face difficulties in managing their older populations [54].

Countries in the European Union are among the oldest in the world. According to data from 2019, the number of people aged 65 or older in EU countries is more than 90 million. By 2050, this number is expected to rise significantly, with more than 130 million people in the European Union projected to be aged 65 and older. An especially high rate of growth is expected among the population aged between 75 and 84, with an expected growth rate of 56.1%. The population aged 85 or older is also expected to rise more than twofold; whereas in 2019, only 12.5 million people were aged 85 or older, by 2050, this number will reach 27 million, showing a rise of 110%. Another group where a notable rise is expected is among people over 100. Only 96,000 people lived past 100 in 2019, but by 2050, this number is expected to exceed 480,000 [55,56].

In the United States, it must be noted that in 1970, almost one in every three people was aged under 18, and only 10% of the population was aged 65 or older. By 2010, only one in every four people were children, and the population of people over the age of 65 had reached 13%. By 2021, the number of people over the age of 65 had reached 40 million, and it is expected that by 2050, this number will rise to 89 million, making up 20% of the population [57,58].

The Asia-Pacific region, like the rest of the world, is facing an aging population. In 2015, the number of people over the age of 60 was counted as 900 million. However, this number is expected to almost double by 2050, reaching a record high of two billion people. China and Japan are the countries where an aging population is most clearly affecting society. In 2019, the number of people over 65 in China was 176 million, but by 2050, it is estimated that this number will reach 356 million, making China as old a country as most European countries. Japan can be seen as the oldest country in the world today, with a median age of 45. By 2050, this median age is expected to reach 52, and Japan will be one of the few countries where population growth is negative, decreasing by 10 million [59].

The Middle East, compared to the Western continents, is a younger region. According to the World Bank's 2012 report, only 4.7% of the population (an estimated 336 million people) in the Middle East and North Africa are over the age of 65. This rate varies between countries; in Lebanon, it is estimated to be 10%, whereas in the United Arab Emirates, it is only 2% [60]. In 1980, life expectancy was 60 years on average for Middle Eastern countries; today, the expectancy has reached 70 years. Projections for the next 30 years suggest that as the region's youthful population grows older, the percentage of elderly people will see a significant rise. WHO estimates that in 11 Arab countries, people over the age of 85 will make up more than 5% of the population by 2050 [61].

Africa is, by most estimates, the youngest continent on Earth. In 1980, the percentage of people over 65 was only 3.1% across the continent. In 2005, while 10% of the world's population was over the age of 60, only 5% of the people in sub-Saharan Africa were in this group. Africa has the lowest life expectancy in the world; in 1990, the average life expectancy was 52.7 years, and in 2010, it had only reached 56 years, falling far behind the rest of the world. In 2010, only 54 million people in Africa were aged 60 or older. It is expected that by 2050, Africa will still remain younger than the rest of the world, with only 12% of the population—226 million people—being aged 60 or older [62].

6.5 THE CURRENT BURDEN: NCDs AND HEALTH SYSTEMS

The interplay between aging populations and the rising burden of NCDs presents substantial challenges for health systems worldwide. Traditional healthcare services, particularly in LMICs, have predominantly focused on communicable diseases, which often involved treating single episodes of acute illness. However, as populations age, there is an urgent need to shift these systems to address the complexities associated with managing NCDs.

The rapid increase in the number of older adults, in addition to the rising prevalence of NCDs, demands that healthy aging becomes a global goal and health systems transition from reactive to proactive care models [63]. This includes increasing health literacy, enhancing access to primary healthcare services, establishing integrated care pathways, creating more surveillance programs, minimizing exposure to risk factors, developing guidelines to deal not only with singular conditions but also with multimorbidities, expanding knowledge and research regarding polypharmacy, and fostering community-based interventions tailored to the unique needs of older populations [64].

Europe, with a life expectancy of 81.3 years in 2021 and a median age of 44.5 in 2023, has the oldest population of any continent in the world. The effects of aging in Europe are most clearly reflected in the finances of countries, with 9.9% of GDP being spent on healthcare. By 2050, estimates show that this percentage will rise to 12.5%. In Germany, 2018 data indicated that 15% of all health expenditures were allocated to the elderly. It is expected that more than 50% of people over age 65 will have at least one chronic condition, while many will have multiple morbidities, leading to a continuous need for medical care. Additionally, the aging population not only creates health needs but also predominantly consists of individuals who are no longer working, presenting a significant burden on social systems.

Estimates suggest that by 2050, the old-age dependency ratio in Europe will reach 60%, meaning there will be 60 dependent people for every 100 working individuals. Not only do health systems need to adapt, but cities must also become more disability-friendly. Social systems need to accommodate an increasing number of retirement pensions, and more retirement homes must be made available. By 2050, estimates indicate that 25% of GDP will be spent on pensions and healthcare [55,56,65].

In the United States, the aging population will place a significant burden on health systems. As the population of people over age 65 rises, current systems, including Medicare and Medicaid, may become unsustainable. Although only 12% of people in the United States are over the age of 60, they account for more than 33% of health expenditures. As the baby boomer generation reaches 65 by 2030, it is expected that the number of older adults needing care will quickly rise [57,58,66].

In Asia, the effects of aging on health systems will be profoundly felt, especially in countries without universal health coverage (UHC). For example, in Sri Lanka, the elderly population is expected to double and reach a record high of 25% by 2040. Out-of-pocket payments currently make up 46% of all health expenditures, and with the increase of NCDs among the elderly, this will lead to limited access to life-saving health services. Inaccessibility to health services is not only a financial issue but also a matter of physical access. For instance, in Hong Kong, studies have revealed that the elderly have difficulty accessing health services due to transportation problems. Research also shows that a significant number of health facilities are not designed to accommodate the needs of the elderly, presenting various physical accessibility challenges, such as a lack of ramps or elevators [59,67].

In Africa, as the youngest continent on Earth and the continent with the least developed health services, the challenges of managing aging populations will be greater compared to the rest of the world. Most countries in Africa, being LMICs, lack the necessary finances to establish integrated and comprehensive health systems [62,68]. However, as the African population ages, the need to address NCDs will become more evident in these regions, where health systems have primarily focused on communicable diseases and are often inadequate. The effects of Africa's underdeveloped health systems were evident during the COVID-19 pandemic, where only 51.8% of the continent's population could be vaccinated, with several countries having vaccination levels well below 40% [69].

6.6 IDENTIFYING CHALLENGES: BARRIERS TO EFFECTIVE NCD MANAGEMENT IN OLDER ADULTS

Accessing healthcare services poses significant challenges for elderly patients, particularly in terms of physical constraints and medication costs. Among these challenges, transportation issues are particularly prominent, especially for elderly patients with disabilities. The loss of close relatives, living far from younger family members, a lack of social support, and the lack of disability-friendly city infrastructure further complicate access to healthcare services. A significant number of older adults, even though not physically disabled, have mobility issues that make it difficult for them to drive themselves, access subway or train stations that don't offer elevators or escalators, or navigate public transportation systems. It is imperative to make public transport disability-friendly and easy to navigate so that people of all ages and health statuses can use it with ease.

The second major problem regarding healthcare access is financial constraints. Even though UHC has been a worldwide goal for over two decades, many countries still require out-of-pocket payments or private insurance. The transition into retirement and the absence of employment opportunities create substantial difficulties for people living in countries without UHC. As the elderly with NCDs require regular checkups and are the group that undergoes hospitalization most frequently, the financial burden of healthcare can be catastrophic for them—especially after long hospitalizations. Thus, the accessibility of quality healthcare remains an economic privilege across the globe [61,70].

The cost of medications required for chronic diseases is another crucial issue that must be addressed. Even when patients have access to healthcare, they may not be able to cover the costs of medications if they are not covered under UHC. As people with chronic illnesses must take their medications consistently, these charges accumulate and create a substantial burden on the already limited finances of individuals [70]. Figure 6.2 highlights the fundamental barriers to effective chronic disease management in older adults.

There are barriers originating from the patients themselves, which may include, as mentioned before, financial difficulties, inability to access medications, lack of sufficient knowledge about their illness, and lack of awareness regarding potential complications.

The second significant factor is the social environment, which may include reasons such as the family's failure to provide necessary financial support, lack of assistance with transportation for the elderly, and downplaying the seriousness of the illness.

Another essential factor is the community. Behaviors from the community may lead patients to avoid seeking medical attention or adhering to their prescribed medications. Communities or families may cause patients to feel ashamed of their illness, trivialize the disease, or exaggerate its severity. The community's traditions regarding illnesses are another significant issue when dealing with NCDs; some societies may rely on traditional remedies or hold prejudices against medications, disrupting treatment.

Finally, the most significant barrier is the health systems themselves, including issues such as inaccessible health facilities, difficulty scheduling appointments due to overburdened doctors, ineffective doctor-patient relationships, healthcare workers' attitudes toward the elderly, or shortages in medication supply.

Every country is undertaking intensive efforts to minimize the burden of NCDs on their healthcare systems, to ensure easier access to treatment for elderly patients, and to alleviate the economic burden of NCDs.

According to a study published by Zong and colleagues in 2018, 80% of deaths in China are attributed to NCDs. Patients with NCDs often face challenges in accessing treatment due to inadequate attention and insufficient funding from the government [71]. In countries with large populations like China, the aging population further increases the prevalence of NCD epidemics [72,73].

China has implemented various programs aimed at preventing and controlling NCDs, including systems for hypertension screening, salt intake reduction, smoking

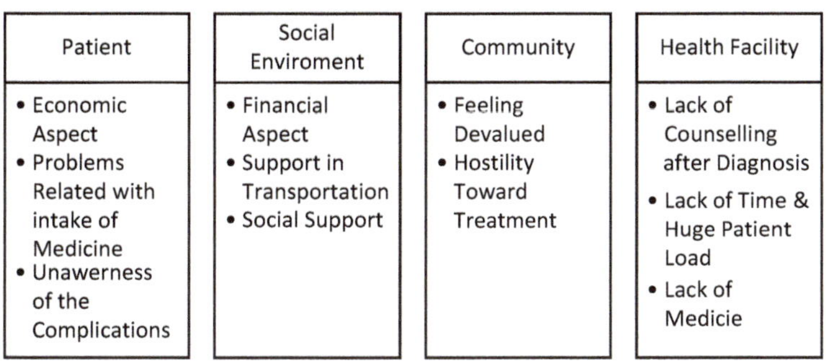

FIGURE 6.2 Barrier to effective NCD management.

cessation centers, and education promoting healthy lifestyles. These initiatives aim to improve the quality of life for those affected by NCDs, help reduce the shortage of healthcare professionals, ease their workload, and result in significant cost savings for the country. With recent policy funding, the management of chronic diseases in China has largely been delegated to village doctors, and this system has proven to be efficient. Between 2017 and 2025, China implemented a medium- and long-term plan for the prevention and treatment of chronic diseases, sharing its results and findings with healthcare workers. The preliminary results have been promising, showing that carefully planned interventions benefit both health outcomes and economics [71].

According to Kamvura [74], the burden of NCDs is disproportionately rising in LMICs. NCDs are attributed to causing 70% of global mortality and premature deaths in these countries [22,32,75]. Cardiovascular risk factors are increasing enormously in sub-Saharan Africa due to malnutrition, reduced physical activity, the rising burden of tobacco use, and the upward trajectory of alcohol consumption. This has also led to the rise of NCDs. It is expected that the burden of NCDs will continue to rise in sub-Saharan Africa, becoming the biggest killer on the continent by 2030 and leaving infectious diseases in second place [76,77].

In their study, Heller et al. report that the growing global burden of NCDs is due in part to overburdened healthcare staff, low patient health literacy levels (e.g., less than one-fifth could interpret a body diagram or identify which quadrants relate to specific organ systems), low adherence rates to medications (leading to poor health outcomes), poor access to medicines and supplies, lack of financial incentives, and indirect costs associated with accessing care, leading to crisis expenditures. Systemic challenges, such as poor policy implementation and weak community engagement related to the integration of NCD management in primary healthcare, are also significant issues. In addition, the absence of proper data collection systems means policymakers are unable to make effective interventions, perpetuating a broken system [78].

Duffy et al. advocate for the importance of addressing access to healthcare services, cost-effective resource use, and public health efforts targeting NCDs, particularly in low- and middle-income settings [79]. In these regions, the rise of NCDs poses a significant challenge. In low-income settings such as sub-Saharan Africa, where health systems remain underdeveloped, McIntyre and colleagues point out that the management of NCDs is shaped by finances and thus remains inadequate. Due to insufficient resources, healthcare workers often work long hours for low wages, operating neglected facilities with inadequate supplies, equipment, and medication. Even the most experienced healthcare professionals are unable to provide adequate care under these constraints.

Most studies suggest that effective interventions must be implemented at an appropriate policy level, adequately funded, and supported with sufficient human resources, tailored to address country-specific challenges in tackling NCDs. The Addis Ababa Declaration [80] urges national governments to allocate 15% of their annual budgets to health, with a significant portion directed toward combating NCDs. Unfortunately, even in HICs, this percentage is not achieved. The Sustainable Development Goals aimed to enable everyone to access essential health services without additional costs by 2030. However, despite progress since the beginning of the century, 4.5 billion people were still not fully covered by essential health services as of 2021. In Zimbabwe, only 21% of the country's total reported health financing needs are covered by the government, with the remainder coming from donors, volunteers, and private health insurance [81]. Unfortunately, this issue extends beyond Zimbabwe to most LMICs.

According to Sikula et al., chronically ill patients account for 80% of primary care consultations, and 30% of all hospitalizations are of these patients. To lower the burden this causes on health systems and better address the rising NCD epidemic, interventions targeting healthcare behavior changes are essential. However, Sikula et al. emphasize that behavior change should not be viewed solely as a personal process but rather as a systemic process. Internal and external factors, as well as their interactions, need to be assessed, and interventions should be designed to address the multifactorial behavioral barriers that arise from family, community, and individual factors. Intervention delivery should be effective across all these levels, and, if necessary, multi-component interventions should be implemented across different domains [82,83].

Sung et al. reported problems in healthy aging among elderly adults and the associated facilitators, which include effective communication with healthcare providers, family support, infrastructure, technical support, and financial resources. Improving health literacy, software usage, and social relationships would help the elderly access healthcare more easily and, if implemented, provide them with the ability to use remote healthcare services [83,84].

Joshi et al. noted that non-physician health workers can perform key diabetes screenings, such as blood pressure and glucose measurements, with numerous trials indicating benefits. Healthcare workers other than physicians can be trained to conduct screenings, record results, and refer at-risk cases to doctors. With the inclusion of non-physician healthcare providers in screenings, not only can a greater number of people be screened, but each patient can also receive more individualized attention. During screenings, health workers are well-positioned to provide behavioral counseling and patient education, increasing health knowledge among the population [85].

Another area where people with non-communicable conditions could access healthcare services is through remote services. In particular, mobile health services offer cost- and time-saving benefits for patients. These interventions present an opportunity to develop innovative methods for improving chronic healthcare in resource-limited environments, such as LMICs. They enhance patient access to healthcare services and drive cost savings [32,86,87]. Cambodia, for example, has a mobile phone usage rate of 94%, demonstrating that mobile health services can be effectively utilized even in underdeveloped countries. Additionally, by using remote health services, patients avoid the risk of contracting communicable diseases commonly found in healthcare facilities—a crucial advantage for individuals with chronic health conditions, as many NCDs are exacerbated by communicable diseases.

When reviewing the literature, it is observed that proactive measures are the most effective in managing NCDs in older adults. Among these measures are increasing physical activity, providing proper dietary programs, and raising public awareness about preventive measures for leading NCDs, such as diabetes and cardiovascular problems. On the other hand, obstacles to disease management include the limited availability of healthcare personnel and the financial and time costs associated with the patient-doctor relationship. Assigning auxiliary healthcare personnel to assist in diagnosis and supporting treatment processes through mobile systems are seen as effective policies.

Many studies report that elderly patients with NCDs often suffer from cardiovascular issues, and one of the key components in managing these conditions is adherence to a healthy diet and regular exercise. With a healthy diet and adequate physical activity, patients can improve both their health and quality of life. While adherence to physical activity is higher in Mediterranean countries, it is lower among adults in Southern and Central European countries and the United States. The importance of personalized counseling in maintaining appropriate levels of physical activity and a balanced diet for individuals with chronic illnesses—and in sustaining their motivation—should be especially emphasized in these regions. The accessibility of exercise and dietary counseling has emerged as a significant factor in improving adherence to behavioral recommendations. This service can easily be provided remotely. By training qualified personnel, designing user-friendly remote systems, and promoting these services, a large number of patients can be reached [88]. This service can benefit not only the ill but also those at risk of illness.

The most important action in dealing with NCDs is taking proactive measures to prevent them. Reducing exposure to risk factors for NCDs is achievable at a low cost, especially through public health education. Easily accessible diet and exercise counseling is one key area where this is possible.

Decreasing the accessibility of tobacco products is another effective policy to prevent or lessen the severity of NCDs. Creating smoke-free environments in public areas, prohibiting tobacco use in closed workplaces and public transportation, and implementing health campaigns are essential. Banning tobacco advertising, regulating the availability of alcohol, and similarly restricting alcohol advertisements and promotions are also important.

Pricing policies to reduce harmful alcohol use, lowering salt intake, adjusting the iodine content in iodized salt when necessary, replacing trans fats with unsaturated fats, and raising public awareness about harmful substances and behaviors are among the most cost-effective interventions. These approaches are particularly impactful in low-income countries and are priority interventions for the efficient use of financial resources [89].

Considering the barriers to disease management, limitations in access to healthcare services, high costs of medications and treatments, complex treatment regimens for certain diseases, physical limitations, functional decline, social isolation, and lack of support systems emerge as major challenges. Low health literacy, the progression of mental health problems alongside NCDs, coordination deficiencies, and systemic barriers further compound these issues. Reviewing the literature suggests that providing mobile health services and increasing the number of village doctors are common solutions, particularly in rural and disadvantaged areas. Expanding health insurance coverage and reducing treatment costs are also among the most appropriate measures for developing countries.

Providing health literacy education to older adults and their families, organizing awareness campaigns within communities, broadcasting public service announcements, and conducting training sessions are global practices. Mobile health systems are emerging as widespread tools to monitor individuals' health conditions and enable early intervention. Indeed, statistical studies in the literature highlight that accessibility to mobile phones and mobile internet has reached widespread levels globally, enhancing the feasibility of mobile systems.

Supporting physical activity and nutrition programs is another method, particularly through organizing sports and exercise programs at community centers to encourage physical activity among older adults. Providing education on healthy eating and running campaigns promoting balanced nutrition are other commonly followed strategies. Integrating health systems to increase information sharing among healthcare providers, creating individual care programs to monitor the health status of older adults, and keeping them updated not only reduce the burden on doctors but also support other healthcare workers.

6.7 STRATEGIC APPROACHES TO MITIGATE THE BURDEN: SOLUTIONS FOR HEALTHCARE SYSTEMS

The analysis of health systems is an important topic for evaluating the current situation. Basic indicators such as access to health services, ease of access, challenges faced during access, quality of services received, and financial sustainability are fundamental classification methods in the analysis of health systems. Developing policies and reform processes is also a crucial aspect for ensuring health systems operate effectively. It is essential to review existing health policies and restructure them to meet the system's needs, including local and national stakeholders in the restructuring processes. Increasing cooperation between the public and private sectors is also significant for policy development and reforms, as it enables resource sharing, reduces costs, and fosters the development of innovative solutions. The key strategies to mitigate the burden include the following:

1. Integration of NCD Services
2. Standardized Protocols
3. Capacity Building
4. Task Distribution Among Health Workers
5. Access to Essential Medicines and Equipment
6. Multi-sectoral Approaches

Focusing on alternative financing models is an important step in developing economic solutions. For example, the development of new models, such as insurance systems that promote healthy lifestyles, can provide an effective framework for reviewing financing models. Education is one of the most fundamental methods to increase the effectiveness of health systems, which includes both the training of health professionals and enhancing community health literacy.

It is crucial for healthcare workers to participate in continuous education programs, acquire knowledge about innovative health practices, and keep up with technology. Increasing community health literacy can be achieved through public campaigns, seminars, and workshops designed to provide education. Enhancing community literacy is vital for educating the population about NCDs and raising awareness about proactive measures they can apply in their lives. In this context, providing consulting services to help patients understand their health status, following processes, and taking preventive measures are also necessary.

In today's world, where technology is continuously advancing, developing online health systems for effective use in health systems is crucial. Telemedicine and digital health systems are already in practice in many countries. Online platforms and mobile applications for remote consultations and monitoring systems can provide online assistance to patients during diagnosis and treatment processes, thus preventing many costs, enabling doctors to use their time effectively and allowing patients to receive quick solutions.

Especially in digital health systems, the inclusion of support staff is essential to reduce the burden on doctors. The application of big data analytics and artificial intelligence to increase efficiency in healthcare services is another method to optimize care as artificial intelligence continues to evolve. Expanding preventive health applications will also play a significant role in alleviating the burden on the health system. Vaccination programs, screening tests, healthy lifestyle promotion, and early intervention strategies can be considered the most important topics in this context.

According to Elezbawy et al., the cost burden of atopic dermatitis on healthcare systems is significant. The most common skin disease in the world, atopic dermatitis, has recently been recognized as a condition prevalent in Middle Eastern and African populations, costing around $460 million annually in direct costs alone. Thus, it is critical to address how to reduce the impact of such a disease on the healthcare system. Some countries and even their healthcare systems have revised their health policies regarding the care of patients suffering from atopic dermatitis. Such alterations respect patients' well-being by alleviating symptoms, preventing disease progression, and lowering the frequency and intensity of flare-ups. In turn, these measures lessen the clinical, humanistic, and economic burden on patients and society. The inclusion of atopic dermatitis drugs in clinical practice guidelines and expanded reimbursement policies have emerged as some of the critical approaches to alleviating the burden of the disease. While this study focused on atopic dermatitis, one can regard the proposed strategy as applicable to lessening stress on the healthcare system for other diseases as well. Nevertheless, it should be remembered, as mentioned in the study, that certain actions may be appropriate in some countries but not in others [90]. Hence, it is absolutely important to customize the recommendations to align with country-specific contexts.

Bello et al. [91] conducted a study investigating health system disruptions using the COVID-19 pandemic as an example. Disruptions are defined as unforeseen events that affect the provision of healthcare goods and services. For instance, during the COVID-19 pandemic, disruptions occurred in essential health services across health systems, ranging from HICs to low-income ones. In Europe, cancer screenings were reduced, and attention shifted to the diagnosis and treatment of COVID-19 [92]. Similarly, in Africa, many health programs, such as those for diabetes and hypertension, were deprioritized during the malaria elimination program, and history repeated itself during the Ebola outbreak. It was shown that during the Ebola outbreak in West Africa, the number of deaths attributed to measles, malaria, and tuberculosis due to health system failures exceeded those from Ebola, while deaths due to reduced care for NCDs remained unclear [88–91]. Health system performance during crises depends on baseline capacity and the magnitude of the crisis. Developed countries are generally anticipated to perform better than underdeveloped and developing countries, as proven during the COVID-19 pandemic. A well-prepared health system must maintain the delivery of essential health services during all types of emergencies; otherwise, significant increases in morbidity and mortality will result.

Additionally, during the COVID-19 pandemic, difficulties in accessing medicines arose due to high costs and imbalances in supply and demand. HICs proved more capable of addressing these challenges, while in LMICs, even basic necessities like surgical masks were limited. Mortality due to lack of medicine access was not a significant issue in HICs, further highlighting health disparities across regions. Increasing interactions between health systems, particularly encouraging support from developed to developing countries, is an important barrier that needs tackling [93–96].

Rudd et al. [97] conducted a study investigating the impact of sepsis on health burden and presenting strategies to mitigate it. Although this study primarily focuses on sepsis, the proposed strategies are also applicable to NCDs. The study pointed out that in 2016 in LMICs, annual health expenditure per capita was $266, whereas it was $5,226 in HICs. Additionally, it was noted that 83 countries—all of which were in Latin America, Africa, and Asia—did not meet the WHO standards for minimum healthcare worker-to-population ratios. Both of these factors were identified as significant obstacles to adequate care.

The strategies proposed to lower the burden of sepsis include several that are also relevant to NCDs. The first is the establishment of definitions and guidelines: implementing clear and cohesive definitions and internationally applicable, step-by-step clinical guidelines is essential to avoid misdiagnosis and inadequate treatment. Additionally, evidence-based guidelines for low-resource settings must also be developed. Public health practices aimed at preventing illnesses should be maximized. These practices include vaccination, improved nutrition, maternal education, promoting healthy living environments, and, above all, fostering health equity as a core value.

Mercer et al. [98] emphasized in their study that the health burden of NCDs is quite significant, particularly noting that diabetes, hypertension, obesity, and smoking are major contributors to deaths caused by NCDs. They highlighted that diabetes not only increases the risk of other non-communicable conditions, such as cardiovascular and renal diseases, but also raises the risk of communicable diseases like pneumonia and tuberculosis. Thus, the burden on the health system arises not from one aspect but from multiple interlinked fronts.

This multifaceted disease burden requires successful management, which incurs high costs. The integration of management, financing, workforce, information systems, and service delivery is essential. The study suggests that health systems can be strengthened through components such as leadership and governance, financing, health workforce development, health information systems, supply chain optimization, and service delivery enhancements. This comprehensive approach has the potential not only to improve biological outcomes but also to achieve better social outcomes for patients.

NCDs pose a significant risk to global health and threaten social and economic development in countries worldwide. The issue was highlighted at the United Nations High-Level Meeting held in New York in 2011, which was subsequently followed by the WHO Global Action Plan that established a timeline for the prevention and control of NCDs. Additionally, a United Nations working group was formed to address the prevention and control of chronic diseases. While guiding principles are still being developed, efforts to address this global challenge are ongoing [22,32,99,100].

In 2010, the WHO published a report containing current evidence-based interventions for NCDs. This report emphasized the importance of integrating services within health systems. The main focuses on NCDs are listed as follows: these diseases are becoming increasingly widespread due to the effects of globalization. Preliminary data confirm that they contribute to an epidemiological transition where communicable diseases and NCDs coexist.

NCDs are further exacerbated by modifiable risk factors, such as alcohol consumption, smoking, physical inactivity, and unhealthy diets, which can be reduced through behavioral changes. Diseases like hypertension, chronic respiratory obstruction, diabetes, and obesity can be detected using simple tests in primary care settings, particularly in low-income countries [101].

The benefits of prevention and care often extend to other public health issues, such as chronic kidney disease, which is frequently caused by hypertension and diabetes. As mentioned by Strong et al. [102], the global target for the prevention and control of NCDs is to reduce the death rate from NCDs by 2% annually. At this point, the primary care response recommended by the WHO is a correct method. However, the primary care response is often unstructured and inadequate. Maher et al. emphasized the urgent need for an effective and affordable framework that can be adapted by countries to improve interventions delivered by primary care providers, such as Ministry of Health services, social security schemes, prisons, military services, and non-governmental organizations [50].

When examining the strategies and approaches aimed at alleviating the burden of NCDs in the healthcare system, the integration of NCD services emerges as a critical priority. Primary care is often the first point of contact for many patients, and establishing a system capable of managing common NCDs such as hypertension, diabetes, and CRDs is considered necessary, particularly in developing and underdeveloped countries. The WHO also continues to advocate for the inclusion of NCD management in primary healthcare services.

Creating standard protocols for the diagnosis and management of NCDs in primary healthcare is another key strategy to reduce the burden on the healthcare system. These protocols enable auxiliary health personnel to contribute effectively within the system, reducing the workload on doctors. Capacity building and training healthcare workers are crucial components of this process. Comprehensive training programs for doctors, nurses, and other healthcare professionals will enhance their ability to diagnose and treat NCDs early, enabling timely intervention.

Task-shifting among healthcare workers is another solution to extend care to more people without overburdening the system. For instance, in areas with limited doctors, delegating responsibilities to community health workers can help alleviate systemic strain. Additionally, sustainable access to essential medications and equipment is critical for the continuous management of chronic diseases.

To combat NCDs, a multi-sectoral approach must be adopted. For example, agricultural policies can encourage healthy eating, while ministries of health and sports can promote physical activity and social engagement. Educational policies can provide the younger generation with the tools for a long and healthy life. Policies aimed at reducing the consumption of alcohol and tobacco are also essential components of this holistic approach.

The establishment of both national and international policies for the prevention, treatment, and management of NCDs is essential. The WHO, in particular, has been actively setting international targets and working intensively in the fight against NCDs. One of the most critical approaches is educating the public about NCD prevention and management. Raising awareness and encouraging proactive measures can significantly reduce the prevalence and impact of these diseases.

6.8 CONCLUSION

Health is significantly influenced by social, economic, political, and cultural factors. As a result, the state of being "healthy" or "unhealthy" does not stem from a single cause. Changes in any of these factors or processes can profoundly impact health. For this reason, a holistic approach is required when addressing health-related issues.

Numerous efforts are being made to improve or enhance health. Some of these efforts are national in scope, while others have international dimensions. However, these efforts often fall short. The reasons for these shortcomings are numerous and multidimensional, including resource shortages, policy gaps, implementation challenges, health inequities, and low levels of health literacy within communities. Furthermore, a lack of coordination among stakeholders and weak intersectoral collaboration significantly contribute to these failures.

The burden of NCDs, especially in aging populations, is intensifying the strain on health systems worldwide. Traditional healthcare models—primarily designed to treat acute and infectious diseases—have proven insufficient in addressing chronic, multifactorial NCDs that require long-term care and continuous management. LMICs face the greatest challenges, experiencing higher rates of premature mortality and limited access to health services. Projections indicate that this crisis will worsen in the coming years as societies grow older.

Health systems must urgently transition toward integrated models, patient-centered care, proactive prevention strategies, and policies aimed at reducing behavioral risk factors and socioeconomic disparities. The first and most essential step remains UHC: ensuring that every person, regardless of age, gender, or race, has access to essential health services.

To address these challenges effectively, health systems must also be reshaped to handle the complications of multi-morbidity and polypharmacy, which are becoming increasingly common. Achieving this requires a multidisciplinary approach across multiple sectors. Key priorities include:

1. Minimizing environmental risk factors and ensuring access to safe housing, clean water, and essential food for all.
2. Reducing risks posed by tobacco, alcohol, unhealthy diets, and physical inactivity. Public awareness campaigns and accessible counseling services are crucial in this regard.
3. Improving access to all aspects of healthcare, including essential medicines, diagnostic tools, and treatment services.
4. Substantially increasing health literacy among people of all ages to empower communities with knowledge about NCD prevention and management.
5. Enhancing the training of healthcare workers worldwide in the management of NCDs, focusing on prevention, early detection, and long-term care.
6. Developing easy-to-use telehealth systems that capitalize on the growing number of healthcare personnel other than physicians. These systems can provide remote consultations, monitoring, and support, expanding access to care, particularly in underserved areas, and alleviating the burden on overstrained healthcare facilities.

The path forward, against the backdrop of an aging global population, depends on multidisciplinary collaboration among policymakers, healthcare providers, and communities to tackle the dual challenges of NCDs and population aging.

REFERENCES

1. Calcaterra V, Zuccotti G (2022). Non-communicable diseases and rare diseases: A current and future public health challenge within pediatrics. *Children*, 9(10), 1491. doi:10.3390/children9101491
2. World Health Organization WHO (2019, June 12). *Noncommunicable Diseases.* https://www.who.int/health-topics/noncommunicable-diseases
3. NCDs|NCD Alliance (2022, July 25). NCD Alliance. https://ncdalliance.org/why-ncds/NCDs
4. Noncommunicable Diseases (2018). *Western Pacific Health Data Platform*, n.d. https://data.wpro.who.int/noncommunicable-diseases-2018
5. Pedroso CF, Pereira CC, Cavalcante AMRZ, Guimarães RA (2023). Magnitude of risk factors for chronic noncommunicable diseases in adolescents and young adults in Brazil: A population-based study. *PLoS One*, 18(10), e0292612. doi:10.1371/journal.pone.0292612
6. NCD Countdown 2030 Collaborators (2018). NCD countdown 2030: Worldwide trends in non-communicable disease mortality and progress towards sustainable development goal target 3.4. *Lancet (London, England)*, 392(10152), 1072–1088. doi:10.1016/S0140-6736(18)31992-5
7. Pan American Health Organization (2019). *NCDs at a Glance: NCD Mortality and Risk Factor Prevalence in the Americas.* Washington, DC: PAHO.
8. WHO (2023). *Fact Sheet: Tobacco.* Geneva: WHO.
9. U.S. Department of Health and Human Services (2014). *The Health Consequences of Smoking—50 Years of Progress. A Report of the Surgeon General.* Atlanta: US Department of Health and Human Services, Centers for Disease Control and Prevention, National Center for Chronic Disease Prevention and Health Promotion, Office on Smoking and Health.

10. Centers for Disease Control and Prevention (2013). QuickStats: Number of deaths from 10 leading causes—national vital statistics system, United States, 2010. *Morbidity and Mortality Weekly Report,* 62(8), 155.
11. Jha P (2009). Avoidable global cancer deaths and total deaths from smoking. *Nature Reviews Cancer,* 9(9), 655.
12. Jha P (2012). Avoidable deaths from smoking: A global perspective. *Public Health Reviews*, 33, 569–600.
13. Lee IM, Shiroma EJ, Lobelo F, Puska P, Blair SN, Katzmarzyk PT, Lancet Physical Activity Series Working Group (2012). Effect of physical inactivity on major non-communicable diseases worldwide: An analysis of burden of disease and life expectancy. *Lancet (London, England)*, 380(9838), 219. doi:10.1016/S0140-6736(12)61031-9
14. Franco OH, de Laet C, Peeters A, Jonker J, Mackenbach J, Nusselder W (2005). Effects of physical activity on life expectancy with cardiovascular disease. *Archives of Internal Medicine,* 165, 2355–2360.
15. Paffenbarger RS Jr, Hyde RT, Wing AL, Hsieh CC (1986). Physical activity, all-cause mortality, and longevity of college alumni. *The New England Journal of Medicine,* 314, 605–613.
16. Wen CP, Wai JPM, Tsai MK, Yang YC, Cheng TYD, Lee M-C et al. (2011). Minimum amount of physical activity for reduced mortality and extended life expectancy: A prospective cohort study. *Lancet*, 378, 1244–1253.
17. Santos AC, Willumsen J, Meheus F, Ilbawi A, Bull FC (2022). The cost of inaction on physical inactivity to public health-care systems: A population-attributable fraction analysis. *The Lancet Global Health*, 11(1), e32–e39. doi:10.1016/s2214-109x(22)00464-8
18. GBD 2017 Diet Collaborators (2019). Health effects of dietary risks in 195 countries, 1990–2017: A systematic analysis for the Global Burden of Disease Study 2017. *Lancet (London, England)*, 393(10184), 1958–1972. doi:10.1016/S0140-6736(19)30041-8
19. Melaku YA, Temesgen AM, Deribew A, Tessema GA, Deribe K, Sahle BW, Abera SF, Bekele T, Lemma F, Amare AT, Seid O, Endris K, Hiruye A, Worku A, Adams R, Taylor AW, Gill TK, Shi Z, Afshin A, Forouzanfar MH (2016). The impact of dietary risk factors on the burden of non-communicable diseases in Ethiopia: Findings from the Global Burden of Disease study 2013. *The International Journal of Behavioral Nutrition and Physical Activity*, 13(1), 122. doi:10.1186/s12966-016-0447-x
20. Melaku YA, Renzaho A, Gill TK, Taylor AW, Dal Grande E, de Courten B, Baye E, Gonzalez-Chica D, Hyppönen E, Shi Z, Riley M, Adams R, Kinfu Y (2019). Burden and trend of diet-related non-communicable diseases in Australia and comparison with 34 OECD countries, 1990–2015: Findings from the Global Burden of Disease Study 2015. *European Journal of Nutrition*, 58(3), 1299–1313. doi:10.1007/s00394-018-1656-7
21. Rehm J, Room R, Monteiro M, Gmel G, Graham K, Rehn N et al. (2003). Alcohol as a risk factor for global burden of disease. *European Addiction Research,* 9, 157–164.
22. World Health Organization. (2013). *Global Action Plan for the Prevention and Control of NCDs* 2013–2020. Geneva, Switzerland: World Health Organization.
23. Navarro HJ, Doran CM, Shakeshaft AP. (2010). Measuring costs of alcohol harm to others: A review of the literature. *Drug and Alcohol Dependence,* 114, 2–3.
24. Connor J, Casswell S (2012). Alcohol-related harm to others in New Zealand: Evidence of the burden and gaps in knowledge. *The New Zealand Medical Journal*, 125(1360), 11–27.
25. Parry CD, Patra J, Rehm J (2011). Alcohol consumption and non-communicable diseases: Epidemiology and policy implications. *Addiction (Abingdon, England)*, 106(10), 1718–1724. doi:10.1111/j.1360-0443.2011.03605.x
26. Micha R, Kalantarian S, Wirojratana P (2012). Estimating the global and regional burden of suboptimal nutrition on chronic disease: Methods and inputs to the analysis. *European Journal of Clinical Nutrition,* 66, 119–129.

27. Yogesh M, Kagathara N, Ram R, Misra S, Kagathara J (2023). Exploring behavioral risk factors for non-communicable diseases among undergraduate medical students in Western Gujarat: A cross-sectional study. *Cureus*, 15(11), e49188. doi:10.7759/cureus.49188
28. Sapkota BP, Baral KP, Rehfuess EA, Parhofer KG, Berger U (2023). Effects of age on non-communicable disease risk factors among Nepalese adults. *PLoS One*, 18(6), e0281028. doi:10.1371/journal.pone.0281028
29. Peltzer K, Azirou DN, Phalane E, Seloka MA, Phaswana-Mafuya RN (2024). Behavioral and biological risk factors of non-communicable diseases: Results of a nationally representative cross-sectional survey in Algeria. *Population Medicine*, 6(June), 1–9. doi:10.18332/popmed/189491
30. Calkins E (1999). *New Ways to Care for Older People : Building Systems based on Evidence*. New York: Springer. https://ci.nii.ac.jp/ncid/BA41396981
31. Banthin JS, Cohen JW (1999). *Changes in the Medicaid Community Population:* 1987–96. Rockville, MD: Agency for Health Care Policy and Research. MEPS Research Findings No. 9. AHCPR Pub. No. 99-0042.
32. World Health Organization (2010). *Global Status Report on Noncommunicable Diseases* 2010. Geneva: World Health Organization.
33. Roth GA, Mensah GA, Johnson CO, Addolorato G, Ammirati E, Baddour LM, Barengo NC, Beaton AZ, Benjamin EJ, Benziger CP, Bonny A, Brauer M, Brodmann M, Cahill TJ, Carapetis J, Catapano AL, Chugh SS, Cooper LT, Coresh J, Criqui M, GBD-NHLBI-JACC Global Burden of Cardiovascular Diseases Writing Group (2020). Global burden of cardiovascular diseases and risk Factors, 1990–2019: Update from the GBD 2019 study. *Journal of the American College of Cardiology*, 76(25), 2982–3021. doi:10.1016/j.jacc.2020.11.010
34. WorldHealth Organization. (2018). *Global Status Report on Alcohol and Health* 2018. Geneva: World Health Organization.
35. Cherla A, Kyriopoulosa I, Pearcya P, Tsangalidoub Z, Hajrulahovicc H, Theodorakisc P et al. Trends in avoidable mortality from cardiovascular diseases in the European Union, 1995–2020: A retrospective secondary data analysis. The Lancet Regional Health. *Europe*, 47, 101079.
36. Common Cancer Sites—Cancer Stat Facts (n.d.). SEER. https://seer.cancer.gov/statfacts/html/common.html
37. Ferlay J, Ervik M, Lam F, Laversanne M, Colombet M, Mery L, Piñeros M, Znaor A, Soerjomataram I, Bray F (2024). *Global Cancer Observatory: Cancer Today*. Lyon, France: International Agency for Research on Cancer. https://gco.iarc.who.int
38. Sung H, Ferlay J, Siegel RL, Laversanne M, Soerjomataram I, Jemal A, Bray F (2021). Global cancer statistics 2020: GLOBOCAN estimates of incidence and mortality worldwide for 36 cancers in 185 countries. *CA: A Cancer Journal for Clinicians*. doi:10.3322/caac.21660
39. CI5 (n.d.). *Cancer Incidence in Five Continents*. https://ci5.iarc.fr/
40. WHO Mortality Database (n.d.). https://www.who.int/data/data-collection-tools/who-mortality-database
41. OECD (2019). Avoidable mortality (preventable and treatable). In: *Health at a Glance* 2019*: OECD Indicators*. Paris: OECD Publishing. https://doi.org/10.1787/4dd50c09-en
42. Stone MA, Charpentier G, Doggen K, Kuss O, Lindblad U, Kellner C et al. Quality of care of people with type 2 diabetes in eight European countries: Findings from the Guideline Adherence to Enhance Care (GUIDANCE) study. *Diabetes Care*, 36(9), 2628–2638.
43. News & Views|Diabetes UK (n.d.). https://www.diabetes.org.uk/about_us/news/premature-deaths-diabetes

44. International Diabetes Federation (2021). *IDF Diabetes Atlas*, 10th edn. Brussels, Belgium: International Diabetes Federation. https://www.diabetesatlas.org
45. International Diabetes Federation (2023). *Type 2 Diabetes: A Preventable Catastrophe? A Call to Action by IDF Europe*. Brussels, Belgium: International Diabetes Federation.
46. Navarro-Torné A, Vidal M, Trzaska DK, Passante L, Crisafulli A, Laang H, Van De Loo J, Berkouk K, Draghia-Akli R (2015). Chronic respiratory diseases and lung cancer research: A perspective from the European Union. *European Respiratory Journal*, 46(5), 1270–1280. doi:10.1183/13993003.00395-2015
47. Soriano JB, Kendrick PJ, Paulson KR, Gupta V, Abrams EM, Adedoyin RA, Adhikari TB, Advani SM, Agrawal A, Ahmadian E, Alahdab F, Aljunid SM, Altirkawi KA, Alvis-Guzman N, Anber NH, Andrei CL, Anjomshoa M, Ansari F, Antó JM, … Kefale AT (2020). Prevalence and attributable health burden of chronic respiratory diseases, 1990–2017: A systematic analysis for the Global Burden of Disease Study 2017. *The Lancet Respiratory Medicine*, 8(6), 585–596. doi:10.1016/s2213-2600(20)30105-3
48. European Respiratory Society (2021). *Forum of International Respiratory Societies: The Global Impact of Respiratory Disease*, 3rd edn. European Respiratory Society. firsnet. https://www.knowledge-action-portal.com/en/content/forum-international-respiratory-societies-global-impact-respiratory-disease-3rd-edition-2021 (accessed 22 September 2021)
49. Vos T, Lim SS, Abbafati C, Abbas KM, Abbasi M, Abbasifard M et al. (2020). Diseases and injuries collaborators. Global burden of 369 diseases and injuries in 204 countries and territories, 1990–2019: A systematic analysis for the global burden of disease study 2019. *Lancet*, 396(10258), P1204–P1222.
50. Maher D, Harries AD, Zachariah R, Enarson D (2009). A global framework for action to improve the primary care response to chronic non-communicable diseases: A solution to a neglected problem. *BMC Public Health*, 9, 355. doi:10.1186/1471-2458-9-355
51. Prype L, Da Silva M, Melchior M (2017) Mental Health and Global Strategies to reduce NCDS and premature mortality. *The Lancet Public Health*, 2(8), e350–e351.
52. Riley JC (2005). Estimates of regional and global life expectancy, 1800–2001. *Population and Development Review*, 31(3), 537–543.
53. Aburto JM, Villavicencio F, Basellini U, Kjærgaard S, Vaupel JW (2020). Dynamics of life expectancy and life span equality. *Proceedings of the National Academy of Sciences*, 117(10), 5250–5259. doi:10.1073/pnas.1915884117
54. Vaupel JW, Zhang Z, Van Raalte AA (2011). Life expectancy and disparity: An international comparison of life table data. *BMJ Open*, 1(1), e000128–e000128. doi:10.1136/bmjopen-2011-000128
55. Eurostat (2023). *Ageing Europe—Statistics on Population Developments*. https://ec.europa.eu/eurostat/statistics-explained/index.php?title=Ageing_Europe_-_statistics_on_population_developments
56. Eurostat (2024). *Eurostat Regional Yearbook* 2024. Brussels, Belgium: European Union.
57. Jacobsen LA, Mather M, Lee M, Kent M (2011). America's aging population. *Population Bulletin*, 66(1), 1–16.
58. National Academy of Sciences (n.d.). *Improving Data on America's Aging Population: Summary of a Workshop*. https://www.nap.edu/catalog/5481.html
59. Chomik R, Piggott J (2013). *Asia in the Ageing Century: Part I—Population Trends (CEPAR Research Brief* 2013/01). New South Wales: Australian School of Business, University of New South Wales.
60. World Bank (2012). *The World Bank Annual Report* 2012, *Main Report,* Vol. 1. Washington, DC: World Bank. https://openknowledge.worldbank.org/handle/10986/11844 (accessed 22 October 2024).

61. Economic and Social Affairs of the United Nations Secretariat (2024). *World Population Prospects: The* 2006 *Revision.* https://digitallibrary.un.org/record/3924313?v=pdf (accessed 22 October 2024).
62. African Development Bank (2011). Aging population challenges in Africa. *African Development Bank*, 1(1), 1–19.
63. Marengoni A, Angleman S, Melis R, Mangialasche F, Karp A, Garmen A, Meinow B, Fratiglioni L (2011). Aging with multimorbidity: A systematic review of the literature. *Ageing Research Reviews*, 10(4), 430–439. doi:10.1016/j.arr.2011.03.003
64. Monaco A, Palmer K, Marengoni A, Maggi S, Hassan TA, Donde S (2020). Integrated care for the management of ageing-related non-communicable diseases: Current gaps and future directions. *Aging Clinical and Experimental Research*, 32(7), 1353–1358. doi:10.1007/s40520-020-01533-z
65. Eurostat (2023). *Ageing Europe—Looking at the Lives of Older People in the EU.* https://ec.europa.eu/eurostat/statistics-explained/index.php?title=Ageing_Europe
66. Hambleton IR, Caixeta R, Jeyaseelan SM, Luciani S, Hennis AJM (2023). The rising burden of non-communicable diseases in the Americas and the impact of population aging: A secondary analysis of available data. *Lancet Regional Health Americas*, 21, 100483. doi:10.1016/j.lana.2023.100483
67. WorldHealth Organization, Regional Office for South-East Asia (2015). *Population Ageing and Health Systems in Asia: Implications for Noncommunicable Diseases.* New Delhi: Asia Pacific Observatory on Health Systems and Policies.
68. Kahn K, Tollman SM, (1999). Stroke in rural South Afrida - contributing to the little known about a big problem. *South African Medical Journal*, 89(1), 63–65.
69. Africa Centres for Disease Control and Prevention (2024, July 12). *COVID*-19 *Vaccination—Africa CDC.* https://africacdc.org/covid-19/covid-19-vaccination/
70. World Health Organization (2010) *The World Health Report: Health Systems Financing, The Path to Universal Health Coverage.* Geneva: World Health Organization.
71. Long H, Huang W, Zheng P, Li J, Tao S, Tang S, Abdullah AS (2018). Barriers and facilitators of engaging community health workers in non-communicable disease (NCD) prevention and control in China: A systematic review (2006–2016). *International Journal of Environmental Research and Public Health,* 15(11), 2378. doi:10.3390/ijerph15112378
72. Lewin S, Munabi-Babigumira S, Glenton C, Daniels K, Bosch-Capblanch X, van Wyk BE et al. (2010). Lay health workers in primary and community health care for maternal and child health and the management of infectious diseases. *Cochrane Database System Review*, 2010(3), CD004015. doi: 10.1002/14651858.CD004015.pub3
73. Tang S, Ehiri J, Long Q (2013). China's biggest, most neglected health challenge: Non-communicable diseases. *Infectious Diseases of Poverty*, 2, 7.
74. Kamvura TT, Dambi JM, Chiriseri E, Turner J, Verhey R, Chibanda D et al. (2022). Barriers to the provision of non-communicable disease care in Zimbabwe: A qualitative study of primary health care nurses. *BMC Nursing,* 21, 64. doi:10.1186/s12912-022-00841-1
75. Miranda JJ, Kinra S, Casas JP, Smith GD, Ebrahim S (2008). Non-communicable diseases in low- and middle-income countries: Context, determinants and health policy. *Tropical Medicine & International Health,* 13, 1225–1234.
76. Yaya S, Reddy KS, Belizán JM, Pingray V (2020). Non-communicable diseases and reproductive health in sub-Saharan Africa: Bridging the policy-implementation gaps. *Reproductive Health,* 17, 8. doi:10.1186/s12978-020-0857-8
77. Mudie K, Jin MM, Tan Kendall L, Addo J, dosSantos-Silva I, Quint J et al. (2019). Non-communicable diseases in sub-Saharan Africa: A scoping review of large cohort studies. *Journal of Global Health,* 9(2), 20409.

78. Heller DJ, Kumar A, Kishore SP, Horowitz CR, Joshi R, Vedanthan R. (2019). Assessment of barriers and facilitators to the delivery of care for noncommunicable diseases by nonphysician health workers in low- and middle-income Countries. *JAMA Netwen Open*, 2(12), e1916545.
79. Duffy M, Ojikutu B, Andrian S, Sohng E, Minior T, Hirschhorn LR (2017). Non-communicable diseases and HIV care and treatment: Models of integrated service delivery. *Tropical Medicine & International Health,* 22(8), 926–937.
80. Asnake M, Bishaw T. The Addis Ababa declaration on global health equity: A call to action. *The Ethiopian Journal of Health Development*, 26(1), eISSN: 1021-6790.
81. Ray SC, Masuka N (2017). Facilitators and barriers to effective primary health care in Zimbabwe. *African Journal of Primary Health Care & Family Medicine,* 9, 2.
82. Duda-Sikuła M, Kurpas D (2023). Barriers and facilitators in the implementation of prevention strategies for chronic disease patients—Best practice guidelines and policies' systematic review. *Journal of Personalized Medicine*, 13(2), 288.
83. Poitras M-E, Maltais M-E, Bestard-Denommé L, Stewart M, Fortin M (2018). What are the effective elements in patient-centered and multimorbidity care? A scoping review. *BMC Health Services Research*, 18, 446.
84. Sung M, He J, Zhou Q, Chen Y, Ji JS, Chen H, Li Z (2022). Using an integrated framework to investigate the facilitators and barriers of health information technology implementation in noncommunicable disease management: Systematic review. *Journal of Medical Internet Research,* 24(7). doi:10.2196/37338
85. Joshi R, Alim M, Kengne AP, Jan S, Maulik PK, Peiris D et al. (2014). Task shifting for non-communicable disease management in low and middle income countries: A systematic review. *PLoS ONE,* 9(8), e103754.
86. WorldHealth Organization (2010). *World Health Statistics* 2010. Geneva: World Health Organization.
87. International Telecommunication Union (ITU) (2019). *The World in* 2013*: ICT Facts and Figures.* https://www.itu.int/en/ITU-D/Statistics/Documents/facts/ICTFactsFigures2013 e.pdf (accessed 2019 January 24)
88. Cavallo M, Morgana G, Dozzani I, Gatti A, Vandoni M, Pippi R, Pucci G, Vaudo G, Fanelli CG (2023). Unraveling barriers to a healthy lifestyle: Understanding barriers to diet and physical activity in patients with chronic non-communicable diseases. *Nutrients*, 15(15), 3473. doi:10.3390/nu15153473
89. United Nations (2013). *Report of the Director-General of the World Health Organization on the Prevention and Control of Non-Communicable Diseases.* A/68/650, General Assembly, Sixty-Eighth Session, Item 118. Distr.: General, 10 December 2013.
90. Elezbawy B, Farghaly M, Al Lafi A, Gamal M, Metni M, Visser W, Al-Abdulkarim H, Hedibel M, Fasseeh AN, Abaza S, Kaló Z (2024). Strategic approaches to reducing the burden of atopic dermatitis in the Middle East and Africa region. *Policy Perspective,* 42, 100987. https://doi.org/10.1016/j.vhri.2024.100987
91. Bello S, Neill R, Jegede AS, Bamgboye EA, Salawu MM, Afolabi RF, Nzelu C, Azodo N, Adoghe A, Ogunlayi M, Yaradua SU, Wang W, Liu A, Fawole OI (2024). Sustainable health systems challenges, mitigation strategies and adaptations to maintain essential health services during the COVID-19 pandemic: Learnings from the six geopolitical regions in Nigeria. *BMC Health Services Research*, 24, 625. doi:10.1186/s12913-024-11072-2
92. World Health Organization (25 March 2020). *COVID-19: Operational Guidance for Maintaining Essential Health Services During an Outbreak: Interim Guidance.* https://apps.who.int/iris/handle/10665/331561

93. Elston JW, Cartwright C, Ndumbi P, Wright J (2017). The health impact of the 2014–15 Ebola outbreak. *Public Health*, 143, 60–70.
94. Parpia AS, Ndeffo-Mbah ML, Wenzel NS, Galvani AP (2016). Effects of response to 2014–2015 Ebola outbreak on deaths from Malaria, HIV/AIDS, and tuberculosis, West Africa. *Emerging Infectious Diseases,* 22(3), 433–441.
95. Plucinski MM, Guilavogui T, Sidikiba S, Diakité N, Diakité S, Dioubaté M et al. (2015). Effect of the Ebola-virus-disease epidemic on malaria case management in Guinea, 2014: A cross-sectional survey of health facilities. *Lancet Infectious Diseases,* 15(9), 1017–1023.
96. Walker PG, White MT, Griffin JT, Reynolds A, Ferguson NM, Ghani AC (2015). Malaria morbidity and mortality in Ebola-affected countries caused by decreased health-care capacity, and the potential effect of mitigation strategies: A modelling analysis. *Lancet Infectious Diseases,* 15(7), 825–832.
97. Rudd KE, Kissoon N, Limmathurotsakul D, Bory S, Mutahunga B, Seymour CW, Angus DC, West TE (2018). The global burden of sepsis: Barriers and potential solutions. *Critical Care*, 22, 232. doi:10.1186/s13613-018-1047-6
98. Mercer T, Chang AC, Fischer L, Gardner A, Kerubo I, Tran DN, Laktabai J, Pastakia S (2019). Mitigating the burden of diabetes in sub-Saharan Africa through an integrated diagonal health systems approach. *Diabetes, Metabolic Syndrome and Obesity: Targets and Therapy*, 12, 2261–2272. doi:10.2147/DMSO.S207427
99. WorldHealth Organization (2009). 20082013 *Action Plan for the Global Strategy for the Prevention and Control of Noncommunicable Diseases.* Geneva: World Health Organization.
100. United Nations (2013). *Note by the Secretary-General Transmitting the Report of the Director-General of the World Health Organization on the Prevention and Control of Noncommunicable Diseases.* New York: General Assembly. Contract No: A/68/650.
101. Demaio AR, Nielsen KK, Tersbøl BP, Kallestrup P, Meyrowitsch DW (2014). Primary Health Care: A strategic framework for the prevention and control of chronic non-communicable disease. *Global Health Action*, 7, 1. doi:10.3402/gha.v7.24504
102. Strong K, Mathers C, Leeder S, Beaglehole R (2005). Preventing chronic diseases: How many lives can we save? *Lancet,* 366, 1578–1582.

7 A New Option for the Treatment of Neuropsychiatric Diseases

Fecal Microbiota Transplantation?

Alper Evrensel

7.1 INTRODUCTION

Compared to thousands of years of medical history, the last century is full of revolutionary developments. If the discovery of penicillin and vaccines plays an important role in improving human health and extending life, the emergence of psychopharmacology is undoubtedly just as important [1]. The term "psychopharmacology" was introduced into medical literature a century ago (pharmacologist David Macht) [2]. Although the discovery of many psychopharmacological molecules (morphine, codeine, cocaine, bromine, barbiturates, and amphetamines) dates back much further, the modern discipline of psychopharmacology was born in 1951 [3]. The discovery of chlorpromazine undoubtedly started the era of modern psychopharmacology. In the following years, the discovery of neurotransmitters and the understanding of synaptic transmission provided psychopharmacotherapy with a scientific and experimental basis [4].

These developments, which emerged in a few decades compared to the 2,500 years since Aristotle and even Hippocrates, are the first paradigm shift in psychopharmacology. In this chapter, we share our views on the possibility of a change in the modern psychiatric treatment paradigm in the light of the information that emerged in the last 20 years.

7.2 PHILOSOPHICAL BACKGROUND

The term "paradigm shift" was first used by philosopher of science Thomas Samuel Kuhn in his book *The Structure of Scientific Revolutions* [5]. The book, published in 1962, had a wide impact in scientific circles. According to Kuhn, a "paradigm" is "different competing scientific approaches" and its conceptual foundation is

DOI: 10.1201/9781003513834-7

well-established. The accepted methods, explicit or implicit beliefs, rules, values, and conceptual/experimental tools, used to determine order in nature were called the "scientific approach" by Kuhn. This approach was adopted by scientists as the "absolute truth" for a certain period of time.

According to Kuhn, science is dogmatic by nature. Scientists are closed to information other than the scientific methods and theories they have adopted. Over time, when old methods of doing science become inadequate to explain questions and problems, they are abandoned and new ones are adopted. The philosopher, who called this painful process "paradigm shift", argued that scientific revolutions only occur when this change occurs.

Kuhn's brilliant claim implies that the modern understanding of science that developed after the Age of Enlightenment will become dogmatic over time, because previous understandings of science followed a similar path and at some point began to block the path of scientific development. According to his theory, the ideas that science will constantly progress, that we will get closer to the truth accordingly, that there is a single and absolute reality that explains the facts, and that the scientific criteria that will determine this are universal are all just assumptions. Through Kuhn, the post-modern understanding of science has been adopted.

Thomas Samuel Kuhn's philosophy of science can be applied to economics, politics, international relations, and social life today. When perspectives and methods change, perceptions of the world change accordingly. Thus, many factors that were previously overlooked are included in the theory and a broader vision emerges.

Today, our perspective on the etiopathogenesis and treatment of psychiatric disorders is being questioned. The paradigm that existed after 1951 is discussed, and a new paradigm is proposed that explains the mechanisms that create resistance to standard pharmacological treatment. We call this the "microbiome-brain interaction". In this chapter, we will try to reveal the foundations of the paradigm necessary to take the kind of revolutionary step advocated by Kuhn in the field of psychiatric treatment and discuss its rationale.

7.3 THE FOUNDATION OF THE NEW PARADIGM IN NEUROPSYCHIATRIC DISORDERS

Neuropsychiatric disorders, especially depression, affect millions of people. This disease cluster has high morbidity and mortality rates [6]. The etiopathological basis of neuropsychiatric disorders is still uncertain. These diseases often appear on a multifactorial basis. Previous studies have shown that primarily the brain monoaminergic neurotransmitter systems do not function properly, autoimmune inflammatory reactions accompany the process, there are problems in the hypothalamic-pituitary-adrenal (HPA) axis, and neurotrophic functions are also impaired [7]. Current treatment approaches are based on these findings. In recent years, the commensal microbiome attracted the attention of not only neuroscientists but also researchers from all branches of biology. This interest led to a focus on the brain-gut interaction and, in particular, the gut microbiome in the pathology and therapy of neuropsychiatric disorders [8,9].

The conclusion reached in this context is roughly that the microbiome has a mutual regulatory function through neuroimmune, neuroanatomical, and neuroendocrine pathways. It seems that the microbiome plays an important role in all biological and physiological processes in the human body, especially neuronal, from the embryonic period until death [10,11]. More than other body regions, the gut microbiome plays an active role in the synthesis of neurotransmitters and other neuroactive molecules, which then pass into systemic circulation and reach the brain. This development seems to have the potential to affect neuronal functions [12].

Numerous studies reported an increase in the proportion of bacterial families such as *Streptococcus*, *Bacteroidales*, *Proteobacteria*, *Actinobacteria*, *Eggerthella*, *Alistipes*, etc., in the intestinal flora of patients with major depressive disorder (MDD). In contrast, a decreased prevalence of bacterial taxa such as *Faecalibacterium*, *Lactobacillus*, and *Bifidobacterium* were found in individuals with MDD [13,14]. Why is there such a difference in bacterial colonization rates when comparing healthy individuals and individuals with MDD? There may be many reasons for this.

There are also speculations that the gut microbiome disrupts the stress tolerance of eukaryotic cells. Chronic stress is already a known risk for MDD. Long-term psychological stress may cause dysbiosis, which in turn may cause various toxic bacterial metabolites to proliferate first in the intestinal lumen and then in the systemic circulation. These toxic metabolites may trigger an autoimmune reaction, affect the enteric nervous system, and alter neuronal physiology, potentially leading to the development of MDD [15,16]. Many studies have shown that an unbalanced gut microbiome can increase the synthesis of stress hormones and subsequently modulate the immune system [14,17,18].

7.4 PROKARYOTE-EUKARYOTE INTERACTION

Although the paradigm shift in psychiatric disorders was observable in the early 21st century, the most significant evidence emerged in the last 20 years with the increase of laboratory facilities. This preclinical and clinical evidence regarding the pathophysiology of mental disorders suggests that there may be a causal relationship between the microbiome and psychopathology [19].

In the "superorganism" consisting of human eukaryotes and prokaryotes of the microbiome, things are not as uniform as it seems. First of all, it is very difficult to measure the basic relationships between microbes and eukaryotic cells in the human ecosystem. However, the most difficult conditions can be modeled in animal experiments. Thus, many clues have been obtained about the mechanisms between the microbiome and the brain [20–24].

Critical studies continue to be published that reveal potential mechanistic pathways and processes, including neuroinflammation, autoimmunity, oxidative stress, mitochondrial dysfunction, tryptophan-kynurenine metabolism disorder, neuroendocrine problems, intestinal leakage, and neurotransmitter production [19,25,26]. In these studies, the determinant has always been bacteria. However, recently it is determined that other microorganisms (viruses, fungi, archaea, and parasites) also have complex internal and external interactions with both the eukaryotic host and each other [27,28].

Studies on the other microorganisms mentioned above are relatively few. But where do these other guests of the microbiome fit into the equation? The answer to this question is of vital importance. In the following section, we have tried to provide an overview of some of these lesser-studied organisms and how they may be related to neuropsychiatric disorders.

Viruses that colonize the human intestines (virome) are generally composed of plant viruses. They enter the body through diet. There are two possible dangers of these viruses. The first of these is that they infect the host human. Perhaps more importantly for our topic, they damage other colonized microbial cells [29]. These types of viruses, also called bacteriophages, have the potential to alter the intestinal bacterial colonization profile.

The proportion of viromes in different parts of the body varies. However, the majority of viruses are found in the gastrointestinal tract [30]. It is estimated that the number of viruses colonizing the intestines may be 10 times greater than commensal bacteria [29–31]. The most numerous members of the virome are bacteriophages. They constitute 95% of the entire intestinal virome [32–34]. The diversity of bacteriophage viruses is highest in the postpartum period and resembles an adult situation after the age of two. This is interesting because the course of bacterial colonies is exactly the opposite. In other words, bacterial diversity is lower in newborns and becomes richer as they age [34]. As we mentioned in the previous paragraph, bacteriophages shape the intestinal bacteriome and affect bacterial metabolism [35].

Differences in the intestinal virome composition of rodents exposed to a depression model were observed. A correlation was found between these differences and the tryptophan metabolism, fecal neurotransmitter, and metabolite levels of the experimental animals [36]. Similar findings were obtained in an experiment conducted on primates. The researchers who conducted this study attributed the differences to changes in lipid metabolism in the brain and periphery [37].

A study conducted on humans is also parallel to the findings obtained from animal experiments. Therefore, it can be said that there are significant differences in the intestinal flora of healthy individuals and individuals with depressive disorders in terms of both bacteriome and virome diversity [38].

In the literature, no study was found investigating the gut virome in a bipolar disorder sample. However, if the virome and bacteriome can be decisive in the pathophysiology of MDD, they may also play the same role in mood disorders. This is probably achieved through the immune system [39,40].

Another important component of the gut microbiome is fungi. The term "fungome" refers to fungal components [41]. Although fungi make up only 0.1% of the microbes found in the gut, they can occupy space up to 100 times larger than bacteria. This mass difference is the exact opposite of what we see in viruses. Fungi may be few in number, but their huge size clearly dominates the biomass compared to bacteria and viruses [42].

The intestinal fungome (mycobiome), like other microorganisms, begins working immediately after birth and is colonized by fungal species. Perhaps the most significant development affecting the intestinal fungome composition is the baby's transition to solid food [43]. Intestinal fungome in adulthood shows high interindividual variability. The "core fungome" continues to be shaped by environmental factors [44,45].

These factors are body mass index (both mother and baby), antibacterial/antifungal drug use, diet, etc. All these parameters are important for both general body health and neuronal performance [46,47].

An interesting finding is that there is an interaction between intestinal bacteria and fungi and this correlates with fecal metabolites [44]. The association of commensal fungome with inflammatory bowel diseases is long known. In Crohn's disease, antibody levels against the fungus *Saccharomyces cerevisiae*, a common intestinal parasite especially in children, are high [48–50]. It may initially be assumed that the passage of this fungus into the systemic circulation is due to leaky gut. However, some researchers have called this possibility dubious [51,52] because *S. cerevisiae* antibodies have also been found to be high in many neuropsychiatric diseases (Parkinson's disease, schizophrenia, bipolar disorder) [53–55]. A similar situation applies to another disease (MDD) for another fungus (*Candida albicans*) [56]. Is it possible to conclude from this? The intestinal fungome modulates both the human immune system and the composition and functioning of the bacteriome. Zhang answers this question with "possible" [57].

Another component of the intestinal microbiota is the archaea. Archaea are more primitive and evolutionarily earlier organisms than bacteria [58]. Archaea are generally adapted to withstand harsh conditions that are not conducive to life, such as lack of oxygen and high levels of salt and methane [59,60]. These difficult conditions are also present in the intestines. Archaea living in the intestines are called archaeomes. Like other components of the intestinal microbiome, many environmental factors affect the archaeome [61]. Changing intestinal lumen conditions will naturally affect the activities of archaea. The most dominant species in the archaeome is Methanobrevibacter. These archaea produce methane using the hydrogen produced by bacteria (methanogens) [62]. Methane accelerates the passage of feces through the intestine and has a lethal effect on the bacteriome. These are pathological effects and therefore play a role in the pathophysiology of inflammatory bowel disease and irritable bowel syndrome (IBS) [63].

There are few studies on the relationship between archaeome and neuropsychiatric disorders. Depression-themed studies have shown that archaea play a role in mechanisms related to the metabolism of biliary acids (trimethylamine and trimethylamine-*N*-oxide) [63,64]. These studies have suggested that bile acids may have a protective potential against depression. In the opposite direction, trimethylamine-*N*-oxide can also cross the blood-brain barrier and have a depressant effect on neurons [65]. Therefore, it can be said that the intestinal archaeome affects neuronal functions through methane production, changing bacteriome demographics and metabolites.

Symbiotic and probiotic protozoa (amoeba) and eukaryotic parasites (helminths) are also found in the human intestine [66,67]. Although the definition of parasite is often considered harmful to health, some may have immune benefits as an exception [68].

Interactions between archaeome, fungome, parasitome, and virome play an important role in the balance of gut microbiota demography. Parasites, which are part of this interaction network, can also affect bacterial composition [66,67,69]. Considering that the rate of parasitic infestation is lower in developed countries than in underdeveloped countries, this is an advantage in favor of the intestinal bacterial diversity of the people of developed countries [66].

Numerous clinical studies were conducted to determine the safety and applicability of helminth therapy in various diseases (allergy, inflammatory bowel diseases, multiple sclerosis, neuropsychiatric disorders, and rheumatoid arthritis) [70,71]. In these studies, an inverse correlation was found between the frequency of helminth infestation and autoimmune diseases [70,71]. This finding suggests that each microbiota component plays a role in the reorganization of the immune system using some pathways that we cannot yet clearly explain.

It is known that in some (especially underdeveloped) countries, people try to treat themselves with helminths [72]. This effort may have roots in ancient medical traditions. If parasitic infestations are endemic and carry a risk of death, patients should receive anthelmintic therapy. However, looking at the other side of the coin, there are also concerns that it may contribute to an increase in inflammatory and autoimmune diseases in these countries over time [71]. More clinical studies are needed in this area to better understand the safety, effectiveness, and, if any, mechanism of action of helminth treatment [72].

Unlike autoimmune diseases, there is a positive correlation between parasitic infestation and the prevalence of psychiatric disorders [73]. Parasites can even increase the risk of psychiatric disorders [74]. Given the potential of helminth therapy for immunological disorders, the contribution of parasites to human health, including mental health, is an important area of research. However, the medical literature mostly includes studies on the intestinal bacteriome. Although the dataset focusing on the virome [34,75,76], fungome [48], and archaeome [62] is expanding, there are still a lack of new and sufficient studies for the intestinal parasitome [77].

The microbiome of the small intestine (ileum) is harder to access than that of the large intestine. For this reason, it may have attracted less attention from researchers because it is more laborious to investigate and examine [78].

Although the bacterial composition in the ileum is less diverse than in the large intestine, the small intestinal microbiome is more dynamic (faster transit time and earlier exposure to nutrients, etc.). In addition, most of the digestion and nutrient absorption occurs in the ileum. For these reasons, the composition and dysbiosis of the ileum microbiome may be more important for human health [78,79].

The ileum microbiome plays a role in nutrient/bile acid metabolism and mucosal immunity [80]. In one study examining stool samples from patients with ileostomies, the ileum microbiome was found to be richer than the colon microbiome (probably as a result of carbohydrate metabolism) [79]. In one study, duodenal samples from underweight and overweight individuals were analyzed metagenomically. In obese individuals, genes related to carbohydrate metabolism were found to be at lower levels, while genes related to lipid metabolism were found to be at higher levels [81]. Dietary fiber level is also one of the determining factors on ileum microbiome diversity [82].

A healthy diet reduces the risk of depression [83,84]. Even just a change in diet can improve depressive symptoms [85–87]. Patients with bipolar disorder often have unhealthy eating habits [88]. Adding unsaturated fatty acids to the diet improves symptoms of bipolar disorder [89].

Dietary interventions naturally alter gut microbiota composition and function [90,91]. The gut microbiome is therefore an intermediate link in the diet-mental health chain [92]. As the diet-microbiome-brain interaction becomes clearer over time, the importance of the ileum microbiome may increase. However, it is clear that much more advanced technology and methodological breakthroughs are needed to conduct these studies.

To date, most of the research on the microbiome has focused on the intestine. However, it can be said that other microbiota also play a role in human health. The following section discusses the findings on the oral microbiota, which is the beginning of the gastrointestinal system.

The oral microbiome contains more than 700 microbial taxa, mostly consisting of bacteria. As such, it has less diversity than the large intestine [93]. The composition of the oral microbiome underwent significant changes with the food industry and oral hygiene practices [94]. However, the oral microbiome is more resistant to change than other parts of the gastrointestinal tract, with the exception of fermentable carbohydrates [95–97].

The oral microbiome was also heavily linked to mood disorders and other brain diseases. Bacterial diversity in the saliva of youth with symptoms of depression and anxiety correlates with baseline C-reactive protein (CRP) and cortisol levels [98,99]. Differences have also been detected in the oral bacterial composition of Behçet's patients [100]. This evidence may point to a link between the immune system and the oral microbiome.

Despite all these efforts, data to explain the causal relationship are unclear and insufficient. Plausible mechanisms for the interaction between mood disorders and the oral microbiome were proposed. Direct microbial translocation from the oral cavity to the central nervous system via the facial and olfactory nerves may be involved. In addition, the immunomodulatory functions of the oral microbiota may activate proinflammatory cytokines and cause neuroinflammation [101]. This hypothesis was even shown as a mechanism contributing to the pathogenesis of Alzheimer's disease [102–104].

Research on these different microorganisms requires specific methods (sample collection, processing, sequencing, and bioinformatics) [105–107]. These problems make it difficult to conduct studies. However, guidelines for standardizing microbiome research shall be prepared in order to reach a common interpretation and a generally accepted scientific reality [108]. However, despite the tedious challenges of microbiota studies, a multidisciplinary approach will help overcome these obstacles.

7.5 FECAL MICROBIOTA TRANSPLANTATION AS A RESTORER OF MICROBIOTA DYSBIOSIS

The microbiota can become dysbiotic due to reasons such as nutrition, antibiotic use, stress, and aging. Dysbiosis can be restored with fecal microbiota transplantation (FMT) [109]. The main goal of FMT is to repair the disturbed floral balance in the intestines through the cultivation of healthy bacterial flora [110].

7.5.1 History of FMT

There are speculations that the first FMT application was made in China 1,700 years ago [111]. In this practice, a suspension obtained from feces was given orally to treat diarrhea and food poisoning. The Chinese physician Ge Hong probably came to this conclusion intuitively. There is no record in medical texts of the use of FMT for the following centuries. There are records of another traditional Chinese physician (Li Shizhen) in the 16th century using FMT to treat complaints such as constipation, diarrhea, and vomiting [111]. Fecal suspension first appeared in the 18th century under the name "transfaunation" (Fabricius Aquapendente). The aim here was to treat sick animals [112]. It is in medical records that this information reached the Bedouins living in Africa and was used in the treatment of German soldiers who caught dysentery during World War 2 [113].

7.5.2 FMT's Main Usage Area

FMT first appeared in modern medical literature in 1958. In this experimental study, four cases of pseudomembranous enterocolitis caused by *Clostridium difficile* were treated with fecal transplantation. The author reported that his efforts were successful [114]. The second case series of *C. difficile* infection (CDI) treated with FMT dates back to 1981 [115]. Following these publications, FMT was investigated in depth and its mechanism of action was better understood. Today, FMT is indicated in cases of recurrent CDI [116]. Although there are no randomized controlled trials (RCTs) on its use in the treatment of psychiatric disorders, developments are promising [28].

7.5.3 FMT Application

The Amsterdam Protocol is now generally accepted to standardize the implementation of FMT [113]. As with any medical treatment, ethical approvals shall be obtained before FMT [117]. In the past, the stool to be transplanted to the patient was obtained from a healthy person in the patient's immediate circle. In recent years, it has been recommended to obtain it from a "stool bank" or a permanent stool donor. Because in this way, it becomes possible to use fresh stool from reliable and healthy donors who have frequent health screenings [118]. Naturally, donors shall eat healthy, not use any medication, take care of their physical health, and live a largely routine life [113].

About 150–250 g of stool is sufficient for transport. The stool shall be obtained immediately before FMT, that is, it shall be fresh [113]. After FMT, the patient's bowel movement reflex can be stimulated. However, in order to increase the success rate of the procedure, it is recommended that the patient does not defecate for at least 4 hours after the transplant. For this purpose, an antidiarrheal drug, loperamide, is given before FMT [109].

Before FMT, stool suspension shall be prepared. Water, physiological serum, or milk can be used to dilute the stool. The stool suspension is filtered to remove solid particles and taken into 60 mL syringes [113,119]. The ideal method for preparing stool suspension is not yet determined. It is determined that the success rate is lower when stool is diluted with physiological serum compared to water. It is argued that when an electric mixer is used, the oxygen mixed into the suspension reduces the number of anaerobic bacteria and the treatment effectiveness decreases [113].

Fecal suspension can be administered to the patient in two ways. It can be delivered to the upper gastrointestinal tract via esophagogastroduodenoscopy or nasogastric tube. It can be administered to the lower gastrointestinal tract via colonoscopy [113]. Colonoscopy was used in 3/4 of the cases and esophagogastroduodenoscopy was used in 1/4 of the cases [120]. Patient demand may have also played a role in this because some patients have a negative view of FMT. Women are more reluctant than men, and young people are more reluctant than old people. Colonoscopy is more preferred. One-third of patients think the procedure should be free of charge [121].

FMT may be rarely applied due to its disturbing aspects for the patient. In cases where the transplant needs to be done urgently, donor health screenings take time and FMT may be delayed. For this reason, an alternative method to FMT was tried [122]. The stool sample taken from the donor was centrifuged and placed in swallowable capsules. The capsules were stored at −80°. Fifteen doses per day were administered to the patients perorally for 2 days. In 70% of the cases, complete remission was achieved after 3 days, and the same procedure was repeated once more in the others [123]. The oral capsule method is non-invasive and more comfortable. It is foreseeable that its use will become widespread in the future and will be used to restore the intestinal microbiota after antibiotic treatments [124].

Studies are being conducted to standardize the application of FMT with the same procedure worldwide. In this direction, a meeting was organized by the International Alliance for Biological Standardization (IABS) and the BIOASTER Microbiology Technology Institute in 2022. This meeting focused on safety, efficacy, clinical trial design, reproducibility and accuracy in microbiome measurements and data reporting, and standardization [125].

7.5.4 Reliability and Side Effects of FMT

The main indications for FMT are inflammatory bowel diseases such as CDI, ulcerative colitis, and Crohn's disease. Although the general medical condition of patients who have stool transplants is quite poor, FMT is a reliable application. Rarely diarrhea, constipation, gas, and abdominal pain may be observed on the day of FMT [113]. In a series of 317 cases, only three cases of enteritis, bleeding, and peritonitis were reported [126]. One case of colitis exacerbation was reported [127]. Peritonitis that developed after transplantation caused the death of one patient [128]. Brandt et al. reported no adverse effects in a long-term follow-up study [121].

Although the history of FMT dates back to 17 centuries, its use became widespread in the last 30–40 years. Therefore, there are many points that are not clear [129]. It is not known in which disorders the intestinal microbiota composition changes. Although it is easier and cheaper to obtain stool to be transplanted from a donor, it is risky. Therefore, it may be recommended to produce probiotic bacteria in culture. It is not known whether fresh stool and stool obtained from a stool bank are different in terms of effectiveness. Using water, physiological serum, or milk to dilute stool may have different results on the effectiveness of the treatment. It may be appropriate to use a different diluent for each indication. There is no consensus on the ideal amount of stool. It is necessary to clarify whether transplantation is more effective when done orally or anally. The changes in the immune and metabolic systems in the short and long term after FMT shall be revealed in detail. No serious risks have been reported in patients with poor physical health. However, the risks that may be encountered when applied with psychiatric indications are not yet known. Large case series and RCTs are needed to determine these risks and clarify the dark points.

7.5.5 Ethical Issues

As with every treatment method, the ethical aspects of FMT should be thoroughly addressed. In this context, one of the important articles was published in 2019. In this article, which is included in the section I edited [129], the authors drew attention to roughly five areas: (i) informed consent and the vulnerability of patients; (ii) determining what a "suitable healthy donor" is; (iii) safety and risk; (iv) commercialization and potential exploitation of vulnerable patients; and (v) public health implications [130]. However, it should not be forgotten that a clear framework for the use of FMT in neuropsychiatric indications does not yet exist. Therefore, the procedures for the definition and resolution of ethical issues will become clear over time [131].

7.6 FMT AS A TREATMENT TOOL FOR PSYCHIATRIC DISORDERS

FMT has been studied mostly in CDI. Antibiotic use can cause dysbiosis and *C. difficile* can become dominant in the microbiota. FMT repairs the damaged flora [132]. FMT may be a beacon of hope in the treatment of treatment-resistant psychiatric disorders such as CDI.

We can now make more definitive statements about the relationship between depression and microbiota [28,133]. An animal model of depression can be obtained through exposure to bacterial lipopolysaccharide (LPS) [134]. In numerous animal experiments, positive changes in immune parameters occurred with intestinal microbiota repair. In one of these experiments, it was determined that interleukin (IL)-10 levels increased after probiotic bacteria were given to germ-free (GF) mice [135]. In another GF mouse study, *Bifidobacterium infantis* led to reduced anxiety and depression scores [136]. *B. infantis* is called "psychobiotic bacteria" because of its antidepressant-like effect [137]. Probiotic bacteria such as *Bifidobacterium longum* and *Lactobacillus helveticus* reduced anxiety scores in rats [138]. In an RCT conducted on healthy volunteers, subjects were given *L. helveticus* with *B. longum* or placebo for 1 month. Anxiety scores and levels of anxiety-related blood parameters decreased in subjects receiving probiotic bacteria [139]. In another animal experiment, FMT from mice fed a high-fat diet was applied to mice fed a normal diet. Following FMT, the mice fed a normal diet developed leaky gut, neuroinflammation, and behavioral disorders [140].

Autistic behaviors regressed in mice given *Bacteroides fragilis*, which repaired the gut and reduced leakiness [141]. In one study conducted on stool samples, more *Clostridium* species were detected in the stools of autistic children [142,143]. It is quite interesting that autistic symptoms regressed in a child diagnosed with autism who underwent FMT [120].

The amount of *Lactobacillus* in the stools of psychotic and healthy individuals is significantly different. This difference also correlates with symptom severity and treatment response [144]. Another study with a similar design compared the stool microbiota analysis of 46 depressed patients with 30 healthy individuals. *Bacteroidetes*, *Proteobacteria*, and *Actinobacteria* levels were found to be higher and *Firmicutes* levels were lower in the stools of depressed patients. Harmful bacterial groups were more in depressed patients and beneficial bacteria were less [145]. In light of these findings, it can be said that probiotic bacteria are beneficial in the treatment of depression [146].

The gut microbiota composition of depressed patients can be modulated with FMT as well as probiotics. In the experiment conducted by Zheng et al., feces from individuals with depression were transplanted into GF mice. It is quite interesting that depression-like behaviors were observed in the mice after the transplant [147]. This observation implies that "depression can be transplanted". If depression can be transplanted with FMT, perhaps its treatment can be transplanted as well. Chronic alcoholism also causes dysbiosis. Probiotics may be useful in the treatment of alcoholism by restoring the intestinal barrier [148]. Therefore, FMT may also provide a similar effect on alcoholics.

With aging, the composition of the microbiota changes and cognitive impairment may occur as a result [149]. Western-type diet can also disrupt microbiota composition. The resulting dysbiosis can lead to hippocampal dysfunction and cognitive impairment [150]. It was determined that *B. longum* 1714 reduces stress levels and has a positive effect on memory in healthy individuals [151]. However, in the RCT conducted by the same team on healthy individuals the following year, the application of *Lactobacillius rhamnosus*, a probiotic bacterium, was not found to be superior to placebo on anxiety, stress-related measures, HPA response, and cognitive performance [152]. Despite this, publications indicating that intestinal leakage and bacterial LPS-induced neuroinflammation are involved in the etiopathogenesis of Alzheimer's disease are increasing [153].

These studies show that it is possible to restore the disrupted gut microbiota through FMT, and that this mechanism has the potential to be used in the treatment of neuropsychiatric disorders. However, it is obvious that we are only at the beginning of the journey.

Numerous studies have examined the possibility of FMT as a therapeutic intervention for MDD [154]. However, it is obvious that we are only at the beginning of the journey [155–157].

In one study, it was found that depressive symptoms were alleviated when FMT containing healthy feces was applied to rats exposed to stress. Detailed biochemical analyses on rats revealed significant differences in the levels of neurotransmitters, inflammatory markers, and neurotrophic factors before and after FMT [158]. Treatment with FMT is thought to be effective in improving clinical symptoms in physical diseases as well as in intestinal diseases [159]. The gut microbiota appears to have the potential to influence brain function and behavior through a variety of pathways, including neuroendocrine, neuroimmune, neuronal, and humoral mechanisms

[160]. Restoring dysbiotic gut microbiota composition with FMT appears to be beneficial in the treatment of neuropsychiatric diseases [161].

It is very interesting that when microbiota from MDD patients was transplanted into GF mice via FMT, the mice exhibited MDD symptoms. In addition to this observation, changes in the gut microbiota, behavior, immune system, and neurotransmitter metabolism were noted in the mice [152]. Other findings from this study include that depressed patients exhibited significantly increased levels of inflammation, altered tryptophan metabolism, increased cortisol levels, and decreased bacterial flora diversity compared to healthy controls. The researchers who conducted the experiment argued that manipulating the gut microbiota via FMT could be a practical approach for creating new antidepressant treatments and strategies to prevent depression [152].

Microbiota dysbiosis may lead to disruptions in proline metabolism, leading to the development of MDD. In a 2022 study, fecal microbiota obtained from depressed patients were transplanted into 20 mice treated with antibiotics, and then mood changes in the mice were monitored. According to the study results, it was determined that the severity of MDD in mice had a significant and positive correlation with diet and plasma proline levels. Plasma proline levels seem to vary depending on the composition and function of the gut microbiota. As a result, the researchers argued that manipulating the gut microbiota and adding proline to the diet may be effective in the treatment of MDD, emphasizing the importance of proline-glutamate-GABA-microbiota interactions [162].

By examining changes in the intestinal microbiota composition through FMT, new information about depression can be obtained in both mouse models and human samples [163,164]. In this context, three clinical cases were reported in humans regarding the potential efficacy of FMT in MDD. In the first of these interesting cases, a 79-year-old woman who was treated with FMT using stool from her 6-year-old grandson after stopping antidepressant treatment was examined. After the procedure, the patient's cognitive functions and depression scores improved for 6 months. In another article, two patients in their 50s experienced improvement in their depressive symptoms within 4 weeks of FMT, but this positive effect lasted for 2 months [165,166].

IBS is a disease with a multifactorial etiology, resulting from a complex interaction of genetic, immunological, microbiological, and environmental variables. Therefore, it is obviously difficult to find a simple and effective treatment option for this disease [167,168]. Comorbid anxiety and depression are also common in IBS cases and pose significant challenges for individuals [169]. It was noted that there is a similarity between the fecal microbiota profiles of individuals diagnosed with depression and IBS with diarrhea (IBS-D) [72]. These studies suggest that FMT may help relieve symptoms of IBS as well as comorbid mood disorders. The study team's other research also suggests that, by regulating the gut microecology, FMT treatment holds significant promise for relieving clinical symptoms for people with IBS-D who experience anxiety and depression [170].

In our own study published in 2020, we obtained similar results on a sample with inflammatory bowel disease [171]. In this study, we found that patients' pre-FMT obsessive and depressive scores decreased after FMT.

The above examples led researchers to be optimistic about the development of innovative treatments for MDD. However, it is essential for a new treatment to pass extremely rigorous tests, especially in terms of reliability.

An 8-week study was designed to evaluate the feasibility and safety of FMT in the indication of MDD. A total of 15 participants were included in the sample consisting of adults diagnosed with moderate and severe MDD, 10 of whom received stool enema containing healthy microbiota, and five of whom received only enema (placebo group). According to the study results, it was concluded that FMT treatment could potentially lead to improvements in gastrointestinal symptoms and quality of life in individuals with MDD and IBS. No serious complications were reported after the procedure. It can be said that FMT applied via colonoscopy has a satisfactory level of safety and tolerance [172]. Although the sample size is small, preliminary findings suggest that FMT is a valid, satisfactory, well-tolerated, and safe treatment option for individuals diagnosed with MDD.

One of the new terms added to the literature is "postbiotic". If the components secreted by microbiota microorganisms or the microbe's own components are molecules that are beneficial for the host, they are called postbiotic [173]. This definition is different from the definition of "prebiotic", which refers to nutrients that beneficial microorganisms must consume in order to survive. These nonliving microbial components perform functions such as modulation of resident intestinal microorganisms, intestinal barrier integrity, optimization of local and systemic immune response, organization of systemic metabolic response, and regulation of the central nervous system [173].

Closely related to the concept of postbiotics are bioactive metabolites produced by bacteria during microbial fermentation processes. These metabolites contribute to the probiotic activity of foods such as sauerkraut, kombucha, kefir, and yogurt. These fermentation products include vitamins (such as B vitamins), bioactive peptides (such as lactotripeptides), bacteriocins (which help bacteria survive), short-chain fatty acids (such as butyric acid), and neurotransmitters (such as gamma-aminobutyric acid/GABA and serotonin) [174]. These postbiotic metabolites are neuroactive and have a direct positive effect on mental health [175,176].

Postbiotics also cause mild changes in the composition of the gut microbiota that improves socialization in healthy mice and has a potential anxiolytic effect [177]. In rodent models, postbiotic use prevented [178] and ameliorated [41,179,180] depression and anxiety-like behaviors. Two RCTs were conducted on its effectiveness in humans. In these studies, postbiotic supplementation in medical students during exam periods reported improvements in general health, sleep, and gastrointestinal symptoms. But anxiety and depression scores did not change [181,182]. However, the possibility of using fermented foods therapeutically in mood and anxiety disorders is still important. Further research is needed to determine the effects of fermented foods on brain structure and function.

We have touched upon published articles in our chapter. In addition, there are ongoing clinical studies. According to www.clinicaltrials.gov records, studies on depression (NCT04805879), obsessive-compulsive disorder (NCT05720793), attention-deficit/hyperactivity disorder (NCT06376331), bipolar affective disorder (NCT03279224), and anorexia nervosa (NCT05834010) are ongoing [183].

7.7 POTENTIAL RESPONSE TO TREATMENT

It is exciting to use the gut microbiome to uncover new horizons for precise medicine strategies. Microbiota research holds great promise for the field of neuropsychiatry. Differences in gut microbiome composition, particularly in individuals with mood disorders, are frequently reported [14]. Data from large populations also point to a relationship between the gut microbiome and quality of life and depression. A clinical study conducted on a female sample found similar results in those diagnosed with MDD compared to healthy volunteers [184]. According to this study, increased rates of *Escherichia*, *Shigella*, and *Alistipes* bacterial families in MDD may cause inflammatory effects [184].

In general, most studies examining differences in gut microbiome composition between those with and without mood disorders have only focused on differences between taxa, whereas different strains within a taxon may have opposing functions [185]. Data along these lines make the already complex microbiota puzzle even more difficult to interpret. Moreover, mood disorders do not have a monoblock homogeneous structure from a clinical perspective. These diseases have a highly heterogeneous appearance due to multifactorial etiopathogenesis. Therefore, it is probably not rational to recommend a single probiotic treatment for depression or another neuropsychiatric disorder. However, perhaps different treatment approaches designed to be "personalized", such as psychotherapy or therapeutic drug monitoring (TDM) approaches, can be discussed [186].

In addition, there is no biomarker that can be considered as "signature of depression" yet. In order to find the possibility of using probiotics or FMT in the treatment of depression, it may be necessary to determine the gut microbiome profiles of patients in order to define individual risks and predict treatment responses. In this direction, efforts are currently being made to determine the gut microbiome composition of individuals in order to predict chemotherapeutic and antibiotic responses [184,185]. In fact, many studies have observed differences in the composition of the core gut microbiome between individuals with MDD who respond to antidepressant treatment and those who do not. Furthermore, changes in the composition of the gut bacteriome have also been reported after initiation of psychotropic drug treatment in MDD [186]. We cannot see this as a surprising result because the antibiotic activity of antidepressants is a known fact [187].

We have previously stated that there are interactions between psychiatric drugs and the gut microbiome. The gut bacteriome affects the bioavailability and metabolism of drugs [188–191]. Considering that psychiatric drugs have antimicrobial effects, it can be understood how complex the interaction is.

In fact, drugs are perhaps one of the factors that most confound the composition of the gut microbiome [192–195]. Therefore, medication use (non-drug-naive sample) is a very important confounding factor in clinical trials of microbiome-modulating treatments in psychiatry. However, understanding how psychotropic medications may affect microbiome-targeting adjunctive therapies such as probiotics or FMT may provide critical information that improves therapeutic success. Thus, if the role of gut microbes in mediating individual variability in drug response is better understood, a step forward in clarifying personalized dosage recommendations can be achieved.

7.8 CONCLUSION

In recent years, detailed research opportunities have developed and the number of studies on the gut-brain axis has increased significantly. In this way, the bidirectional interaction between microbiota-immune system-psychotropics and neuronal functions will become clearer day by day. If the mechanisms underlying mental health and disorders are better understood, methods of modulating microbiota composition (probiotics and FMT) will also make more sense. Intestinal microbiota is involved in all stages from etiopathogenesis to treatment of all neuropsychiatric disorders, especially depression. In addition, antidepressant drugs also have microbiota-mediated activities. However, perhaps the most important obstacle in front of us is ethics because the Food and Drug Administration (FDA) has not yet licensed FMT for use in the treatment of any neuropsychiatric disorders. This situation makes it difficult to conduct research on FMT. However, there are relatively fewer difficulties in animal experiments. There are more studies in the open literature testing the effectiveness of probiotics compared to FMT. Although these studies do not produce very consistent results, preliminary data indicate that microbiota-based treatment applications may be used in the treatment of neuropsychiatric disorders. More RCTs with large samples are needed in this area to make more definitive comments. Of course, the therapeutic approach will be shaped after these interpretations.

REFERENCES

1. Köknel O. At the fiftieth anniversary the history of modern psychopharmacology and psychopharmacological researches in Turkey and in the world. *Bulletin Clin Psychopharmacol.* 2002;12:201–10.
2. Macht DL. Contributions to psychopharmacology. *Johns Hopkins Hospital Bulletin.* 1920;31:167–73.
3. Ban TA. Fifty years chlorpromazine: A historical perspective. *Neuropsychiatric Dis Treat.* 2007;3:495–500.
4. Ban TA. Pharmacotherapy of mental illness: A historical analysis. *Prog Neuropsychopharmacol Biol Psychiatry.* 2001;25:709–27.
5. Kuhn TS. *The Structure of Scientific Revolutions.* University of Chicago Press: Chicago, 1962.
6. Schramm E, Klein DN, Elsaesser M, Furukawa TA, Domschke K. Review of dysthymia and persistent depressive disorder: History, correlates, and clinical implications. *Lancet Psychiatry.* 2020;7:801–12.
7. Monroe SM, Harkness KL. Major depression and its recurrences: Life course matters. *Annu Rev Clin Psychol.* 2022;18:329–57.
8. Kelly JR, Kennedy PJ, Cryan JF, Dinan TG, Clarke G, Hyland NP. Breaking down the barriers: The gut microbiome, intestinal permeability and stress-related psychiatric disorders. *Front Cell Neurosci.* 2015;9:392.
9. Xi C, Li A, Lai J et al. Brain-gut microbiota multimodal predictive model in patients with bipolar depression. *J Affect Disord.* 2023;323:140–52.
10. Agirman G, Yu KB, Hsiao EY. Signaling inflammation across the gut-brain axis. *Science.* 2021;374:1087–92.
11. Mayer EA, Nance K, Chen S. The gut-brain axis. *Annu Rev Med.* 2022;73:439–53.
12. Hashimoto K. Molecular mechanisms of the rapid-acting and long-lasting antidepressant actions of (R)-ketamine. *Biochem Pharmacol.* 2020;177:113935.

13. McGuinness AJ, Davis JA, Dawson SL et al. A systematic review of gut microbiota composition in observational studies of major depressive disorder, bipolar disorder and schizophrenia. *Mol Psychiatry.* 2022;27:1920–35.
14. Nikolova VL, Smith MRB, Hall LJ, Cleare AJ, Stone JM, Young AH. Perturbations in gut microbiota composition in psychiatric disorders: A review and meta-analysis. *JAMA Psychiatry.* 2021;78:1343–54.
15. Simpson CA, Diaz-Arteche C, Eliby D, Schwartz OS, Simmons JG, Cowan CSM. The gut microbiota in anxiety and depression: A systematic review. *Clin Psychol Rev* 2021;83:101943.
16. Tian P, Chen Y, Zhu H et al. Bifidobacterium breve CCFM1025 attenuates major depression disorder via regulating gut microbiome and tryptophan metabolism: A randomized clinical trial. *Brain Behav Immunity* 2022;100:233–41.
17. Bisgaard TH, Allin KH, Keefer L, Ananthakrishnan AN, Jess T. Depression and anxiety in inflammatory bowel disease: Epidemiology, mechanisms and treatment. *Nat Rev Gastroenterol Hepatol.* 2022;19:717–26.
18. Chang L, Wei Y, Hashimoto K. Brain-gut-microbiota axis in depression: A historical overview and future directions. *Brain Res Bull.* 2022;182:44–56.
19. Cryan JF, O'Riordan KJ, Cowan CSM et al. The microbiota-gut-brain axis. *Physiol Rev.* 2019;99:1877–2013.
20. Blacher E, Bashiardes S, Shapiro H et al. Potential roles of gut microbiome and metabolites in modulating ALS in mice. *Nature.* 2019;572:474–80.
21. Foster JA. Modulating brain function with microbiota. *Science.* 2022;376(6596):936–37.
22. Needham BD, Adame MD, Serena G et al. Plasma and fecal metabolite profiles in autism spectrum disorder. *Biol Psychiatry.* 2021;89:451–62.
23. Needham BD, Funabashi M, Adame MD et al. A gut-derived metabolite alters brain activity and anxiety behaviour in mice. *Nature.* 2022;602:647–53.
24. Neufeld KM, Kang N, Bienenstock J, Foster JA. Reduced anxiety-like behavior and central neurochemical change in germ-free mice. *Neurogastroenterol Motil.* 2011;23:255–64.
25. Ortega MA, Alvarez-Mon MA, Garcia-Montero C et al. Microbiota-gut-brain axis mechanisms in the complex network of bipolar disorders: Potential clinical implications and translational opportunities. *Mol Psychiatry.* 2023;28:2645–73.
26. Evrensel A, Ünsalver BÖ, Ceylan ME. Immune-kynurenine pathways and the gut microbiota-brain axis in anxiety disorders. *Adv Exp Med Biol.* 2020;1191:155–67.
27. Rao C, Coyte KZ, Bainter W, Geha RS, Martin CR, Rakoff-Nahoum S. Multi-kingdom ecological drivers of microbiota assembly in preterm infants. *Nature.* 2021; 591:633–38.
28. Evrensel A. Probiotics and fecal microbiota transplantation in major depression: Doxa or episteme? *Adv Exp Med Biol.* 2024;1456:67–83.
29. Cao Z, Sugimura N, Burgermeister E, Ebert MP, Zuo T, Lan P. The gut virome: A new microbiome component in health and disease. *EBioMedicine.* 2022;81:104113.
30. Liang G, Bushman FD. The human virome: Assembly, composition and host interactions. *Nat Rev Microbiol.* 2021;19:514–27.
31. Shkoporov AN, Hill C. Bacteriophages of the human gut: The "known unknown" of the microbiome. *Cell Host Microbe.* 2019;25:195–209.
32. Dutilh BE, Cassman N, McNair K et al. A highly abundant bacteriophage discovered in the unknown sequences of human faecal metagenomes. *Nat Commun.* 2014;5:4498.
33. Guerin E, Shkoporov A, Stockdale SR et al. Biology and taxonomy of crass-like bacteriophages, the most abundant virus in the human gut. *Cell Host Microbe.* 2018;24:653–64.
34. Gregory AC, Zablocki O, Zayed AA, Howell A, Bolduc B, Sullivan MB. The gut virome database reveals age-dependent patterns of virome diversity in the human gut. *Cell Host Microbe.* 2020;28:724–40.

35. De Sordi L, Lourenço M, Debarbieux L. The battle within: Interactions of bacteriophages and bacteria in the gastrointestinal tract. *Cell Host Microbe.* 2019;25:210–18.
36. Duan J, Wang W, Jiang T, Bai X, Liu C. Viral metagenomics combined with metabolomics reveals the role of gut viruses in mouse model of depression. *Front Microbiol.* 2022;13:1046894.
37. Wu J, Chai T, Zhang H et al. Changes in gut viral and bacterial species correlate with altered 1,2-diacylglyceride levels and structure in the prefrontal cortex in a depression-like non-human primate model. *Transl Psychiatry.* 2022;12:74.
38. Yang J, Zheng P, Li Y et al. Landscapes of bacterial and metabolic signatures and their interaction in major depressive disorders. *Sci Adv.* 2020;6:eaba8555.
39. Popescu M, Van Belleghem JD, Khosravi A, Bollyky PL. Bacteriophages and the immune system. *Annu Rev Virol.* 2021;8:415–35.
40. Foster JA, Baker GB, Dursun SM. The relationship between the gut microbiome-immune system-brain axis and major depressive disorder. *Front Neurol.* 2021;12:721126.
41. Zhang F, Aschenbrenner D, Yoo JY, Zuo T. The gut mycobiome in health, disease, and clinical applications in association with the gut bacterial microbiome assembly. *Lancet Microbe.* 2022;3:e969–83.
42. Richard ML, Sokol H. The gut mycobiota: Insights into analysis, environmental interactions and role in gastrointestinal diseases. *Nat Rev Gastroenterol Hepatol.* 16:331–345.
43. Schei K, Avershina E, Oien T, Rudi K et al. Early gut mycobiota and mother-offspring transfer. *Microbiome.* 2017;5:107.
44. Shuai M, Fu Y, Zhong HL et al. Mapping the human gut mycobiome in middle-aged and elderly adults: Multiomics insights and implications for host metabolic health. *Gut.* 2022;71:1812–20.
45. Szostak N, Handschuh L, Samelak-Czajka A, Tomela K, Schmidt M, Pruss L et al. Host factors associated with gut mycobiome structure. *mSystems.* 2023;8:e0098622.
46. Cattane N, Räikkönen K, Anniverno R et al. Depression, obesity and their comorbidity during pregnancy: Effects on the offspring's mental and physical health. *Mol Psychiatry.* 2021;26:462–81.
47. Gutierrez MW, Mercer EM, Moossavi S et al. Maturational patterns of the infant gut mycobiome are associated with early-life body mass index. *Cell Rep Med.* 2023;4:100928.
48. Nash AK, Auchtung TA, Wong MC et al. The gut mycobiome of the Human Microbiome Project healthy cohort. *Microbiome.* 2017;5:153.
49. Bodecker-Zingmark L, Widbom L, Hultdin J, Eriksson C, Karling P. Anti-saccharomyces cerevisiae antibodies are only modestly more common in subjects later developing Crohn's disease. *Dig Dis Sci.* 2023;68:608–15.
50. Chandrakumar A, Georgy M, Agarwal P, 't Jong GW, El-Matary W. Anti-saccharomyces cerevisiae antibodies as a prognostic biomarker in children with Crohn disease. *J Pediatr Gastroenterol Nutr.* 2019;69:82–87.
51. Benjamin J, Makharia GK, Joshi YK. Association between intestinal permeability and anti-Saccharomyces cerevisiae antibodies in patients with Crohn's disease. *Inflammatory Bowel Diseases.* 2008;14:1610.
52. Vermeire S, Peeters M, Vlietinck R et al. Anti-Saccharomyces cerevisiae antibodies (ASCA), phenotypes of IBD, and intestinal permeability: A study in IBD families. *Inflamm Bowel Dis.* 2001;7:8–15.
53. Chen Y, Zhang LY, Fang Y et al. Elevated serum anti-Saccharomyces cerevisiae antibody accompanied by gut mycobiota dysbiosis as a biomarker of diagnosis in patients with de novo Parkinson disease. *Eur J Neurol.* 2023;30:3462–70.
54. Severance EG, Alaedini A, Yang S et al. Gastrointestinal inflammation and associated immune activation in schizophrenia. *Schizophr Res.* 2012;138:48–53.
55. Severance EG, Gressitt KL, Yang S et al. Seroreactive marker for inflammatory bowel disease and associations with antibodies to dietary proteins in bipolar disorder. *Bipolar Disord.* 2014;16:230–40.

56. Jiang HY, Pan LY, Zhang X, Zhang Z, Zhou YY, Ruan B. Altered gut bacterial-fungal interkingdom networks in patients with current depressive episode. *Brain Behav.* 2020;10:e01677.
57. Zhang Y, Liang H, Wang Y et al. Heat-inactivated Lacticaseibacillus paracasei N1115 alleviates the damage due to brain function caused by long term antibiotic cocktail exposure in mice. *BMC Neurosci.* 2022;23:38.
58. Eme L, Doolittle WF. Archaea. Curr Biol. 2015;25:R851–5.
59. Thomas CM, Desmond-Le Quemener E, Gribaldo S, Borrel G. Factors shaping the abundance and diversity of the gut archaeome across the animal kingdom. *Nat Commun.* 2022;13:3358.
60. Kim JY, Whon TW, Lim MY et al. The human gut archaeome: Identification of diverse haloarchaea in Korean subjects. *Microbiome.* 2020;8:114.
61. Bai X, Sun Y, Li Y et al. Landscape of the gut archaeome in association with geography, ethnicity, urbanization, and diet in the Chinese population. *Microbiome.* 2022;10:147.
62. Chibani CM, Mahnert A, Borrel G et al. A catalogue of 1,167 genomes from the human gut archaeome. *Nat Microbiol.* 2022:7:48–61.
63. Ortega MA, Alvarez-Mon MA, Garcia-Montero C et al. Gut microbiota metabolites in major depressive disorder-deep insights into their pathophysiological role and potential translational applications. *Metabolites.* 2022;12:50.
64. Ramezani A, Nolin TD, Barrows IR et al. Gut colonization with methanogenic archaea lowers plasma trimethylamine n-oxide concentrations in apolipoprotein e-/- mice. *Sci Rep.* 2018;8:14752.
65. Liu L, Wang H, Chen X, Zhang Y, Zhang H, Xie P. Gut microbiota and its metabolites in depression: From pathogenesis to treatment. *EBioMedicine.* 2023;90:104527.
66. Chabe M, Lokmer A, Segurel L. Gut protozoa: Friends or foes of the human gut microbiota? *Trends Parasitol.* 2017;33:925–34.
67. Ianiro G, Iorio A, Porcari S et al. How the gut parasitome affects human health. *Therap Adv Gastroenterol.* 2022;15:17562848221091524.
68. Bach JF. The hygiene hypothesis in autoimmunity: The role of pathogens and commensals. *Nat Rev Immunol.* 2018;18:105–20.
69. Stensvold CR, van der Giezen M. Associations between gut microbiota and common luminal intestinal parasites. *Trends Parasitol.* 2018;34:369–77.
70. Abdoli A, Mirzaian Ardakani H. Potential application of helminth therapy for resolution of neuroinflammation in neuropsychiatric disorders. *Metab Brain Dis.* 2020;35:95–110.
71. Wammes LJ, Mpairwe H, Elliott AM, Yazdanbakhsh M. Helminth therapy or elimination: Epidemiological, immunological, and clinical considerations. *Lancet Infect Dis.* 2014;14:1150–62.
72. Liu J, Morey RA, Wilson JK, Parker W. Practices and outcomes of self-treatment with helminths based on physicians' observations. *J Helminthol.* 2017;91:267–77.
73. Lampard-Scotford AR, McCauley A, Kuebel JA, Ibbott R, Mutapi F. Impact of parasitic infection on mental health and illness in humans in Africa: A systematic review. *Parasitology.* 2022;149:1003–18.
74. Lin HC, Huang KY, Chung CH et al. Infection with Trichomonas vaginalis increases the risk of psychiatric disorders in women: A nationwide population-based cohort study. *Parasit Vectors.* 2019;12:88.
75. Camarillo-Guerrero LF, Almeida A, Rangel-Pineros G, Finn RD, Lawley TD. Massive expansion of human gut bacteriophage diversity. *Cell.* 2021;184:1098–1109.
76. Nayfach S, Paez-Espino D, Call L et al. Metagenomic compendium of 189,680 DNA viruses from the human gut microbiome. *Nat Microbiol.* 2021;6:960–70.
77. Marzano V, Mancinelli L, Bracaglia G et al. "Omic" investigations of protozoa and worms for a deeper understanding of the human gut "parasitome". *PLoS Negl Trop Dis.* 2017;11:e0005916.

78. Kastl AJ, Jr., Terry NA, Wu GD, Albenberg LG. The structure and function of the human small intestinal microbiota: Current understanding and future directions. *Cell Mol Gastroenterol Hepatol.* 2020;9:33–45.
79. Zoetendal EG, Raes J, van den Bogert B et al. The human small intestinal microbiota is driven by rapid uptake and conversion of simple carbohydrates. *ISME J.* 2012;6:1415–26.
80. Martinez-Guryn K, Leone V, Chang EB. Regional diversity of the gastrointestinal microbiome. *Cell Host Microbe.* 2019;26:314–24.
81. Angelakis E, Armougom F, Carriere F et al. A metagenomic investigation of the duodenal microbiota reveals links with obesity. *PLoS One.* 2015;10:e0137784.
82. Saffouri GB, Shields-Cutler RR, Chen J et al. Small intestinal microbial dysbiosis underlies symptoms associated with functional gastrointestinal disorders. *Nat Commun.* 2019;10:2012.
83. Lassale C, Batty GD, Baghdadli A et al. Healthy dietary indices and risk of depressive outcomes: A systematic review and meta-analysis of observational studies. *Mol Psychiatry.* 2019;24:965–86.
84. Nicolaou M, Colpo M, Vermeulen E et al. Association of a priori dietary patterns with depressive symptoms: A harmonised meta-analysis of observational studies. *Psychol Med.* 2020;50:1872–83.
85. Firth J, Marx W, Dash S et al. The effects of dietary improvement on symptoms of depression and anxiety: A meta-analysis of randomized controlled trials. *Psychosom Med.* 2019;81:265–80.
86. Bayes J, Schloss J, Sibbritt D. The effect of a Mediterranean diet on the symptoms of depression in young males (the "AMMEND: A mediterranean diet in MEN with depression" study): A randomized controlled trial. *Am J Clin Nutr.* 2022;116:572–80.
87. Jacka FN, O'Neil A, Opie R et al. A randomised controlled trial of dietary improvement for adults with major depression (the 'SMILES' trial). *BMC Med.* 2017;15:23.
88. Jacka FN, Pasco JA, Mykletun A et al. Diet quality in bipolar disorder in a population-based sample of women. *J Affect Disord.* 2011;129:332–37.
89. Gabriel FC, Oliveira M, Martella BM et al. Nutrition and bipolar disorder: A systematic review. *Nutr Neurosci.* 2023;26:637–51.
90. Wilson AS, Koller KR, Ramaboli MC et al. Diet and the human gut microbiome: An international review. *Dig Dis Sci.* 2020;65:723–40.
91. Ghosh TS, Rampelli S, Jeffery IB et al. Mediterranean diet intervention alters the gut microbiome in older people reducing frailty and improving health status: The NU-AGE 1-year dietary intervention across five European countries. *Gut.* 2020;69:1218–28.
92. Marx W, Lane M, Hockey M et al. Diet and depression: Exploring the biological mechanisms of action. *Mol Psychiatry.* 2021;26:134–50.
93. Dewhirst FE, Chen T, Izard J et al. The human oral microbiome. *J Bacteriol.* 2010;192:5002–17.
94. Adler CJ, Dobney K, Weyrich LS et al. Sequencing ancient calcified dental plaque shows changes in oral microbiota with dietary shifts of the Neolithic and Industrial revolutions. *Nature Genetics.* 2013;45:450–55.
95. Nearing Jacob T, DeClercq V, Van Limbergen J, Langille Morgan GI. Assessing the variation within the oral microbiome of healthy adults. *mSphere.* 2020;5:e00451.
96. Wade WG. Resilience of the oral microbiome. *Periodontal.* 2000. 2021;86:113–22.
97. Sedghi L, DiMassa V, Harrington A, Lynch SV, Kapila YL. The oral microbiome: Role of key organisms and complex networks in oral health and disease. *Periodontol.* 2000. 2021;87:107–31.
98. Simpson CA, Adler C, du Plessis MR et al. Oral microbiome composition, but not diversity, is associated with adolescent anxiety and depression symptoms. *Physiol Behav.* 2020;226:113126.

99. Wingfield B, Lapsley C, McDowell A et al. Variations in the oral microbiome are associated with depression in young adults. *Sci Rep.* 2021;11:15009.
100. Cunha FA, Cota LOM, Cortelli SC et al. Periodontal condition and levels of bacteria associated with periodontitis in individuals with bipolar affective disorders: A case-control study. *J Periodontal Res.* 2019;54:63–72.
101. Kleinstein SE, Nelson KE, Freire M. Inflammatory networks linking oral microbiome with systemic health and disease. *J Dent Res.* 2020;99:1131–39.
102. Kristensson K. Microbes' roadmap to neurons. *Nat Rev Neurosci.* 2011;12:345–57.
103. Loughman A, Adler CJ, Macpherson H. Unlocking modifiable risk factors for Alzheimer's disease: Does the oral microbiome hold some of the keys? *J Alzheimer's Dis.* 2023;92:1111–29.
104. Scassellati C, Marizzoni M, Cattane N et al. The complex molecular picture of gut and oral microbiota-brain-depression system: What we know and what we need to know. *Front Psychiatry.* 2021;12:722335.
105. Khan Mirzaei M, Xue J, Costa R et al. Challenges of studying the human virome: Relevant emerging technologies. *Trends Microbiol.* 2021;29:171–81.
106. Mahnert A, Blohs M, Pausan MR, Moissl-Eichinger C. The human archaeome: Methodological pitfalls and knowledge gaps. *Emerg Top Life Sci.* 2018;2:469–82.
107. Thielemann N, Herz M, Kurzai O, Martin R. Analyzing the human gut mycobiome. A short guide for beginners. *Comput Struct Biotechnol J.* 2022;20:608–14.
108. Mirzayi C, Renson A, Genomic Standards C et al. Reporting guidelines for human microbiome research: The STORMS checklist. *Nat Med.* 2021;27:1885–92.
109. Evrensel A, Ceylan ME. Fecal microbiota transplantation and its usage in neuropsychiatric disorders. *Clin Psychopharmacol Neurosci.* 2016;14(3):231–37.
110. Vindigni SM, Surawicz CM. Fecal microbiota transplantation. *Gastroenterol Clinics North Am.* 2017;46(1):171–85.
111. Zhang F, Luo W, Shi Y, Fan Z, Ji G. Should we standardize the 1,700-year-old fecal microbiota transplantation? *Am J Gastroenterol.* 2012;107(11):1755.
112. Borody TJ, Warren EF, Leis SM, Surace R, Ashman O, Siarakas S. Bacteriotherapy using fecal flora: Toying with human motions. *J Clin Gastroenterol.* 2004;38(6):475–83.
113. Smits LP, Bouter KE, de Vos WM, Borody TJ, Nieuwdorp M. Therapeutic potential of fecal microbiota transplantation. *Gastroenterology.* 2013;145(5):946–53.
114. Eiseman B, Silen W, Bascom GS, Kauvar AJ. Fecal enema as an adjunct in the treatment of pseudomembranous enterocolitis. *Surgery.* 1958;44(5):854–59.
115. Bowden TA, Mansberger AR, Lykins LE. Pseudomembranous enterocolitis: Mechanism of restoring floral homeostasis. *Am Surgeon.* 1981;47(4):178–83.
116. Brandt LJ, Aroniadis OC, Mellow M Kanatzar A et al. Long-term follow-up of colonoscopic fecal microbiota transplantation for recurrent Clostridium difficile infection. *Am J Gastroenterol.* 2012;107(7):1079–87.
117. Ma Y, Liu J, Rhodes C, Nie Y, Zhang F. Ethical issues in fecal microbiota transplantation in practice. *Am J Bioethics.* 2017;17:34–45.
118. Di Bella S, Drapeau C, García-Almodóvar E, Petrosillo N. Fecal microbiota transplantation: The state of the art. *Infect Dis Rep.* 2013;5(2):e13.
119. Evrensel A, Ceylan ME. The role of fecal microbiota transplantation in psychiatric treatment. *Anadolu Psikiyatri Dergisi.* 2015;16(5):380.
120. Aroniadis OC, Brandt LJ. Fecal microbiota transplantation: Past, present and future. *Curr Opin Gastroenterol.* 2013;29(1):79–84.
121. Brandt LJ, Aroniadis OC. An overview of fecal microbiota transplantation: Techniques, indications, and outcomes. *Gastrointest Endosc.* 2013;78(2):240–49.
122. Youngster I, Gerding DN. Editorial: Making fecal microbiota transplantation easier to swallow: Freeze-dried preparation for recurrent clostridium difficile infections. *Am J Gastroenterol.* 2017;112(6):948–50.

123. Youngster I, Russell GH, Pindar C, Ziv-Baran T, Sauk J, Hohmann EL. Oral, capsulized, frozen fecal microbiota transplantation for relapsing Clostridium difficile infection. *JAMA*. 2014;312(17):1772–78.
124. Borody TJ, Brandt LJ, Paramsothy S. Therapeutic faecal microbiota transplantation: Current status and future developments. *Curr Opin Gastroenterol*. 2014;30(1):97–105.
125. Belotserkovsky I, Stabryla LM, Hunter M, Allegretti J, Callahan BJ, Carlson PE, Daschner PJ, Goudarzi M, Guyard C, Jackson SA, Rao K, Servetas SL, Sokol H, Wargo JA, Novick S. Standards for fecal microbiota transplant: Tools and therapeutic advances. *Biologicals*. 2024;86:101758.
126. Gough E, Shaikh H, Manges AR. Systematic review of intestinal microbiota transplantation (fecal bacteriotherapy) for recurrent Clostridium difficile infection. *Clin Infect Dis*. 2011;53(10):994–1002.
127. De Leon LM, Watson JB, Kelly CR. Transient flare of ulcerative colitis after fecal microbiota transplantation for recurrent Clostridium difficile infection. *Clin Gastroenterol Hepatol*. 2013;11(8):1036–38.
128. Aas J, Gessert CE, Bakken JS. Recurrent Clostridium difficile colitis: Case series involving 18 patients treated with donor stool administered via a nasogastric tube. *Clin Infect Dis*. 2003;36(5):580–85.
129. Vandenplas Y, Pierard D, De Greef E. Fecal microbiota transplantation: Just a fancy trend? *J Pediatr Gastroenterol Nutr*. 2015;61(1):4–7.
130. Evrensel A, Ceylan ME. Editorial overview: The gut microbiome: Its role in disorders of the GI tract and metabolic homeostasis. *Curr Opin Pharmacol*. 2019;49:iii–v.
131. Zhang F, Zhang T, Zhu H, Borody TJ. Evolution of fecal microbiota transplantation in methodology and ethical issues. *Curr Opin Pharmacol*. 2019;49:11–16.
132. Bakken JS, Borody T, Brandt LJ et al. Treating Clostridium difficile infection with fecal microbiota transplantation. *Clin Gastroenterol Hepatol*. 2011;9(12):1044–1049.
133. Evrensel A, Ceylan ME. The gut-brain axis: The missing link in depression. *Clin Psychopharmacol Neurosci*. 2015;13(3):239–244
134. Kubera M, Curzytek K, Duda W et al. A new animal model of (chronic) depression induced by repeated and intermittent lipopolysaccharide administration for 4 months. *Brain Behav Immunity*. 2013;31:96–104.
135. Macpherson AJ, Uhr T. Gut flora-mechanisms of regulation. *Eur J Surg Suppl*. 2002;587:3–7.
136. Desbonnet L, Garrett L, Clarke G Kiely B, Cryan JF, Dinan TG. Effects of the probiotic Bifidobacterium infantis in the maternal separation model of depression. *Neuroscience*. 2010;170(4):1179–88.
137. Dinan TG, Quigley EM. Probiotics in the treatment of depression: Science or science fiction? *Aust New Zealand J Psychiatry*. 2011;45(12):1023–25.
138. Messaoudi M, Lalonde R, Violle N et al. Assessment of psychotropic-like properties of a probiotic formulation (Lactobacillus helveticus R0052 and Bifidobacterium longum R0175) in rats and human subjects. *Br J Nutr*. 2011;105(5):755–64.
139. Messaoudi M, Violle N, Bisson JF, Desor D, Javelot H, Rougeot C. Beneficial psychological effects of a probiotic formulation (Lactobacillus helveticus R0052 and Bifidobacterium longum R0175) in healthy human volunteers. *Gut Microbes*. 2011;2(4):256–61.
140. Bruce-Keller AJ, Salbaum JM, Luo M et al. Obese-type gut microbiota induced neurobehavioral changes in the absence of obesity. *Biol Psychiatry*. 2015;77(7):607–15.
141. Hsiao EY, McBride SW, Hsien S et al. Microbiota modulate behavioral and physiological abnormalities associated with neurodevelopmental disorders. *Cell*. 2013;155(7):1451–63.
142. Finegold SM, Molitoris D, Song Y, et al. Gastrointestinal microflora studies in late-onset autism. *Clin Infect Dis*. 2002;35(Suppl 1):6–16.

143. Song Y, Liu C, Finegold SM. Real-time PCR quantitation of clostridia in feces of autistic children. *Appl Environ Microbiol.* 2004;70(11):6459–65.
144. Schwarz E, Maukonen J, Hyytiäinen T, Kieseppä T, Orešič M, Sabunciyan S, Mantere O, Saarela M, Yolken R, Suvisaari J. Analysis of microbiota in first episode psychosis identifies preliminary associations with symptom severity and treatment response. *Schizophr Res.* 2018;192:398–403.
145. Jiang H, Ling Z, Zhang Y, et al. Altered fecal microbiota composition in patients with major depressive disorder. *Brain Behav Immunity.* 2015;48:186–94.
146. Wallace CJK, Milev R. The effects of probiotics on depressive symptoms in humans: A systematic review. *Ann General Psychiatry.* 2017;16:14.
147. Zheng P, Zeng B, Zhou C et al. Gut microbiome remodeling induces depressive-like behaviors through a pathway mediated by the host's metabolism. *Mol Psychiatry.* 2016;21(6):786–96.
148. Leclercq S, de Timary P, Delzenne NM, Stärkel P. The link between inflammation, bugs, the intestine and the brain in alcohol dependence. *Transl Psychiatry.* 2017;7(2):e1048. doi:10.1038/tp.2017.15.
149. Scott KA, Ida M, Peterson VL et al. Revisiting Metchnikoff: Age-related alterations in microbiota-gut-brain axis in the mouse. *Brain Behav Immunity.* 2017;65:20–32.
150. Noble EE, Hsu TM, Kanoski SE. Gut to brain dysbiosis: Mechanisms linking western diet consumption, the microbiome, and cognitive impairment. *Front Behav Neurosc.* 2017;11:9.
151. Allen AP, Hutch W, Borre YE et al. Bifidobacterium longum 1714 as a translational psychobiotic: Modulation of stress, electrophysiology and neurocognition in healthy volunteers. *Transl Psychiatry.* 2016;6(11):e939.
152. Kelly JR, Allen AP, Temko A et al. Lost in translation? The potential psychobiotic Lactobacillus rhamnosus (JB-1) fails to modulate stress or cognitive performance in healthy male subjects. *Brain Behav Immunity.* 2017;61:50–59.
153. Jiang C, Li G, Huang P, Liu Z, Zhao B. The gut microbiota and Alzheimer's disease. *J Alzheimer's Dis.* 2017;58(1):1–15.
154. Settanni CR, Ianiro G, Bibbo S, Cammarota G, Gasbarrini A. Gut microbiota alteration and modulation in psychiatric disorders: Current evidence on fecal microbiota transplantation. *Prog Neuropsychopharmacol Biol Psychiatry.* 2021;109:110258.
155. Kuijer EJ, Steenbergen L. The microbiota-gut-brain axis in hippocampus-dependent learning and memory: Current state and future challenges. *Neurosci Biobehav Rev.* 2023;152:105296.
156. Liu Z, Chen X, Cui H et al. Green space exposure on depression and anxiety outcomes: A meta-analysis. *Environ Res.* 2023;231:116303.
157. Rutsch A, Kantsjö JB, Ronchi F. The gut-brain axis: How microbiota and host inflammasome influence brain physiology and pathology. *Front Immunol.* 2020; 10;11:604179.
158. Cai T, Zheng SP, Shi X et al. Therapeutic effect of fecal microbiota transplantation on chronic unpredictable mild stress-induced depression. *Front Cell Infect Microbiol.* 2022;12:900652.
159. Costello SP, Hughes PA, Waters O et al. Effect of fecal microbiota transplantation on 8-week remission in patients with ulcerative colitis: A randomized clinical trial. *JAMA.* 2019;321:156–64.
160. Anza S, Schneider D, Daniel R et al. The long-term gut bacterial signature of a wild primate is associated with a timing effect of pre- and postnatal maternal glucocorticoid levels. *Microbiome.* 2023;11:165.
161. Wang S, Ishima T, Qu Y et al. Ingestion of Faecalibaculum rodentium causes depression-like phenotypes in resilient Ephx2 knock-out mice: A role of brain-gut-microbiota axis via the subdiaphragmatic vagus nerve. *J Affect Disord.* 2021;292:565–73.

162. Mayneris-Perxachs J, Castells-Nobau A, Arnoriaga-Rodriguez M et al. Microbiota alterations in proline metabolism impact depression. *Cell Metab.* 2022;34:681–701.
163. Donoso F, Cryan, JF, Olavarria-Ramirez L, Nolan YM, Clarke G. Inflammation, lifestyle factors, and the microbiome-gut-brain axis: Relevance to depression and antidepressant action. *Clin Pharmacol Ther.* 2023;113:246–59.
164. Evrensel A, Tarhan KN. 2021. Emerging role of gut-microbiota-brain axis in depression and therapeutic implication. *Prog Neuropsychopharmacol Biol Psychiatry.* 2021;106:110138.
165. Cai T, Shi X, Yuan LZ, Tang D, Wang F. Fecal microbiota transplantation in an elderly patient with mental depression. *Int Psychogeriatr.* 2019;31;1525–26.
166. Doll JPK, Vazquez-Castellanos JF, Schaub AC et al. Fecal microbiota transplantation (FMT) as an adjunctive therapy for depression-case report. *Front Psychiatry.* 2022;13:815422.
167. Camilleri M. Diagnosis and treatment of irritable bowel syndrome: A review. *JAMA.* 2021;325:865–77.
168. Ford AC, Sperber AD, Corsetti M, Camilleri M. Irritable bowel syndrome. *Lancet.* 2020;396;1675–88.
169. Staudacher HM, Mikocka-Walus A, Ford AC. Common mental disorders in irritable bowel syndrome: Pathophysiology, management, and considerations for future randomised controlled trials. *Lancet Gastroenterol Hepatol.* 2021;6:401–10.
170. Guo Q, Lin H, Chen P et al. Dynamic changes of intestinal flora in patients with irritable bowel syndrome combined with anxiety and depression after oral administration of enterobacteria capsules. *Bioengineered.* 2021;12;11885–97.
171. Kilinçarslan S, Evrensel A. The effect of fecal microbiota transplantation on psychiatric symptoms among patients with inflammatory bowel disease: An experimental study. *Actas Esp Psiquiatr.* 2020;48:1–7.
172. Greer JB, Dalsky EM, Lane RF, Hansen JD. Tire-derived transformation product 6ppd-quinone induces mortality and transcriptionally disrupts vascular permeability pathways in developing coho salmon. *Environ Sci Technol.* 2023;57:10940–50.
173. Salminen S, Collado MC, Endo A et al. The International Scientific Association of Probiotics and Prebiotics (ISAPP) consensus statement on the definition and scope of postbiotics. *Nat Rev Gastroenterol Hepatol.* 2021;18:649–67.
174. Indira M, Venkateswarulu TC, Abraham Peele K, Nazneen Bobby M, Krupanidhi S. Bioactive molecules of probiotic bacteria and their mechanism of action: A review. 3 Biotech. 2019;9:306.
175. Caspani G, Kennedy S, Foster JA, Swann J. Gut microbial metabolites in depression: Understanding the biochemical mechanisms. *Microb Cell.* 2019;6:454–81.
176. Aslam H, Green J, Jacka FN et al. Fermented foods, the gut and mental health: A mechanistic overview with implications for depression and anxiety. *Nutr Neurosci.* 2020;23:659–71.
177. Warda AK, Rea K, Fitzgerald P, Hueston C, Gonzalez-Tortuero E, Dinan TG, Hill C. Heat-killed lactobacilli alter both microbiota composition and behaviour. *Behav Brain Res.* 2019;362:213–23.
178. Kosuge A, Kunisawa K, Arai S et al. Heat-sterilized Bifidobacterium breve prevents depression-like behavior and interleukin-1beta expression in mice exposed to chronic social defeat stress. *Brain Behav Immunity.* 2021;96:200–11.
179. Maehata H, Kobayashi Y, Mitsuyama E et al. Heat-killed Lactobacillus helveticus strain MCC1848 confers resilience to anxiety or depression-like symptoms caused by subchronic social defeat stress in mice. *Biosci Biotechnol Biochem.* 2019;83:1239–47.
180. Reber SO, Siebler PH, Donner NC et al. Immunization with a heat-killed preparation of the environmental bacterium Mycobacterium vaccae promotes stress resilience in mice. *Proc Natl Acad Sci USA.* 2016;113:E3130–39.

181. Nishida K, Sawada D, Kawai T, Kuwano Y, Fujiwara S, Rokutan K. Para-psychobiotic Lactobacillus gasseri CP2305 ameliorates stress-related symptoms and sleep quality. *J Appl Microbiol.* 2017;123:1561–70.
182. Nishida K, Sawada D, Kuwano Y, Tanaka H, Rokutan K. Health benefits of lactobacillus gasseri cp2305 tablets in young adults exposed to chronic stress: A randomized, double-blind, placebo-controlled study. *Nutrients.* 2019;11:1859.
183. www.clinicaltrials.gov (Accessed date 25 December 2024).
184. Heshiki Y, Vazquez-Uribe R, Li J et al. Predictable modulation of cancer treatment outcomes by the gut microbiota. *Microbiome.* 2020;8:28.
185. Rashidi A, Ebadi M, Rehman TU et al. Gut microbiota response to antibiotics is personalized and depends on baseline microbiota. *Microbiome.* 2021;9:211.
186. Dong Z, Shen X, Hao Y et al. Gut microbiome: A potential indicator for predicting treatment outcomes in major depressive disorder. *Front Neurosci.* 2022;16:813075.
187. Maier L, Pruteanu M, Kuhn M et al. Extensive impact of non-antibiotic drugs on human gut bacteria. *Nature.* 2018;555:623–28.
188. Flowers SA, Bhat S, Lee JC. Potential implications of gut microbiota in drug pharmacokinetics and bioavailability. *Pharmacotherapy.* 2020;40:704–12.
189. Cussotto S, Clarke G, Dinan TG, Cryan JF. Psychotropics and the microbiome: A chamber of secrets. *Psychopharmacology (Berl).* 2019;236:1411–32.
190. Sjostedt P, Enander J, Isung J. Serotonin reuptake inhibitors and the gut microbiome: Significance of the gut microbiome in relation to mechanism of action, treatment response, side effects, and tachyphylaxis. *Front Psychiatry.* 2021;12:682868.
191. Seeman MV. The gut microbiome and antipsychotic treatment response. *Behav Brain Res.* 2021;396:112886.
192. Eckenberger J, Butler JC, Bernstein CN, Shanahan F, Claesson MJ. Interactions between medications and the gut microbiome in inflammatory bowel disease. *Microorganisms.* 2022;10:1963.
193. Falony G, Joossens M, Vieira-Silva S et al. Population-level analysis of gut microbiome variation. *Science.* 2016;352:560–64.
194. Forslund K, Hildebrand F, Nielsen T et al. Disentangling type 2 diabetes and metformin treatment signatures in the human gut microbiota. *Nature.* 2015;528:262–6.
195. Nagata N, Nishijima S, Miyoshi-Akiyama T et al. Population-level metagenomics uncovers distinct effects of multiple medications on the human gut microbiome. *Gastroenterology.* 2022;163:1038–52.

8 Elevating Wellness
Integrating Health, Sustainability, and Urban Vitality in Tall Building Design

Kheir M. Al-Kodmany

8.1 INTRODUCTION

As cities worldwide face rapid urbanization and densification, tall buildings have become indispensable elements of the modern urban landscape. These vertical structures are no longer confined to their roles as office spaces or residential towers; they represent a convergence of architectural innovation, environmental responsibility, and urban resilience (Ali & Moon, 2007). In addressing challenges such as population growth, limited land availability, and escalating environmental pressures, tall buildings offer opportunities to redefine urban living, contributing to healthier, more sustainable, and vibrant city environments (Du et al., 2024; Emre Ilgın, 2021; Iqbal, 2021; Oldfield, 2019).

At the intersection of health and architecture, the design of tall buildings plays a transformative role in influencing occupant well-being, ecological sustainability, and urban health. By integrating principles of biophilic design, thermal comfort, and indoor air quality optimization, these structures foster physical and mental wellness, reduce stress, and encourage community engagement. Features such as sky gardens, green walls, and dynamic shading systems demonstrate how thoughtful design can harmonize human comfort with environmental stewardship (Kellert et al., 2008; Oldfield, 2017). Moreover, these buildings are not just environments for living and working but ecosystems that actively contribute to the health and vitality of their surroundings (Davern et al., 2017).

Environmental sustainability remains a cornerstone of tall building design, addressing the urgent need to combat climate change and reduce resource consumption. Innovations such as geothermal heating and cooling (Manitoba Hydro Place (MHP); Rempel et al., 2024), rainwater harvesting (Shanghai Tower; Xia et al., 2010), and energy-efficient façades (Attia, 2017; Emre Ilgın, 2021) exemplify the strides being made in minimizing ecological footprints. These features underscore the capacity of tall buildings to serve as benchmarks for resource-efficient design while advancing broader urban sustainability goals (Parker & Wood, 2013). Simultaneously,

DOI: 10.1201/9781003513834-8

urban health is elevated through strategies that integrate tall buildings into public transit networks, reduce urban heat islands (UHIs), and prioritize pedestrian-friendly environments, as seen in One World Trade Center (1WTC)'s seamless connectivity with New York's transit systems (Al-Kodmany, 2024; Lewis & Holt, 2011).

This chapter explores how tall buildings can prioritize occupant well-being, environmental sustainability, and urban health by analyzing real-world case studies such as MHP, 1WTC, Shanghai Tower, and Al Bahar Towers. These projects illustrate how innovative architectural practices can address contemporary urban challenges while setting new standards for design and functionality. Through a detailed examination of design principles and strategies, the chapter emphasizes the potential of tall buildings to serve as transformative models of sustainable, inclusive, and health-focused urban development. By aligning architectural aspirations with societal needs, tall buildings can evolve into vital contributors to resilient and equitable urban futures (Habash, 2022).

8.1.1 Purpose

This research addresses a critical gap in the literature concerning the intersection of health and the architecture of tall buildings. While extensive studies have examined technical aspects such as structural engineering, mechanical and electrical systems, vertical transportation, aesthetics, and placemaking (Parker & Wood, 2013; Gonçalves & Umakoshi, 2010), the health-centric dimensions of tall building design remain insufficiently explored. Existing discourse often emphasizes skyscrapers' technical and visual elements, overlooking their potential to actively contribute to occupant well-being, environmental sustainability, and urban health (Oldfield, 2019; Habash, 2022).

This study seeks to bridge this gap by integrating health-oriented design principles and reimagining tall buildings as holistic environments prioritizing physical and mental wellness. By exploring strategies such as biophilic integration (Kellert et al., 2008), advanced ventilation systems (Rempel et al., 2024), and urban connectivity (Davern et al., 2017), this research highlights how tall buildings can serve as critical assets in addressing urban challenges such as climate change, resource scarcity, and declining public health.

This study offers actionable insights and innovative frameworks for integrating health considerations into the design of tall buildings, contributing to a broader dialogue on sustainable and health-focused urban development. By aligning design practices with the pressing demands of urbanization and sustainability, this research underscores the transformative potential of tall buildings as models of resilience, inclusivity, and environmental stewardship (Oldfield, 2017; Al-Kodmany, 2024).

8.1.2 Goals and Objectives

This chapter investigates how tall buildings can be designed to prioritize occupant well-being, environmental sustainability, and urban health, addressing the interconnected challenges of rapid urbanization, climate change, and growing public health concerns. In an era of increasing urban density, tall buildings have the potential to transcend traditional functionality, evolving into transformative environments that foster healthier, more sustainable, and socially vibrant urban ecosystems (Al-Kodmany, 2024; Oldfield, 2019).

The research emphasizes health-focused design principles, highlighting strategies that enhance physical and mental wellness. Natural ventilation, abundant daylighting, and biophilic features such as sky gardens, green walls, and indoor plants are explored as critical components for improving indoor air quality, thermal comfort, and psychological well-being. These features demonstrate how tall buildings can create supportive environments for healthier lifestyles and stronger community connections (Habash, 2022; Oldfield, 2017).

Environmental sustainability is another cornerstone of this research, focusing on reducing the ecological footprint of tall buildings while addressing urban demands. The chapter examines the role of energy-efficient technologies, renewable energy integration, and innovative water conservation systems, demonstrating how these elements can create resource-efficient and climate-resilient structures. By adopting lifecycle sustainability approaches, tall buildings can serve as models for green design in dense urban contexts, setting new benchmarks for energy and resource efficiency (Du et al., 2015; Oldfield et al., 2009; Gonçalves & Umakoshi, 2010).

The chapter also underscores the pivotal role of tall buildings in promoting urban health. By enhancing connectivity with public transportation, improving walkability, and integrating vibrant public spaces, tall buildings can mitigate UHI effects, foster inclusive communities, and strengthen the social fabric of cities. These strategies position tall buildings as dynamic agents of urban revitalization, capable of addressing the complex intersections of human well-being, environmental sustainability, and urban development (Lewis & Holt, 2011; Parker & Wood, 2013).

By framing tall buildings as solutions to and reflections of contemporary urban challenges, this chapter provides architects, urban planners, and policymakers with actionable strategies to align tall building design with the demand for healthier and more sustainable cities. The findings emphasize the transformative potential of tall buildings to shape resilient, inclusive, and health-oriented urban futures, inspiring innovation and equity in urban development (Al-Kodmany, 2024; Parker & Wood, 2013).

8.1.3 Contextualizing Wellness and Urban Vitality in Tall Building Design

Wellness in the built environment extends beyond essential comfort to encompass holistic physical, mental, and social well-being. According to the WELL Building Standard, wellness in architecture includes optimized indoor air quality, access to natural light, biophilic design, active design elements, and thermal comfort. These factors reduce stress, enhance cognitive function, and foster healthier lifestyles within tall buildings (Kellert et al., 2008). Similarly, the International WELL Building Institute (IWBI) underscores the role of human-centric architecture in improving workplace productivity, sleep quality, and overall life satisfaction.

Biophilic design plays a significant role in wellness-oriented tall buildings. This design philosophy, which integrates natural elements such as sky gardens, green walls, and open terraces, has been shown to improve mental health, lower stress levels, and promote social connectivity (Ulrich, 1984; Kellert et al., 2008). Projects like the Shanghai Tower, which incorporates vertical sky gardens, and MHP, which features winter gardens and passive ventilation, exemplify the application of biophilic principles to enhance occupant well-being (Gong, 2017).

Indoor air quality is another critical determinant of wellness in tall buildings. The ASHRAE 62.1 Standard provides guidelines for ventilation and indoor air quality, emphasizing the importance of pollutant filtration, CO_2 monitoring, and access to fresh air. 1WTC exemplifies these principles by using 3,000 air quality sensors, ensuring continuous fresh air circulation while maintaining energy efficiency (Friedman et al., 2011).

Urban vitality refers to the degree of social interaction, economic activity, and environmental health within an urban space. Tall buildings contribute to urban vitality by promoting mixed-use environments, increasing density near transit hubs, and integrating pedestrian-friendly design. Research highlights that well-integrated tall buildings can reduce urban sprawl, enhance walkability, and create dynamic public spaces (Al-Kodmany & Ali, 2013).

Transit-oriented development (TOD) is a key driver of urban vitality. Case studies such as Shanghai Tower, directly connected to the metro system, and 1WTC, integrated with New York's extensive transit network, illustrate how tall buildings can encourage public transportation while reducing reliance on cars (Lewis & Holt, 2011). MHP has also successfully revitalized downtown Winnipeg by relocating 2,000 employees to the city core, catalyzing economic growth and social engagement (Rempel et al., 2024).

Tall buildings also reduce the UHI effect, a major environmental challenge in dense cities. Features like green roofs, permeable surfaces, and vegetative façades help to mitigate heat absorption while improving urban biodiversity (Davern et al., 2017). For instance, the Al Bahar Towers' mashrabiyya system reduces solar gain by 50%, contributing to a cooler microclimate and lowering energy demand (Attia, 2017).

8.2 METHODS: EXAMINING CASE STUDIES TO DEFINE HEALTH DESIGN PRINCIPLES FOR TALL BUILDINGS

This study employs a qualitative, case study-based methodology to extract and articulate health-centric design principles for tall buildings. Given the limited existing research on the intersection of health and architecture in the context of tall buildings, this method allows for in-depth analysis of exemplary projects to derive actionable insights. The study bridges the gap between theory and practice by focusing on real-world examples of architectural excellence, offering a robust framework for integrating health considerations into tall building design.

8.2.1 Selection of Case Studies

The selection process for case studies was rigorous, prioritizing buildings with international recognition for their innovative and health-focused designs. Criteria included:

- **Prominence and Recognition**: Only projects with international acclaim, such as awards from reputable architectural organizations and LEED certifications, were considered (Canadian Architect, 2012; SOM Architects, 2016).
- **Geographic and Cultural Diversity**: Case studies span the United States, Canada, China, and the Middle East—regions with significant skyscraper construction activity and leading urban innovation (Lewis & Holt, 2011; Gong, 2017).
- **Varied Typologies**: The case studies include a mix of office towers, mixed-use developments, and urban-integrated complexes, offering a broad perspective on design approaches across different functions and urban contexts (Parker & Wood, 2013).

This diversity ensures that the principles derived from these projects adapt to varying geographic, cultural, and environmental conditions, enhancing their applicability to various urban scenarios.

8.2.2 Analytical Framework

A structured analytical framework was developed to evaluate the selected case studies systematically. This framework focuses on three core dimensions that align with the nexus of health and architecture:

1. **Occupant Well-Being**:
    - Strategies to enhance physical and mental health, including natural ventilation, daylighting, biophilic integration, and the creation of communal spaces (Attia, 2017; Kellert et al., 2008).
    - Emphasis on occupant comfort through optimized indoor air quality, thermal regulation, and acoustic design (Habash, 2022).
2. **Environmental Sustainability**:
    - Adoption of energy-efficient systems, renewable energy technologies, and innovative water conservation measures (GhaffarianHoseini et al., 2013; Oldfield et al., 2009).
    - Assessment of material sustainability, including the use of recycled content and lifecycle considerations to minimize ecological footprints (De Wolf et al., 2017).
3. **Urban Health**:
    - Exploration of tall buildings' interactions with the urban fabric, such as mitigating UHIs, enhancing connectivity, and integrating vibrant public spaces (Lewis & Holt, 2011; Al-Kodmany & Ali, 2013).
    - Consideration of their role in fostering inclusive, walkable, and transit-oriented urban environments (Du et al., 2015).

Table 8.1 presents a structured framework that outlines the essential design principles for constructing healthy tall buildings, emphasizing three fundamental dimensions:

TABLE 8.1
Design Principles for Constructing Healthy Tall Buildings

Design Principle	Strategies and Approaches
1. Design Features Promoting Health and Well-Being	
Optimized indoor air quality	• Advanced HVAC systems to monitor and regulate air quality, ensuring fresh, filtered air. • Use of low-emission materials to minimize VOCs and indoor pollutants.
Natural light and visual comfort	• Maximize natural daylight penetration while reducing glare. • Provide outdoor views to enhance mental well-being and a connection with nature.
Thermal comfort	• Adaptive thermal systems such as radiant heating and cooling. • Optimize temperature control by using dynamic shading devices, double-skin façades, and thermal buffers.
Acoustic comfort	• Soundproofing materials and designs to minimize noise pollution from both external and internal sources.
Biophilic design	• Integrate natural elements such as green walls, sky gardens, and indoor plants to reduce stress, improve air quality, and enhance aesthetics.
Active design features	• Include accessible staircases, fitness centers, and walking tracks to encourage physical activity.
Healthy materials	• Use non-toxic, hypoallergenic, and sustainable materials to promote occupant health.
Community-oriented spaces	• Create multi-use spaces like shared lounges, co-working areas, and sky gardens to foster community engagement.
2. Environmental Sustainability and Energy Efficiency	
Energy efficiency	• Incorporate renewable energy sources like solar panels and wind turbines. • Design high-performance building envelopes to minimize energy loss and reduce heating and cooling loads.
Water management	• Utilize rainwater harvesting and graywater recycling for irrigation, cooling, and non-potable uses. • Employ low-flow plumbing fixtures to reduce water consumption.
Resource efficiency	• Select materials with high recycled content and ensure responsible sourcing. • Incorporate flexible and adaptable designs to extend the building's lifespan.
Green spaces	• Design vegetative roofs and green façades to mitigate urban heat island effects, enhance biodiversity, and improve insulation.
Data-driven building management	• Use smart building systems to optimize energy use, monitor indoor air quality, and adjust lighting or temperature in real time.

(*Continued*)

TABLE 8.1 (*Continued*)
Design Principles for Constructing Healthy Tall Buildings

Design Principle	Strategies and Approaches
Sustainable construction practices	• Employ waste recycling, low-impact site preparation, and clean energy during construction to minimize environmental impacts.
	3. Urban Health and Community Revitalization
Sustainable site planning	• Position tall buildings near transit nodes and walkable urban areas to reduce car dependency. • Design pedestrian-friendly ground levels with public plazas, parks, or open spaces to promote social interaction and physical activity.
Climate responsiveness	• Tailor building designs to local climatic conditions, employing passive strategies to reduce energy consumption and improve occupant comfort.
Urban integration	• Enhance neighborhood connectivity and integrate with the streetscape at a human scale.
Disaster resilience	• Design resilient structural systems to withstand natural disasters. • Include emergency features like refuge floors, widened stairwells, and backup power systems to ensure safety.
Access to nature	• Ensure that all occupants, regardless of their location within the building, have access to green spaces, daylight, and fresh air.
Affordability and inclusivity	• Incorporate a mix of affordable and market-rate spaces to foster diversity and accessibility.

Source: Author.

Occupant Well-Being, Environmental Sustainability and Energy Efficiency, and Urban Health and Community Revitalization. These principles are based on key strategies that ensure tall buildings are functional and efficient and contribute positively to human health, environmental resilience, and urban vitality.

The first dimension, Occupant Well-Being, details strategies prioritizing indoor air quality, thermal comfort, access to natural light, and biophilic design, all crucial in enhancing physical and mental health. Measures such as advanced heating, ventilation, and air-conditioning (HVAC) filtration systems, dynamic shading devices, and the integration of indoor green spaces help mitigate stress, improve indoor environmental quality, and foster a sense of well-being. Community-oriented spaces and active design features, such as fitness centers and pedestrian-friendly staircases, also encourage physical activity and social engagement.

The second dimension, Environmental Sustainability and Energy Efficiency, focuses on minimizing the ecological footprint of tall buildings. Strategies include energy-efficient building envelopes, renewable energy integration, water conservation methods, and sustainable material sourcing. Green roofs and vegetative façades further enhance building performance by reducing the UHI effect, supporting biodiversity, and improving stormwater management. Smart building management systems (BMSs) also leverage real-time data to optimize resource consumption, ensuring long-term sustainability.

The third dimension, Urban Health and Community Revitalization, explores how tall buildings contribute to the broader urban fabric. Emphasizing sustainable site planning, climate responsiveness, disaster resilience, and accessibility, this section underscores the importance of integrating high-rise developments into walkable, transit-oriented environments. Thoughtfully designed public plazas, green corridors, and mixed-use spaces enhance social cohesion, improve pedestrian experiences, and foster urban inclusivity. Ensuring affordability and access to natural elements further supports a diverse and equitable urban ecosystem.

By organizing these principles into a clear and actionable framework, Table 8.1 serves as a practical guide for architects, planners, and policymakers seeking to design tall buildings that are sustainable and resilient and foster human-centered urban environments.

8.2.3 Methodological Approach

Each case study is dissected through a detailed examination of design features, supported by measurable data where available. Key performance indicators included energy efficiency metrics, water usage reductions, and indoor air quality improvements. The analysis also considered qualitative aspects, such as design strategies' cultural and contextual relevance and their contribution to occupant satisfaction and community engagement (Ruggiero et al., 2014; Oldfield, 2017).

By synthesizing these findings, the study identifies recurring themes and innovative approaches, forming the foundation for comprehensive design principles. These principles are intended to guide architects, planners, and policymakers in creating tall buildings that are functional, sustainable, and deeply attuned to the health and well-being of their occupants and urban environments.

8.3 CASE STUDIES

Case Study 8.1: One World Trade Center

1. OVERVIEW

1WTC, the Freedom Tower, is a powerful emblem of resilience, sustainability, and urban regeneration. Located at the heart of Lower Manhattan, it was conceived as part of the World Trade Center master plan, developed in response to the September 11, 2001, attacks, which destroyed the original Twin Towers. Rising 541 m (1,776 ft)—

a symbolic reference to the year of American independence—the 105-story skyscraper is the tallest building in the Western Hemisphere, redefining the skyline of New York City and serving as a beacon of hope and progress.

The tower is designed by Skidmore, Owings & Merrill (SOM, 2016) and integrates cutting-edge structural innovations, sustainable technologies, and occupant-centered design principles. Its architectural language balances strength and elegance, featuring a reinforced concrete core, high-performance glass façades, and a distinctive tapering form that enhances aesthetics and aerodynamics. The tower's robust structure incorporates advanced blast resistance, fireproofing, and life safety systems, making it one of the safest and most resilient skyscrapers ever constructed.

Beyond its symbolic significance, 1WTC sets new benchmarks in sustainability, achieving LEED Gold certification for its exceptional environmental performance. The building utilizes advanced energy management systems, renewable energy integration, and water conservation measures, significantly reducing its carbon footprint while enhancing operational efficiency. Its strategic location within New York's transit network promotes walkability, accessibility, and multimodal connectivity, reinforcing its role as a centerpiece of urban revitalization.

As a mixed-use skyscraper, 1WTC houses Class A office spaces, observation decks, cultural exhibits, and retail amenities, attracting millions of visitors annually. It exemplifies the future of tall buildings, demonstrating how architecture can embody symbolism, resilience, sustainability, and urban well-being in a rapidly evolving world (Glanz & Lipton, 2003; SOM Architects, 2016).

2. DESIGN FEATURES PROMOTING HEALTH AND WELL-BEING

1WTC integrates a comprehensive range of health-focused design strategies that enhance occupant well-being, indoor environmental quality, and safety. These features reflect a commitment to creating a workspace that prioritizes physical and mental health, comfort, and adaptability, setting a new standard for human-centric skyscraper design.

Abundant Natural Light for Visual Comfort and Energy Efficiency

The ultra-clear glass façade of 1WTC maximizes natural daylight penetration, significantly improving visual comfort and reducing reliance on artificial lighting. The tower's thermally interrupted curtain walls provide insulation and allow for better light diffusion, ensuring even illumination throughout interior spaces. To enhance energy efficiency, automated dimming systems adjust lighting levels in response to natural daylight availability, minimizing energy consumption while maintaining an optimal working environment (Lewis & Holt, 2011). Integrating daylighting strategies fosters circadian rhythm alignment, boosting occupant productivity, mental alertness, and overall well-being.

Optimized Indoor Air Quality through Advanced Ventilation

1WTC features an advanced air quality monitoring system to support a healthy indoor environment with over 3,000 air monitoring stations embedded throughout the building. These sensors, coupled with intelligent building software, continuously monitor carbon dioxide levels, humidity, and air pollutants, ensuring that occupants receive a constant flow of fresh, filtered air. The system automatically adjusts ventilation rates in response to indoor air conditions, reducing stale air accumulation and minimizing exposure to indoor pollutants (Friedman et al., 2011). Additionally, construction used low volatile organic compound (VOC) materials extensively, further promoting occupant respiratory health and reducing harmful chemical off-gassing.

Sustainable and Recycled Materials for a Healthier Built Environment

Sustainability is embedded in 1WTC's material selection, with 75% of construction materials sourced from recycled content. Gypsum boards, ceiling tiles, and structural steel were carefully chosen for their low environmental impact and high durability, reducing the building's embodied carbon footprint. Additionally, all wood products used in the tower's interiors were certified by the Forest Stewardship Council (FSC), ensuring responsible forestry practices. By prioritizing eco-friendly materials, the tower enhances environmental sustainability and fosters healthier indoor spaces with minimal off-gassing and toxicity.

Enhanced Tenant Safety, Emergency Preparedness, and Spatial Flexibility

1WTC incorporates state-of-the-art safety measures, ensuring tenant security and emergency preparedness. The column-free interior layouts provide maximum spatial flexibility, allowing businesses to customize and adapt office configurations to meet evolving workspace needs. In addition, pressurized stairwells and designated refuge floors are strategically designed to facilitate safe evacuation in emergencies, protecting occupants from smoke infiltration and structural hazards (Borg et al., 2003). The tower's reinforced concrete core and high-performance structural materials enhance resilience against seismic events, extreme weather, and potential security threats, making it one of the safest high-rise buildings in the world.

A Benchmark for Health-Focused Skyscraper Design

1WTC represents a pioneering model of human-centered skyscraper design, demonstrating that occupant health, safety, and environmental sustainability can coexist within a single architectural vision. The tower redefines urban high-rise living through abundant natural light, advanced air quality management, sustainable materials, and robust safety systems, offering a healthier, more adaptable, and resilient workspace for its occupants.

3. ENVIRONMENTAL SUSTAINABILITY AND ENERGY EFFICIENCY

1WTC sets a global precedent for sustainable skyscraper design, integrating cutting-edge energy systems, water conservation measures, and recycled materials to minimize its environmental footprint. These green building strategies align with contemporary climate resilience goals and contribute to long-term energy savings, carbon reduction, and responsible resource utilization.

High-Efficiency Energy Systems and Renewable Power Sources

1WTC incorporates innovative energy solutions to achieve greater efficiency and reduced environmental impact. The tower's hydrogen fuel cells generate 4.8 megawatts of on-site power, contributing to a more self-sufficient energy model and reducing dependency on traditional fossil fuels. Complementing this system, a centralized chiller plant utilizes Hudson River water for cooling, significantly lowering the tower's energy demand for air-conditioning while reducing reliance on conventional HVAC systems (Lewis & Holt, 2011). During construction, green concrete containing recycled fly ash was used, effectively lowering carbon emissions associated with cement production and enhancing the building's structural durability. This combination of high-efficiency technologies demonstrates 1WTC's commitment to sustainable energy use and resource optimization.

Comprehensive Water Management and Conservation Strategies

Water conservation is a core aspect of 1WTC's sustainability framework, reflecting a commitment to efficient resource utilization and urban resilience. The building integrates a large-scale rainwater harvesting system, collecting up to 1.2 m (4 ft) of annual rainfall. This harvested water is then used to support critical building functions, including cooling operations, landscape irrigation, and fire suppression systems, reducing demand for municipal water supplies. Additionally, low-flow plumbing fixtures are installed throughout the tower, cutting water consumption by 30% compared to conventional high-rise buildings. These innovative water management strategies significantly lower wastewater output, ensuring that 1WTC operates as an environmentally responsible urban landmark.

Sustainable and Recycled Construction Materials

1WTC emphasizes responsible material sourcing to minimize its embodied carbon footprint and environmental impact. Approximately 75% of the construction materials used in the tower consist of recycled content, including gypsum boards, ceiling tiles, and structural steel. This approach reduces reliance on virgin raw materials, helping preserve natural resources and enhancing material durability. Furthermore, all wood products used in the building's interior spaces were certified by the FSC, ensuring adherence to responsible forestry practices. By prioritizing recycled and eco-friendly materials, 1WTC demonstrates how sustainable construction can seamlessly integrate into high-rise developments without compromising structural integrity or occupant experience.

4. URBAN HEALTH AND COMMUNITY REVITALIZATION

Integration of Green Spaces for Public Well-Being

1WTC is surrounded by an expansive urban plaza featuring over 400 locally sourced trees, offering a serene and accessible green environment in the heart of Lower Manhattan. These public green spaces serve as urban sanctuaries, providing city dwellers with relaxation, social interaction, and mental restoration opportunities.

Additionally, incorporating green roofs enhances the building's environmental performance, improving insulation, reducing energy consumption, and adding to the visual appeal of the skyline. These efforts significantly mitigate the UHI effect, creating a healthier and more comfortable urban environment (Friedman et al., 2011).

TOD and Sustainable Mobility

One of 1WTC's most impactful contributions to urban health is its seamless integration with public transportation networks. The tower is situated within the World Trade Center Transportation Hub and is directly connected to the PATH train system, multiple subway lines, and regional transit services. This ensures efficient, car-free mobility for thousands of commuters daily. By promoting mass transit over private vehicle use, 1WTC plays a crucial role in reducing traffic congestion, lowering greenhouse gas emissions, and improving overall air quality in the city. This sustainable transit approach not only enhances accessibility but also encourages a healthier, pedestrian-friendly urban environment.

Economic Renewal and Commercial Revitalization

Beyond its architectural and environmental contributions, 1WTC catalyzes economic growth, helping to revitalize Lower Manhattan's commercial sector. As a Class A office space, it has attracted global businesses, financial institutions, and technology firms, solidifying its role as a leading corporate hub. The tower's premium retail spaces, cultural venues, and public amenities have further boosted economic activity, drawing visitors, professionals, and tourists to the area. This commercial resurgence has created new job opportunities, increased foot traffic, and fostered a vibrant, 24/7 urban environment, reinforcing the long-term economic sustainability of the district (Borg et al., 2003).

5. AWARDS AND RECOGNITION

1WTC has earned several prestigious accolades for its architectural innovation, sustainability, and resilience:

- **LEED Gold Certification**: Awarded by the U.S. Green Building Council for its exemplary sustainable design and construction practices, making it the tallest LEED-certified building in the Western Hemisphere.
- **Award of Excellence (10-Year Award, 2024)**: Recognized by the Council on Tall Buildings and Urban Habitat (CTBUH) for its enduring significance and performance a decade after completion.
- **IDEAS Award, Presidential Award of Excellence in Engineering (2014)**: Presented by the American Institute of Steel Construction (AISC) for innovative use of structural steel.
- **New Construction of the Year (2014)**: Awarded by the Building Owners and Managers Association (BOMA) of New York for excellence in new construction.

6. CONCLUSION

1WTC stands as a testament to the transformative power of architecture to enhance health, sustainability, and urban vitality. The tower represents resilience and renewal by incorporating occupant-focused features, cutting-edge energy-efficient systems,

TABLE 8.2
One World Trade Center Case Study Summary

Category	Key Features
1. Design features promoting health and well-being	• **Abundant Natural Light**: Ultra-clear glass façade and thermally interrupted curtain walls optimize daylight penetration and energy efficiency. • **Enhanced Air Quality**: 3,000 air monitoring stations regulate carbon dioxide levels; low-VOC materials enhance indoor air quality. • **Sustainable Materials**: 75% recycled content in construction materials, including gypsum boards and ceiling tiles. • **Tenant Safety and Flexibility**: Column-free interior layouts provide adaptable spaces; pressurized stairwells and designated refuge floors enhance emergency safety.
2. Environmental sustainability and energy efficiency	• **Energy Efficiency**: Hydrogen fuel cells generate 4.8 MW of power; Hudson River water used for cooling to reduce energy demand. • **Water Management**: Rainwater harvesting system collects 1.2 m of rainfall annually for irrigation, cooling, and fire protection; low-flow plumbing fixtures reduce water consumption by 30%. • **Recycled Materials**: 75% recycled content in construction; all wood products FSC certified for sustainability.
3. Urban health and community revitalization	• **Green Spaces**: The plaza surrounding 1WTC features over 400 locally sourced trees, mitigating the urban heat island effect and enhancing urban aesthetics. • **Transit-Oriented Development**: Seamless integration with transit networks, including the World Trade Center Transportation Hub and PATH terminal, promoting sustainable commuting. • **Economic Renewal**: Revitalized Lower Manhattan's economy by attracting businesses, providing Class A office spaces, and fostering local community growth.

Source: Author.

and vibrant community-centric spaces. Its innovative design sets a benchmark for future urban development and underscores architecture's role in addressing contemporary urban challenges (Table 8.2). As a beacon of hope, innovation, and environmental responsibility, 1WTC exemplifies the potential of sustainable urban architecture (Glanz & Lipton, 2003; SOM Architects, 2016).

Case Study 8.2: Manitoba Hydro Place

1. OVERVIEW

MHP is a landmark in sustainable high-rise design, redefining how architecture can prioritize occupant well-being, environmental sustainability, and urban health. Located in downtown Winnipeg, Canada, the 21-story, 115-m (377-ft) tower serves as the headquarters of Manitoba Hydro, the province's most prominent energy utility. Uniquely positioned in a city known for its extreme climate conditions, where temperatures fluctuate between –35°C and +34°C (–31°F to +95°F), the building was meticulously designed to operate efficiently in all seasons, using passive design principles and climate-responsive strategies.

Completed in 2009, MHP is recognized as Canada's first large office tower to achieve LEED Platinum certification, establishing itself as a global model for energy-efficient, health-focused urban design. It was developed through an innovative collaboration between Kuwabara Payne McKenna Blumberg Architects (KPMB) in Toronto, Smith Carter Architects and Engineers in Winnipeg, and Transsolar Klima-Engineering, a Germany-based sustainability consultant. The project integrates biophilic design, passive ventilation, geothermal energy, and advanced building automation, setting a new precedent for high-performance workspaces.

MHP's vision extends beyond sustainability; it fosters community engagement, urban renewal, and employee wellness. Designed as an open, transparent, and highly connected workplace, the tower features narrow floor plates, extensive glazing, and winter gardens, ensuring occupants receive maximum daylight and natural ventilation. A solar chimney and automated louvers regulate indoor temperatures year-round, minimizing energy consumption while enhancing comfort. Geothermal heating and cooling, radiant slab technology, and a high-efficiency façade contribute to a 70% reduction in energy use compared to conventional office buildings.

Beyond the workplace, MHP is transformative in downtown Winnipeg's revitalization. The relocation of nearly 2,000 employees from suburban offices has reinvigorated local businesses, cultural spaces, and transit infrastructure. With publicly accessible winter gardens, pedestrian skywalks, and transit-friendly planning, the building represents a holistic approach to urban sustainability, ensuring it not only functions efficiently but also enhances the social and environmental fabric of its surrounding cityscape (ArchDaily, 2009; Canadian Architect, 2012; Rempel et al., 2024).

2. DESIGN FEATURES PROMOTING HEALTH AND WELL-BEING

MHP exemplifies a human-centric design approach, where daylight optimization, passive ventilation, biophilic integration, and thermal comfort systems create a healthy and productive indoor environment. These features enhance occupant well-being while reinforcing the building's commitment to sustainability and urban revitalization.

Maximizing Natural Light for Circadian Health and Energy Efficiency

The architectural design of MHP prioritizes daylight penetration, ensuring that no workspace is more than 9 m (30 ft) away from a window. This strategic design, coupled with high ceilings and floor-to-ceiling glazing, allows for abundant natural light to flood interior spaces, significantly reducing the need for artificial lighting (ArchDaily, 2009). Beyond energy savings, this approach enhances circadian rhythm regulation, improving occupant alertness, productivity, and overall well-being. Research has shown that access to natural daylight reduces eye strain and fatigue, contributing to a healthier indoor work environment (Werbicki, 2019).

Optimizing Indoor Air Quality through Passive Ventilation

MHP integrates an advanced passive ventilation system, enhancing indoor air quality and thermal comfort while minimizing reliance on mechanical HVAC systems. The solar chimney, operable windows, and winter gardens function as a natural air exchange system, continuously drawing fresh air into the building and expelling stale air. This design optimizes airflow and reduces the buildup of carbon dioxide and indoor pollutants, creating a healthier, oxygen-rich work environment (Canadian Architect, 2012).

Biophilic Design: Enhancing Well-Being through Natural Elements

Incorporating biophilic elements, MHP integrates indoor winter gardens featuring 24-m (78-ft) waterfalls, serving as aesthetic and functional components of the building's health-oriented design. These green spaces act as evaporative cooling systems, improving humidity levels, reducing stress, and enhancing mental well-being. Research highlights the psychological benefits of exposure to nature, demonstrating that greenery in workspaces leads to lower stress levels, increased creativity, and improved cognitive performance (Rempel et al., 2024). Additionally, these gardens offer employees a visually stimulating and restorative environment, reinforcing the integration of nature within a high-rise setting, even in Winnipeg's extreme winter climate.

Advanced Thermal Comfort through Geothermal and Radiant Systems

MHP utilizes a state-of-the-art geothermal exchange system comprising 280 boreholes extending 125 m (400 ft) underground, ensuring stable indoor temperatures year-round. This system efficiently captures and redistributes thermal energy, maintaining optimal temperature conditions during harsh winters and hot summers (Rempe et al., 2024). Furthermore, radiant heating and cooling systems embedded within concrete slabs provide even temperature distribution, eliminating localized thermal discomfort while reducing the energy loads of traditional forced-air systems.

Dynamic Shading and Glare Control for Visual and Thermal Comfort

To enhance occupant comfort and energy efficiency further, MHP incorporates automated louver shading systems that adjust to sunlight levels, minimizing glare and heat gain. These dynamic shading devices regulate interior lighting conditions, ensuring visual comfort for occupants while reducing cooling energy demands (Werbicki, 2019). Balancing solar exposure and shading supports an optimal indoor environment, allowing employees to work in naturally lit spaces without the discomfort of excessive brightness or overheating.

3. ENVIRONMENTAL SUSTAINABILITY AND ENERGY EFFICIENCY

MHP sets a global benchmark for sustainable high-rise office design, achieving over 70% energy savings compared to conventional office towers. The building minimizes its carbon footprint by integrating geothermal energy, passive ventilation, green roofs, and advanced energy management systems while ensuring long-term energy efficiency and environmental resilience.

Geothermal Exchange System: A Net-Zero Energy Approach

An advanced geothermal exchange system is at the core of MHP's sustainability strategy, responsible for providing 50% of the building's heating needs and 100% of its cooling requirements. The system consists of 280 underground boreholes drilled 125 m (400 ft), where thermal energy is stored and exchanged between seasons. During winter, heat is extracted from the ground to warm indoor spaces, while in summer, excess heat is dissipated back into the ground, achieving a net-zero energy exchange (ArchDaily, 2009). This low-energy, high-efficiency heating and cooling solution significantly reduces reliance on fossil fuels, lowering operational costs and greenhouse gas emissions.

Solar Chimney: Enhancing Passive Ventilation and Energy Savings

MHP's most iconic sustainability feature is its solar chimney, which is designed to enhance natural ventilation and reduce the need for mechanical air-conditioning. The solar chimney utilizes thermal dynamics to create a continuous airflow system, where warm indoor air rises and exits through the chimney, drawing in fresh, cooler air at lower levels. In winter, this system also functions as a passive solar heating mechanism, preheating incoming air before entering the building, thus reducing heating loads and overall energy demand (Building, 2009). This strategy improves indoor air quality while substantially cutting down energy consumption for heating and cooling.

Green Roofs: Mitigating the UHI Effect

MHP incorporates extensive green roofs planted with native prairie vegetation, which serve multiple environmental functions. These vegetative surfaces provide additional insulation, reducing heating and cooling demands by minimizing winter heat loss and reducing summer heat absorption. Additionally, green roofs improve stormwater management, absorbing excess rainfall and reducing strain on municipal drainage systems. By filtering airborne pollutants, these rooftop gardens contribute to better air quality and mitigate the UHI effect, making Winnipeg's downtown core more climate-resilient (Canadian Architect, 2012).

Advanced Energy Management: Optimizing Performance in Real Time

MHP employs a sophisticated BMS that continuously monitors and optimizes energy performance. This system integrates real-time data analysis to adjust HVAC, lighting, and shading controls, ensuring optimal energy efficiency without compromising occupant comfort. For example, the automated louver system responds to daylight intensity, reducing artificial lighting needs while maintaining comfortable indoor temperatures. Similarly, HVAC operations are fine-tuned based on occupancy levels and external weather conditions, preventing wasted energy and enhancing indoor climate control (Rempel et al., 2003).

4. URBAN HEALTH AND COMMUNITY REVITALIZATION

MHP catalyzes urban renewal, fostering economic revitalization, improved transit accessibility, public engagement, and minimal environmental disruption. By relocating employees, integrating public transportation, and creating dynamic community spaces, MHP strengthens Winnipeg's downtown core, demonstrating how sustainable architecture can contribute to broader urban health and connectivity.

Employee Integration: Revitalizing Downtown Economy

MHP's strategic decision to relocate nearly 2,000 employees from suburban offices to downtown Winnipeg has played a pivotal role in rejuvenating the local economy. The project has boosted economic activity by concentrating on the workforce in the city center, driving demand for local businesses, restaurants, retail shops, and services. The increased foot traffic has revitalized street life, enhancing safety and vibrancy in the downtown area while reinforcing Winnipeg's commitment to mixed-use, sustainable urban growth (Rempel et al., 2024).

Transit Accessibility: Reducing Car Dependency and Emissions

MHP is strategically positioned along major bus routes, making it a model for TOD. The building promotes public transportation, with 68% of its workforce commuting via transit, significantly reducing congestion and private vehicle reliance. This shift has cut carbon emissions, alleviated traffic burdens, and reinforced the importance of sustainable commuting in urban centers. By prioritizing pedestrian and transit access, MHP exemplifies how large-scale office developments can align with climate-conscious urban policies (Werbicki, 2019).

Public Spaces: Enhancing Social Interaction and Cultural Engagement

MHP's commitment to public engagement is evident in its three-story atrium and skywalk connection, which seamlessly link the tower with Winnipeg's existing pedestrian infrastructure. This protected, climate-controlled network facilitates year-round pedestrian mobility, particularly during Winnipeg's harsh winters. The atrium functions as a cultural and community hub, offering space for public events, exhibitions, and social interactions. This integration of shared urban spaces within a commercial high-rise promotes a sense of community and placemaking, reinforcing the building's role as more than just an office tower, but a dynamic part of the city fabric (ArchDaily, 2009).

Minimal Environmental Impact: Preserving the Urban Landscape

MHP's height and streamlined design were meticulously planned to minimize environmental disruptions to the surrounding urban environment. Unlike conventional high-rise structures that can cast oversized shadows and generate wind tunnels, MHP was designed to ensure minimal shading and wind impact on adjacent buildings and public spaces. The adjacent Air Canada Plaza remains well-lit and pedestrian-friendly, allowing continued enjoyment of public outdoor spaces without adverse microclimatic effects. This sensitive approach to high-rise development highlights how large office towers can coexist harmoniously within an urban setting (Building, 2009).

Transforming Winnipeg's Urban Fabric

By reintegrating the workforce into the downtown core, fostering transit accessibility, creating shared public spaces, and maintaining a sensitive urban footprint, MHP demonstrates how tall buildings can contribute positively to urban health and community revitalization. Its pedestrian-friendly design, commitment to public interaction, and focus on reducing environmental impact serve as a model for future urban developments, reinforcing the idea that sustainable high-rises can actively enhance the cities in which they reside.

5. AWARDS AND RECOGNITIONS

MHP has garnered significant recognition for its innovative design and commitment to sustainability, including:

- **LEED Platinum Certification (2012)**: The Canada Green Building Council certified MHP as Canada's first large office tower to achieve LEED Platinum (Canadian Architect, 2012).
- **Best Tall Building Americas Award (2009)**: CTBUH awarded MHP for its site-specific, sustainable design (Building, 2009).
- **AIA COTE Top Ten Green Projects (2010)**: Recognized for environmental performance and design excellence.
- **RAIC National Urban Design Award (2010)**: Awarded for its urban design contributions (Canadian Architect, 2012).
- **ArchDaily Building of the Year—Office Category (2009)**: Honored for its architectural innovation (ArchDaily, 2009).
- **SAB Canadian Green Building Award (2010)**: Celebrated for exemplary sustainable design (Building, 2009).
- **Engineers Canada National Project Achievement Award (2010)**: Recognized for engineering excellence in design and construction (Rempel et al., 2003).
- **Consulting Engineers of Manitoba Keystone Award (2010)**: Awarded for outstanding engineering achievements in Manitoba.

These awards underscore MHP's role as a benchmark in sustainable design and its impact on advancing green building practices in North America.

6. CONCLUSION

MHP is a model of how tall buildings can integrate health, sustainability, and urban revitalization. By incorporating biophilic design, advanced climate-responsive systems, and energy-efficient strategies, MHP meets occupant needs and transforms Winnipeg's urban landscape. This case study demonstrates the transformative potential of sustainable architecture in creating healthier, more resilient cities (Table 8.3).

TABLE 8.3
Manitoba Hydro Place (MHP) Case Study Summary

Category	Key Features
1. Design features promoting health and well-being	1. **Daylight Optimization**: Narrow floor plates, high ceilings, and floor-to-ceiling glazing enhance natural light penetration. 2. **Indoor Air Quality and Passive Ventilation**: Solar chimney, operable windows, and winter gardens improve air quality and ventilation. 3. **Biophilic Elements**: Indoor winter gardens with 24-m waterfalls enhance mental well-being. 4. **Thermal Comfort**: Geothermal system with 280 boreholes ensures stable indoor temperatures. 5. **Dynamic Shading and Glare Control**: Automated louver shading systems optimize lighting and reduce energy use.
2. Environmental sustainability and energy efficiency	1. **Geothermal Exchange System**: Provides 50% of heating and 100% of cooling through a net-zero energy exchange system. 2. **Solar Chimney**: Supports natural ventilation and reduces energy demand. 3. **Green Roofs**: Native prairie plants enhance stormwater management and insulation. 4. **Energy Management**: Advanced BMS optimizes HVAC, lighting, and shading systems in real time.
3. Urban health and community revitalization	1. **Employee Integration**: Relocated 2,000 employees to downtown, stimulating local businesses. 2. **Transit Accessibility**: 68% of employees commute via transit, reducing emissions. 3. **Public Spaces**: A three-story gallery connects to Winnipeg's skywalk system for pedestrian-friendly movement. 4. **Minimal Environmental Impact**: Streamlined design ensures minimal shading and wind impact on nearby buildings.

Source: Author.

Case Study 8.3: Shanghai Tower

1. OVERVIEW

The Shanghai Tower, a LEED Platinum-certified skyscraper, is a pinnacle of architectural innovation, redefining sustainability, occupant well-being, and urban vitality in high-density environments. Soaring to 632 m (2,073 ft) across 128 floors, it is China's tallest building and the second tallest globally, reinforcing Shanghai's status as a global financial and architectural hub. The tower is the final component of Lujiazui's iconic supertall trio, alongside the Jin Mao Tower and Shanghai World Financial Center, anchoring the Lujiazui Finance and Trade Zone. This district has undergone a remarkable transformation into a high-density, mixed-use urban hub (Xia et al., 2010).

Designed by Gensler, the Shanghai Tower symbolizes forward-thinking skyscraper development, prioritizing energy efficiency, vertical urbanism, and human-centered design. Its twisting, asymmetrical form reduces wind loads by 24%, decreasing structural demands and material use. The tower incorporates nine stacked vertical zones, creating self-contained neighborhoods that enhance community interaction and well-being—an innovative approach to redefining urban density and live-work integration (Gong, 2017).

The double-skin façade (DSF), an engineering marvel, creates a thermal buffer zone that improves insulation, reduces energy consumption, and enhances indoor air quality. Smart BMSs, harvesting rainwater, and wind turbines further reinforce its commitment to low-carbon urban development. The tower achieves 21% energy savings compared to ASHRAE standards, setting a global benchmark for sustainable supertall buildings (Parker & Wood, 2013).

Beyond its architectural and environmental achievements, the Shanghai Tower embodies urban integration and connectivity. It is directly linked to Shanghai Metro's Line 2, reducing vehicular congestion and promoting TOD. Publicly accessible sky gardens, cultural venues, and a high-rise atrium contribute to a vibrant, inclusive urban environment, enhancing the livability and sustainability of high-rise cities. Through its innovative approach to healthy urbanism, the Shanghai Tower represents the future of sustainable high-density development (Xia et al., 2010; Gong, 2017).

2. DESIGN FEATURES PROMOTING HEALTH AND WELL-BEING

Shanghai Tower exemplifies human-centric skyscraper design, integrating biophilic elements, innovative façade systems, and vertical neighborhoods to enhance occupant health, comfort, and well-being. By prioritizing natural ventilation, daylight access, and community-driven spaces, the tower creates an optimal indoor environment that supports physical and mental wellness while maintaining high energy efficiency.

Vertical Neighborhoods and Sky Gardens: Enhancing Community and Biophilic Wellness

Shanghai Tower is divided into nine distinct vertical neighborhoods, each comprising 12–15 floors, functioning as self-sufficient urban clusters within the supertall structure. This innovative vertical zoning strategy fosters community and social connectivity among occupants, mitigating the potential isolation in large commercial buildings.

At the core of these vertical communities are sky gardens, designed to emulate traditional Chinese courtyards, which historically served as spaces for social interaction, relaxation, and environmental balance. These elevated green spaces provide aesthetic and psychological benefits and serve functional roles in improving indoor air quality and enhancing thermal comfort. They introduce fresh air, abundant natural light, and natural shading, promoting mental well-being, stress reduction, and overall occupant satisfaction. This biophilic approach reaffirms that greenery within tall buildings is not just a luxury but a necessity for long-term wellness and sustainability (Al-Kodmany & Ali, 2013).

Optimized Indoor Environments: Advanced Façade and Natural Ventilation

A key feature of Shanghai Tower's occupant wellness strategy is its DSF, a high-performance climate-responsive system. Unlike conventional high-rise enclosures, the DSF consists of two glass layers—an inner circular façade and an outer twisting skin—creating a dynamic air buffer zone between them. This space naturally insulates the building, significantly reducing temperature fluctuations and energy consumption while ensuring a more stable and comfortable indoor climate.

Additionally, the DSF enables natural ventilation, a rarity in supertall structures. Air is preconditioned and filtered as it moves through the façade's ventilation pathways, reducing reliance on mechanical HVAC systems. This process ensures continuous fresh air circulation, improves indoor air quality, and minimizes airborne pollutants, contributing to a healthier workspace with enhanced respiratory benefits. By integrating passive cooling and ventilation strategies, Shanghai Tower exemplifies how skyscrapers can operate sustainably without compromising indoor comfort (Xia et al., 2010).

3. ENVIRONMENTAL SUSTAINABILITY AND ENERGY EFFICIENCY

Shanghai Tower is a global model for sustainable skyscraper design, integrating advanced energy systems, water conservation strategies, and material sustainability practices. The tower reduces energy consumption by 21% compared to ASHRAE standards, demonstrating its commitment to environmental responsibility while maintaining high-performance efficiency in a dense urban context (Gong, 2017).

Energy Efficiency and Renewable Energy: Harnessing Wind and Cogeneration Systems

Shanghai Tower employs cutting-edge renewable energy solutions, reducing grid dependency and carbon emissions. Wind turbines strategically installed beneath the parapet harness wind energy at high altitudes, generating power for the upper floors and ensuring on-site renewable energy production.

The building also features a 2,130 kW natural gas-fired cogeneration system, which provides electricity and heating, significantly improving energy efficiency. This combined heat and power (CHP) system ensures optimized fuel utilization, reducing energy waste and operational costs. By integrating renewable and efficient energy solutions, Shanghai Tower exemplifies how supertall buildings can achieve high-performance sustainability while maintaining occupant comfort.

Water Conservation: Maximizing Efficiency through Rainwater Harvesting

Water efficiency is a cornerstone of Shanghai Tower's sustainability strategy. The building incorporates a rainwater harvesting system, which reduces water consumption by 38%. This system captures and stores rainwater, redistributing it for irrigation, air-conditioning, and flushing systems.

By reusing water in essential building functions, Shanghai Tower significantly reduces potable water demand, contributing to sustainable urban water management. This approach conserves vital resources and aligns with global best practices for water efficiency in high-rise developments.

Material Sustainability: Reducing Carbon Footprint through Responsible Sourcing

Shanghai Tower adheres to a sustainable material selection process, prioritizing locally sourced and high-recycled-content materials. The project minimizes transportation-related carbon emissions by sourcing materials from regional suppliers, reinforcing environmental stewardship.

Additionally, using high-recycled-content materials, including structural steel, glass, and concrete, further reduces the tower's embodied carbon footprint. These sustainable construction methods support regional economies while ensuring long-term resource efficiency, setting a precedent for future skyscraper developments (Parker & Wood, 2013).

4. URBAN HEALTH AND COMMUNITY REVITALIZATION

Shanghai Tower redefines urban connectivity and environmental integration, contributing to healthier, more sustainable cityscapes. The tower actively supports urban health and revitalization by incorporating green spaces, efficient transit access, and a vertical city model, reinforcing Shanghai's global stature as a leading metropolis.

Green Spaces: Enhancing Air Quality and Urban Well-Being

Shanghai Tower integrates extensive landscaped gardens, connecting urban dwellers with nature in an otherwise dense city environment. These green spaces serve as natural air purifiers, mitigating the UHI effect, absorbing pollutants, and improving air quality.

Beyond environmental benefits, these areas offer tranquil retreats for occupants and visitors, fostering mental well-being, reducing stress, and encouraging social interaction. The strategic placement of these green zones within and around the tower ensures that nature remains an integral component of Shanghai Tower's urban presence (Gong, 2017).

TOD: Encouraging Sustainable Mobility

Positioned in Shanghai's Lujiazui Financial District, Shanghai Tower is seamlessly integrated into the city's extensive mass transit network. Direct access to metro stations, bus routes, and pedestrian pathways reduces automobile dependency, effectively lowering traffic congestion and minimizing urban air pollution.

By prioritizing public transit accessibility, the tower actively supports sustainable commuting practices, encouraging occupants and visitors to opt for eco-friendly travel modes. This TOD approach aligns with global efforts to create more pedestrian-friendly, less car-dependent urban centers.

Vertical City Concept: A Multi-Functional Urban Ecosystem

Shanghai Tower exemplifies the "city within a city" concept, consolidating offices, hotels, retail outlets, cultural venues, and entertainment spaces into one interconnected environment. This multifunctional approach maximizes land use efficiency, ensuring the tower minimizes urban sprawl while enhancing user convenience.

By integrating diverse functions within its vertical structure, the tower fosters a dynamic, self-sustaining urban ecosystem where occupants live, work, and engage with their surroundings in a single high-rise environment. This model enhances urban vibrancy and supports a more sustainable and efficient urban development paradigm (Al-Kodmany & Ali, 2013).

5. AWARDS AND RECOGNITION

The Shanghai Tower has received numerous accolades for its innovative design, sustainability, and occupant-focused features:

- **LEED Platinum Certification**: Recognized for outstanding sustainability strategies and environmental performance.
- **Best Tall Building Worldwide (2016)**: Awarded by the CTBUH.
- **Green Building Award (China)**: Honored by the China Green Building Council for integrating innovative green technologies.
- **Emporis Skyscraper Award (2015)**: Ranked among the world's top skyscrapers for design excellence and sustainability.
- **Shanghai Municipal Green Building Award**: Celebrated for contributing to local green architecture initiatives.

6. CONCLUSION

The Shanghai Tower exemplifies how supertall buildings can prioritize health, sustainability, and urban vitality (Table 8.4). The tower redefines its relationship with the urban context by integrating biophilic design, green technologies, and cultural references. Its innovative features, commitment to occupant well-being, and environmental stewardship establish the Shanghai Tower as a global benchmark for sustainable, human-centered skyscraper design (Xia et al., 2010; Gong, 2017).

TABLE 8.4
Shanghai Tower Case Study Summary

Category	Key Features
1. Design features promoting health and well-being	• **Vertical Neighborhoods and Sky Gardens**: Nine vertical neighborhoods, each spanning 12–15 floors, enhance community engagement and connectivity. Sky gardens, inspired by traditional Chinese courtyards, provide fresh air, natural light, and greenery, promoting mental well-being and improving thermal comfort and air quality (Al-Kodmany & Ali, 2013). • **Optimized Indoor Environments**: Double-skin façade (DSF) with inner circular and outer twisting layers enhances air quality and moderates temperature fluctuations. Natural ventilation pathways precondition and filter incoming air, reducing reliance on mechanical systems (Xia et al., 2010).

(Continued)

TABLE 8.4 (*Continued*)
Shanghai Tower Case Study Summary

Category	Key Features
2. Environmental sustainability and energy efficiency	• **Energy Efficiency and Renewable Energy**: Wind turbines beneath the parapet generate power for the upper floors, while a 2,130 kW natural gas-fired cogeneration system provides electricity and heat. • **Water Conservation**: Rainwater harvesting systems reduce water consumption by 38%, supplying irrigation, air-conditioning, and flushing systems. • **Material Sustainability**: Locally sourced materials with high recycled content minimize the building's carbon footprint and support regional economies, aligning with sustainable construction practices (Parker & Wood, 2013).
3. Urban health and community revitalization	• **Green Spaces**: Landscaped gardens enhance air quality, mitigate urban heat island effects, and provide tranquil spaces for relaxation (Gong, 2017). • **Transit-Oriented Development**: Strategic location near mass transit systems reduces private vehicle reliance, alleviates congestion, and lowers air pollution. • **Vertical City Concept**: The tower consolidates offices, hotels, retail, and cultural venues into a multifunctional hub, maximizing land use efficiency, minimizing urban sprawl, and fostering vibrant urban environments (Al-Kodmany & Ali, 2013).

Source: Author.

Case Study 8.4: Al Bahar Towers

1. OVERVIEW

The Al Bahar Towers, home to the Abu Dhabi Investment Council, stand as a pioneering example of how architectural innovation can harmonize tradition, sustainability, and human well-being. Completed in 2012, these twin 25-story towers rise 150 m (490 ft) above Abu Dhabi Island, covering 70,000 m^2 (753,000 ft^2) of office space. The towers redefine climate-responsive architecture in hot, arid regions by merging Islamic architectural traditions with cutting-edge environmental technologies, creating a benchmark for sustainable and occupant-focused design (Attia, 2017; Al-Kodmany, 2014).

Designed by Aedas Architects, the towers are distinguished by their dynamic mashrabiyya façade, a modern interpretation of traditional Islamic shading screens. This adaptive system, composed of 2,000 polytetrafluoroethylene (PTFE) umbrella-like units, automatically adjusts to sunlight, reducing solar glare and heat gain by 50% while maintaining natural daylighting and thermal comfort. This bioclimatic innovation minimizes the reliance on artificial cooling systems, significantly enhancing energy efficiency and reducing carbon emissions in alignment with Abu Dhabi's 2030 vision for sustainable development (Attia, 2017; Liu, 2016).

Beyond energy efficiency, Al Bahar Towers prioritize occupant health and well-being. The façade design balances daylight penetration, improving visual comfort and productivity while offering panoramic views of the Arabian Gulf and Eastern Mangroves. The high-performance glazing and DSF further enhance thermal regulation, reducing UHI effects. Advanced mechanical ventilation systems optimize indoor air quality, ensuring a healthy workspace while minimizing indoor pollutants (Al-Kodmany, 2014; El-Amrousi & Biln, 2013).

The towers also play a crucial role in urban health and connectivity by promoting walkability and sustainable urban mobility. Located in a mixed-use district with direct access to public transportation and pedestrian pathways, they encourage low-carbon commuting and reduced reliance on private vehicles. With their LEED Silver certification, photovoltaic integration, and smart environmental controls, Al Bahar Towers serve as a model for climate-adaptive, health-centered, and culturally responsive skyscraper design in the Middle East and beyond (El-Amrousi & Biln, 2013; Liu, 2016)

2. DESIGN FEATURES PROMOTING HEALTH AND WELL-BEING

Al Bahar Towers exemplify a health-centric approach to high-rise architecture by integrating climate-responsive innovations and culturally inspired design elements. Situated in the extreme desert climate of Abu Dhabi, the towers prioritize occupant well-being through dynamic shading, optimized daylighting, and advanced air quality systems. These features improve thermal comfort and enhance psychological well-being, making the towers a model for sustainable, human-centered design.

Dynamic Façade for Thermal Comfort and Visual Appeal

A defining feature of Al Bahar Towers is the modernized mashrabiyya system, an adaptive shading mechanism inspired by traditional Islamic architecture. This dynamic façade comprises 2,000 PTFE umbrella-like units that automatically adjust in response to sunlight. The intelligent solar control system significantly reduces solar glare and heat gain, ensuring interior spaces remain comfortable despite the region's high temperatures. This system enhances energy efficiency by minimizing reliance on mechanical cooling while maintaining a visual connection to the urban landscape. The innovative façade is a functional necessity in Abu Dhabi's climate and a tribute to the region's architectural heritage, demonstrating how traditional design principles can be successfully reinterpreted for modern skyscrapers.

Optimized Natural Light and Views

Natural lighting and access to expansive views are fundamental to the well-being of building occupants, and Al Bahar Towers excel in both aspects. The mashrabiyya system strategically balances daylight penetration with shading, ensuring that workspaces are illuminated with natural light without excessive heat gain. This approach minimizes the need for artificial lighting, contributing to energy savings while fostering a more vibrant and visually stimulating indoor environment. The towers' strategic orientation offers panoramic views of the Eastern Mangroves and the Arabian Gulf, reinforcing a connection to nature. Research indicates that exposure to natural light and outdoor scenery enhances mental well-being, improves cognitive function, and supports healthy circadian rhythms, making these design features essential to occupant health.

Indoor Air Quality

Indoor air quality is another critical consideration, particularly in high-rise office environments where prolonged exposure to poor ventilation can impact health and productivity. Al Bahar Towers incorporate advanced mechanical ventilation systems that continuously optimize fresh air intake while maintaining energy efficiency. The efficient circulation of clean air reduces the risk of respiratory issues and minimizes the buildup of indoor pollutants. By reducing reliance on energy-intensive cooling technologies, the design also aligns with the towers' broader sustainability goals, ensuring that health and environmental responsibility go hand in hand.

By integrating climate-responsive shading, optimized daylighting, and superior air quality systems, Al Bahar Towers establish a new benchmark for occupant well-being in high-rise design. The project successfully merges traditional architectural wisdom with cutting-edge technology, creating an environment that is both culturally resonant and inherently supportive of human health. By prioritizing comfort, sustainability, and connectivity to nature, the towers serve as an exemplary model for future tall buildings in hot and arid climates.

3. ENVIRONMENTAL SUSTAINABILITY AND ENERGY EFFICIENCY

Al Bahar Towers incorporate advanced sustainability measures that redefine eco-conscious high-rise design. The towers demonstrate how architectural strategies can minimize energy consumption while enhancing environmental performance through innovative shading, renewable energy integration, and efficient BMSs. Their sustainability-driven approach aligns with Abu Dhabi's broader urban planning goals, such as the Abu Dhabi 2030 Plan, which prioritizes resource-efficient and climate-adaptive development.

Innovative Solar Control System

One of the most distinctive sustainability features of Al Bahar Towers is the mashrabiyya system, which reduces solar gain by 50%. The dynamic façade significantly lowers cooling demand by minimizing direct sunlight exposure to the building's interiors, reducing dependence on energy-intensive air-conditioning. Unlike conventional shading methods that rely on permanently tinted glass, this adaptive system allows ample natural light to enter, creating a bright yet thermally comfortable environment. By regulating indoor temperatures while preserving access to daylight, the mashrabiyya façade plays a crucial role in maintaining energy efficiency while ensuring occupant comfort.

Integration of Photovoltaic Panels

The towers enhance their energy sustainability by integrating photovoltaic panels on south-facing roofs. These solar panels generate renewable energy, which is used to power the automated mashrabiyya shading system. This feature underscores the project's commitment to sustainable energy solutions by reducing reliance on grid electricity. The strategic placement of solar panels maximizes energy harvesting potential, capitalizing on Abu Dhabi's abundant sunlight to offset operational energy consumption. This renewable energy integration highlights how passive and active energy strategies can work together to create a more self-sufficient building system.

Energy Efficiency

In addition to its shading and solar power solutions, Al Bahar Towers employ an advanced BMS that optimizes energy use across multiple functions. Automated controls regulate lighting, cooling, and shading in real time, ensuring energy consumption remains as efficient as possible. The towers' DSF further enhances thermal performance by creating a buffer zone that minimizes heat transfer between the exterior and interior spaces. High-performance glazing complements this system by reducing thermal loads and decreasing cooling requirements in the region's harsh desert climate. The seamless integration of these energy-saving measures improves operational efficiency and extends the lifespan of mechanical systems by reducing strain on heating and cooling infrastructure.

Al Bahar Towers set a new standard for environmentally responsible high-rise design through the strategic use of dynamic shading, solar energy, and intelligent building management. Their emphasis on sustainability demonstrates how adaptive architecture can respond to local climatic challenges while reducing energy consumption and carbon emissions. By merging traditional passive design principles with contemporary technological advancements, the towers serve as an exemplary model for sustainable urban development in hot and arid environments.

4. URBAN HEALTH AND COMMUNITY REVITALIZATION

Al Bahar Towers significantly contribute to urban health and community vitality by integrating cultural responsiveness, environmental sustainability, and enhanced mobility. The towers' design fosters a strong connection to the local climate and heritage while mitigating environmental stressors and promoting sustainable urban movement. As part of a mixed-use district, the towers exemplify how architecture can actively shape healthier and more livable urban environments through pedestrian-friendly planning and climate-responsive strategies.

Cultural and Climatic Responsiveness

Al Bahar Towers serve as a contemporary expression of vernacular architecture, seamlessly merging traditional design elements with modern engineering solutions. Incorporating the mashrabiyya system reflects the rich architectural traditions of the region, enhancing both cultural identity and environmental performance. By integrating passive shading techniques historically used in Middle Eastern architecture, the towers successfully bridge the past and present, creating a contextually appropriate and functionally advanced design. This commitment to cultural continuity fosters a strong sense of place, reinforcing the towers' role as an architectural landmark that respects local identity while addressing the pressing demands of modern urbanization (Attia, 2017; El-Amrousi & Biln, 2013).

Reduced UHI Effect

As part of their broader sustainability agenda, Al Bahar Towers actively contribute to reducing the UHI effect, a common issue in high-density environments. The towers' energy-efficient façade, combined with its adaptive shading system, minimizes excessive heat accumulation, lowering surrounding temperatures. This reduction in surface heat enhances occupant comfort and positively impacts the surrounding microclimate by decreasing ambient temperatures and reducing cooling energy demands. Integrating sustainable design features ensures that the towers do not exacerbate local heat retention, reinforcing their role as environmentally responsible urban structures (Attia, 2017).

Promoting Walkability and Interaction

Strategically located within a mixed-use district, Al Bahar Towers actively promote walkability and interaction, contributing to a healthier and more connected urban fabric. The towers are well-integrated with public transportation networks, offering convenient access to transit systems that encourage sustainable commuting and reduce reliance on private vehicles. Furthermore, the surrounding pedestrian pathways and accessible public spaces enhance walkability, fostering an environment where people can comfortably engage in daily activities on foot. By prioritizing pedestrian-oriented design and connectivity, the towers contribute to improved air quality, lower traffic congestion, and a more dynamic public realm. This emphasis on sustainable mobility aligns with broader urban planning strategies to create healthier, more efficient, and socially engaging cities (Liu, 2016; Al-Kodmany, 2014).

By combining cultural sensitivity, environmental responsibility, and urban connectivity, Al Bahar Towers illustrate how high-rise developments can positively influence urban health. Their holistic design approach highlights the importance of integrating traditional architectural wisdom with contemporary innovations to create vibrant, sustainable, and health-conscious urban spaces.

5. AWARDS AND RECOGNITION

Al Bahar Towers have received numerous accolades for their innovative design and sustainability:

- **LEED Silver Certification**: Recognized by the U.S. Green Building Council for integrating sustainable technologies and reducing energy consumption.
- **Best Overall Project in the Middle East (2013)**: Awarded at the Middle East Architect Awards.
- **Commercial Project of the Year (2013)**: Also recognized at the Middle East Architect Awards for excellence in commercial architecture.

- **Tall Building Innovation Award (2012)**: Presented by the CTBUH for the pioneering dynamic shading system inspired by traditional Islamic architecture.
- **Emporis Skyscraper Award—Second Place (2012)**: Honored for excellence in high-rise design.
- **International Architecture Award (2014)**: Bestowed by the Chicago Athenaeum Museum of Architecture and Design for its contribution to contemporary architecture.

6. CONCLUSION

Al Bahar Towers exemplify how architecture can enhance occupant well-being, integrate cultural heritage, and contribute to environmental and urban health. By prioritizing thermal comfort, sustainability, and cultural identity, the project sets a benchmark for resilient, health-focused urban spaces in the 21st century. The towers redefine high-rise architecture, showcasing how local traditions and advanced technologies can converge to create sustainable, community-oriented designs (Table 8.5).

TABLE 8.5
Al Bahar Towers Case Study Summary

Category	Key Features
1. Design features promoting health and well-being	• **Dynamic Façade for Thermal Comfort and Visual Appeal**: A modernized mashrabiyya system with 2,000 PTFE umbrella-like units that automatically adjust based on sunlight exposure, reducing solar glare and heat gain while maintaining visual connectivity to the urban environment (Attia, 2017; Liu, 2016). • **Optimized Natural Light and Views**: The mashrabiyya system balances daylight penetration and shade, creating well-lit interiors that minimize artificial lighting and promote mental well-being with views of Eastern Mangroves and the Arabian Gulf (Al-Kodmany, 2014; El-Amrousi & Biln, 2013). • **Indoor Air Quality**: Advanced mechanical systems optimize fresh air intake, minimizing stale air buildup and ensuring a healthy indoor environment while reducing reliance on energy-intensive cooling systems (Liu, 2016).
2. Environmental sustainability and energy efficiency	• **Innovative Solar Control System**: The dynamic mashrabiyya façade reduces solar gain by 50%, lowering energy consumption and CO_2 emissions while minimizing the need for heavily tinted glass (Attia, 2017; Liu, 2016). • **Integration of Photovoltaic Panels**: Solar panels on south-facing roofs generate renewable energy to power the façade system, reducing grid dependency (El-Amrousi & Biln, 2013). • **Energy Efficiency**: Automated systems optimize lighting, cooling, and shading. High-performance glazing and a dual-skin façade provide a thermal buffer, reducing cooling loads and supporting the Abu Dhabi 2030 Plan for energy-conscious development (Al-Kodmany, 2014; Liu, 2016).

(Continued)

TABLE 8.5 (*Continued*)
Al Bahar Towers Case Study Summary

Category	Key Features
3. Urban health and community revitalization	• **Cultural and Climatic Responsiveness**: The towers integrate vernacular architectural traditions, fostering a sense of place and community while addressing contemporary urban challenges (Attia, 2017; El-Amrousi & Biln, 2013). • **Reduced Urban Heat Island Effect**: The energy-efficient façade and shading devices lower the building's heat emissions, reducing its impact on Abu Dhabi's urban heat island effect (Attia, 2017). • **Promoting Walkability and Interaction**: Strategically located in a mixed-use district with pedestrian pathways and public transit access, the towers encourage walking, reducing vehicle reliance, emissions, and improving air quality (Liu, 2016; Al-Kodmany, 2014).

Source: Author.

8.4 DISCUSSION

The case studies explored in this chapter—MHP, 1WTC, Shanghai Tower, and Al Bahar Towers—illustrate innovative strategies for prioritizing occupant well-being, environmental sustainability, and urban health. However, alongside celebrating their achievements, a critical examination reveals opportunities for further improvement and broader lessons for architects, urban planners, and policymakers (Al-Kodmany, 2024; Habash, 2022; Oldfield, 2017).

8.4.1 Occupant Well-Being: Celebrating Strengths While Addressing Gaps

These projects showcase the potential of tall buildings to create environments that nurture physical and psychological health:

- *MHP* integrates biophilic elements like winter gardens and a solar chimney to provide fresh air, natural light, and optimal thermal comfort. However, complex passive systems such as the solar chimney require ongoing maintenance and skilled operational management, potentially straining resources in less technically capable regions (Rempel et al., 2024; Werbicki, 2019).
- *Shanghai Tower* emphasizes vertical neighborhoods and sky gardens that foster community interaction and mental well-being while enhancing air quality. Yet, the scale and exclusivity of these spaces may limit accessibility for a broader range of users, raising questions about equity in high-profile structures (Ali & Moon, 2007; Xia, Poon, & Mass, 2010; Gong, 2017).
- *1WTC* uses advanced technologies like automated air quality systems and non-toxic materials to support occupant well-being. Nevertheless, its

dependence on high-tech solutions may pose challenges related to long-term maintenance costs and technological obsolescence (Glanz & Lipton, 2003; SOM Architects, 2016).

- *Al Bahar Towers'* responsive mashrabiyya façade is culturally significant and maintains indoor comfort. However, replicating such complex systems in less resource-intensive projects could present financial and technical challenges (Attia, 2017; Al-Kodmany, 2014).

8.4.2 Environmental Sustainability: Innovations Balanced by Practical Challenges

The environmental strategies employed in these case studies align with global sustainability goals but highlight areas for refinement:

- *MHP* achieves net-zero energy exchange through geothermal heating and cooling systems, demonstrating feasibility for extreme climates. However, significant upfront investment and long payback periods may hinder adoption in less affluent regions (Canadian Architect, 2012; Habash, 2022).
- *1WTC* incorporates hydrogen fuel cells and graywater systems to reduce emissions and water consumption. However, the scalability of hydrogen fuel cells in broader urban contexts remains limited (Borg et al., 2003; SOM Architects, 2016).
- *Shanghai Tower* employs a DSF, wind turbines, and rainwater harvesting systems to reduce energy use, yet the maintenance complexity and associated costs may deter replication in developing economies (Parker & Wood, 2013; Gong, 2017).
- *Al Bahar Towers'* dynamic façade addresses regional environmental challenges but relies heavily on high-performance materials, raising concerns about embodied carbon during construction (Attia, 2017; Liu, 2016).

8.4.3 Urban Health and Connectivity: Strengthening Integration and Accessibility

Tall buildings can significantly enhance urban health by fostering connectivity and improving the public realm. The case studies highlight both successes and challenges:

- *MHP* revitalized downtown Winnipeg by relocating suburban employees, catalyzing economic activity, and reducing car dependency. However, its relatively low height (21 stories) limits its ability to contribute to urban density (Rempel et al., 2024; Werbicki, 2019).
- *1WTC* integrates seamlessly with New York's transit networks, reducing vehicular emissions and enhancing connectivity. Yet, the exclusivity of office spaces and high retail costs may hinder public accessibility (Lewis & Holt, 2011; Glanz & Lipton, 2003).
- *Shanghai Tower's* vertical neighborhoods and public spaces highlight the importance of tall buildings as integral components of urban fabrics.

However, its status as a financial hub risks overshadowing its community-centric features (Xia et al., 2010; Oldfield, 2019).

- *Al Bahar Towers* emphasize cultural and environmental responsiveness, but their mixed-use potential remains underutilized due to limited public amenities or affordable spaces (El-Amrousi & Biln, 2013; Attia, 2017).

8.4.4 Lessons for Future Design: Critique-Informed Strategies

The overarching lesson from these case studies is the necessity of a holistic and adaptable approach to tall building design. While they exemplify the potential for integrating occupant well-being, sustainability, and urban health, several recurring themes emerge (Oldfield et al., 2009; Du et al., 2015):

1. **Equity and Accessibility**: Iconic structures must balance exclusivity with inclusivity, ensuring their benefits extend beyond elite users to the broader community.
2. **Lifecycle Sustainability**: Beyond operational efficiency, future projects must prioritize reducing embodied carbon and ensuring the viability of high-tech systems over their lifespans.
3. **Context-Specific Innovations**: Localized solutions like Al Bahar Towers' mashrabiyya system or MHP's geothermal systems effectively address climatic challenges but must consider cost-efficiency and replicability.
4. **Community Integration**: Tall buildings must become extensions of the urban environment, fostering vibrant, walkable, and equitable communities rather than isolated landmarks.

By integrating these lessons into future projects, architects, urban planners, and policymakers can design tall buildings that push the boundaries of innovation while addressing urban populations and the environment's pressing needs (Al-Kodmany, 2024; Habash, 2022).

8.4.5 Balancing Sustainability with Wellness Goals in Tall Buildings

Achieving a balance between environmental sustainability and occupant wellness in tall buildings requires strategic design choices that optimize energy efficiency while maintaining high standards of comfort and well-being. However, this balance presents inevitable trade-offs:

1. **Energy Efficiency vs. Air Quality**: Many sustainability strategies prioritize reducing energy consumption by minimizing outdoor air intake to decreased heating and cooling loads. While this improves energy performance, it may compromise indoor air quality if ventilation is not properly managed (Habash, 2022). 1WTC addresses this issue by integrating smart air filtration systems that ensure a steady, clean air supply without excessive energy consumption (Friedman et al., 2011).

2. **Daylighting vs. Thermal Comfort**: Maximizing daylight penetration reduces artificial lighting demand, but excessive glass façades can increase solar heat gain. The DSF of Shanghai Tower mitigates this challenge by creating a thermal buffer zone that reduces temperature fluctuations while optimizing daylight use (Xia et al., 2010). Similarly, MHP uses automated louvers to regulate glare and indoor temperature, ensuring visual comfort and energy savings (Canadian Architect, 2012).
3. **Biophilic Features vs. Water Consumption**: Incorporating green spaces and water features enhances well-being, but these elements can increase water consumption, particularly in arid climates. Al Bahar Towers balance this trade-off by integrating rainwater harvesting systems that supply irrigation for the façade's vegetation, reducing overall water demand (El-Amrousi & Biln, 2013).
4. **Resilient Infrastructure vs. Construction Costs**: Integrating renewable energy systems, adaptive façades, and passive ventilation can increase upfront costs, potentially limiting the feasibility of these strategies in budget-constrained projects. MHP addressed this challenge by implementing a geothermal heating system, which, despite high initial costs, has resulted in long-term energy savings and lower operational expenses (Rempel et al., 2024).

8.4.6 Innovative Solutions for Aligning Sustainability with Wellness

Leading-edge solutions in innovative building technologies are bridging the gap between sustainability and wellness in tall buildings. The Internet of Things (IoT) and artificial intelligence (AI)-driven BMS enable real-time monitoring of air quality, energy use, and occupant behavior, ensuring that wellness parameters are maintained without unnecessary resource depletion (GhaffarianHoseini et al., 2013).

Modular and flexible design strategies also allow for future adaptability, ensuring that wellness features remain effective over time. The "vertical neighborhoods" concept seen in Shanghai Tower, where mixed-use zones cater to diverse social needs, exemplifies how adaptability can support long-term occupant well-being while maintaining sustainability goals (Al-Kodmany & Ali, 2013).

As cities expand vertically, a holistic approach to tall building design that integrates occupant health, energy efficiency, and urban connectivity will be critical in shaping sustainable and livable urban futures. This chapter provides a framework for architects, urban planners, and policymakers to align wellness objectives with sustainability imperatives, ensuring that tall buildings serve as resilient, inclusive, and environmentally responsible spaces.

8.5 CONCLUSIONS

Integrating occupant well-being, environmental sustainability, and urban health into the design of tall buildings represents a transformative and necessary shift in architectural practice, one that addresses the multifaceted challenges of contemporary urbanization. This chapter has explored these interconnected dimensions through the critical analysis of case studies, including MHP, 1WTC, Shanghai Tower, and Al Bahar Towers. These iconic buildings demonstrate that tall structures—often celebrated as symbols of technological progress and economic power—can also embody human-centric, culturally sensitive, and environmentally sustainable design (Al-Kodmany, 2024; Parker & Wood, 2013).

Tall buildings are uniquely positioned to tackle urban challenges such as population density, climate change, and resource scarcity. The case studies highlight innovative strategies, such as biophilic integration, advanced renewable energy systems, and responsive façades, that reduce environmental impacts while enhancing the quality of life for occupants. For instance, MHP's geothermal systems and winter gardens effectively integrate biophilic elements to improve air quality and thermal comfort (Rempel et al., 2024), while the Shanghai Tower's vertical neighborhoods and sky gardens create restorative environments that foster mental well-being (Xia, Poon, & Mass, 2010). These examples underscore that prioritizing human health and well-being is a design goal and a cornerstone of sustainable development.

Moreover, these projects emphasize the critical role of tall buildings in shaping urban health and connectivity. By integrating with public transit systems, reducing reliance on private vehicles, and contributing to the revitalization of surrounding communities, tall buildings extend their influence beyond their physical boundaries to enhance urban ecosystems. 1WTC's seamless integration with New York's transit network exemplifies how tall buildings can foster sustainable urban mobility while stimulating local economies (Lewis & Holt, 2011). Similarly, Al Bahar Towers' culturally responsive design demonstrates how tall buildings can resonate with their local context, blending modern innovation with traditional architectural elements (Attia, 2017).

However, the lessons from these projects also highlight areas for improvement. Issues such as equitable access, lifecycle sustainability, and the high costs of advanced technologies must be addressed to ensure that the benefits of tall buildings extend to broader urban populations. Future developments should prioritize reducing embodied carbon, ensuring long-term maintenance feasibility, and fostering inclusivity by integrating affordable spaces and public amenities. Context-sensitive solutions, like Al Bahar Towers' adaptive mashrabiyya façade or MHP's geothermal systems, must also be evaluated for scalability and replicability in diverse global contexts (Habash, 2022; Du et al., 2015).

The path forward requires a collaborative, interdisciplinary approach that unites architects, urban planners, engineers, policymakers, and communities. By aligning design objectives with societal goals such as equity, resilience, and environmental stewardship, tall buildings can evolve into dynamic symbols of sustainable urban living. As the case studies show, such structures are not just vertical expansions of urban form but transformative agents that redefine skylines, foster vibrant communities, and address pressing global challenges (Oldfield, 2017; Al-Kodmany & Ali, 2013).

Ultimately, the health and architecture nexus offers a robust framework for designing tall buildings that harmonize human well-being, ecological sustainability, and urban vitality. By adopting the lessons presented in this chapter, future developments can balance ambition and practicality, creating harmonious spaces where people and nature thrive. This chapter aims to inspire a new generation of tall buildings that reshape cityscapes and serve as beacons of innovation, inclusivity, and resilience in an ever-changing world.

8.6 FUTURE RESEARCH

As the intersection of health, architecture, and sustainability continues to evolve, tall buildings present significant opportunities for deeper exploration and innovation. Future research must address gaps to enhance their potential to respond to urbanization, climate change, and public health challenges.

A critical area for further study is quantifying health outcomes linked to design strategies. While features such as biophilic design, natural ventilation, and optimized air quality are known to benefit occupants, robust longitudinal data on metrics like stress reduction, productivity, and physical activity are limited (Ulrich, 1984; Kellert et al., 2008; Allen & Macomber, 2020). Additionally, comprehensive lifecycle analyses are needed to balance operational energy savings with embodied carbon and the long-term environmental impacts of materials and systems (Oldfield et al., 2009; De Wolf et al., 2017).

Adapting tall buildings for climate resilience is another priority. Studies on materials and adaptive systems that address extreme weather conditions can mitigate climate risks (McGregor & Coley, 2018; Guan et al., 2020). Innovative technologies, including IoT and AI-driven systems, can optimize energy use and occupant comfort while introducing new challenges like data privacy (Habash, 2022; GhaffarianHoseini et al., 2013).

Further, long-term post-occupancy evaluations are vital for assessing occupant experiences and refining designs, ensuring tall buildings evolve as holistic systems promoting health, sustainability, and urban vitality (Mallory-Hill et al., 2012; Ruggiero et al., 2014). These research directions are pivotal for advancing tall buildings as resilient and inclusive urban solutions.

Finally, comparative studies across diverse regions and the modernization of traditional architectural practices could uncover innovative, culturally tailored strategies (Al-Kodmany & Ali, 2013; Parker & Wood, 2013). Furthermore, integrating tall buildings with urban ecosystems to promote biodiversity and air purification offers opportunities to redefine these structures as "vertical ecosystems" (Beatley, 2016; Gonçalves & Umakoshi, 2010).

REFERENCES

Ali, M. M., & Moon, K. S. (2007). Structural developments in tall buildings: Current trends and future prospects. *Architectural Science Review*, *50*(3), 205–223.

Al-Kodmany, K. (2014). Green towers and iconic design: Cases from three continents. *ArchNet-IJAR: International Journal of Architectural Research*, *8*(1), 11.

Al-Kodmany, K. (2024). *Humanizing the High-Rise City: Podiums, Plazas, Parks, Pedestrian Networks, and Public Art*. Taylor & Francis.

Al-Kodmany, K., & Ali, M. M. (2013). *The Future of the City: Tall Buildings and Urban Design*. WIT Press.

Allen, J. G., & Macomber, J. D. (2020). *Healthy Buildings: How Indoor Spaces Drive Performance and Productivity.* Harvard University Press.
ArchDaily. (2009). Manitoba Hydro/KPMB Architects. Retrieved from https://www.archdaily.com/44596/manitoba-hydro-kpmb-architects
Attia, S. (2017). Evaluation of adaptive facades: The case study of Al Bahar Towers in the UAE. *QScience Connect,* 2017(2), 6.
Beatley, T. (2016). *Handbook of Biophilic City Planning and Design.* Island Press.
Borg, R. F., Gambatese, J., Haines Jr, K., Hendrickson, C., Hinze, J., Horvath, A., & Haughney, R. A. (2003). Rebuilding the World Trade Center. *Practice Periodical on Structural Design and Construction, 8*(3), 137–145.
Building. (2009). Manitoba Hydro Place wins Tall Building Award. Retrieved from https://building.ca/manitoba-hydro-place-wins-tall-building-award
Canadian Architect. (2012). Manitoba Hydro Place Sets New Record with LEED Platinum. Retrieved from https://www.canadianarchitect.com/manitoba-hydro-place-sets-new-record-with-leed-platinum
Davern, M., Farrar, A., Kendal, D., & Giles-Corti, B. (2017). Quality green space supporting health, well-being, and biodiversity: A literature review. *Land Use Policy, 69*, 402–412.
De Wolf, C., Pomponi, F., & Moncaster, A. (2017). Measuring embodied carbon dioxide equivalent of buildings: A review and critique of current industry practice. *Energy and Buildings, 140*, 68–80.
Du, P., Al-Kodmany, K., & Ali, M. M. (2024). *The Routledge Handbook on Greening High-Density Cities*. Routledge.
Du, P., Wood, A., Stephens, B., & Song, X. (2015). Life-cycle energy implications of downtown high-rise vs. suburban low-rise living: An overview and quantitative case study for Chicago. *Buildings, 5*(3), 1003–1024.
El-Amrousi, M., & Biln, J. (2013). Abu Dhabi: Global changes and competing visions of modernity. *GSTF Journal of Engineering Technology, 2*(2), 84.
Emre Ilgın, H. (2021). Space efficiency in contemporary supertall office buildings. *Journal of Architectural Engineering*, 27(3), 04021024.
Friedman, S. M., Maslow, C. B., Reibman, J., Pillai, P. S., Goldring, R. M., Farfel, M. R., & Berger, K. I. (2011). Case–control study of lung function in World Trade Center Health Registry area residents and workers. *American Journal of Respiratory and Critical Care Medicine, 184*(5), 582–589.
GhaffarianHoseini, A., Dahlan, N. D., Berardi, U., GhaffarianHoseini, A., Makaremi, N., & GhaffarianHoseini, M. (2013). Sustainable energy performances of green buildings: A review of current theories, implementations, and challenges. *Renewable and Sustainable Energy Reviews, 25*, 1–17.
Glanz, J., & Lipton, E. (2003). *City in the Sky: The Rise and Fall of the World Trade Center.* Macmillan.
Gonçalves, J. C. S., & Umakoshi, É. M. (2010). *The Environmental Performance of Tall Buildings*. Routledge.
Gong, J. (2017). Shanghai tower. *Frontiers of Engineering Management, 4*(1), 106–109.
Guan, X., Wei, H., Lu, S., Dai, Q., & Su, H. (2020). Resilient urban design for adapting to future extreme climates: An integrated assessment framework. *Journal of Cleaner Production, 254*, 120050.
Habash, R. (2022). *Sustainability and Health in Intelligent Buildings*. Woodhead Publishing.
Iqbal, A. (2021). Developments in tall wood and hybrid buildings and environmental impacts. *Sustainability*, *13*(21), 11881.
Kellert, S. R., Heerwagen, J. H., & Mador, M. L. (Eds.). (2008). *Biophilic Design: The Theory, Science, and Practice of Bringing Buildings to Life.* Wiley.
Lewis, K., & Holt, N. (2011). Case study: One World Trade Center, New York. *CTBUH Journal*, *III*, 14–19.

Liu, H. J. (2016). From Nicholas negroponte to Al Bahar tower: The development in theory and technology of responsive architecture. In *Civil Engineering and Urban Planning IV: Proceedings of the 4th International Conference on Civil Engineering and Urban Planning,* Beijing, China, 25–27 July 2015 (p. 161). CRC Press.

Mallory-Hill, S., Preiser, W. F. E., & Watson, C. (Eds.). (2012). *Enhancing Building Performance.* Wiley-Blackwell.

McGregor, J., & Coley, D. (2018). Passive environmental design strategies in tall buildings. *Renewable and Sustainable Energy Reviews, 82*, 4237–4253.

Oldfield, P. (2017). A "fabric-first" approach to sustainable tall building design. *International Journal of High-Rise Buildings, 6*(2), 177–185.

Oldfield, P. (2019). The Sustainable Tall Building. Retrieved from https://books.google.se

Oldfield, P. F. (2012). Tall Buildings and Sustainability. Doctoral Dissertation, University of Nottingham.

Oldfield, P., Trabucco, D., & Wood, A. (2009). Five energy generations of tall buildings: An historical analysis of energy consumption in high-rise buildings. *The Journal of Architecture, 14*(5), 591–613.

Parker, D., & Wood, A. (Eds.). (2013). *The Tall Buildings Reference Book*. Routledge.

Phillips, R., Troup, L., Fannon, D., & Eckelman, M. J. (2020). Triple bottom line sustainability assessment of window-to-wall ratio in US office buildings. *Building and Environment, 182*, 107057.

Rempel, R. G., Eng, P., & Ferguson, C. C. P. N. (2003). Consulting Engineers of Manitoba Holds 4th Annual Awards of Excellence, Celebrates 25 Years. Retrieved from https://heritage.enggeomb.ca/images/6/69/00jun.pdf

Rempel, Z., Harney, N., Hudson, M., Cameron, L., & Aubin, Z. S. (2024). Manitoba Builds Green. Retrieved from https://www.iisd.org/publications/report/manitoba-builds-green

Ruggiero, S., Onkila, T., & Kuittinen, V. (2014). Realizing sustainable development in buildings: Trade-offs in post-occupancy evaluation. *Building Research & Information, 42*(4), 410–423.

SOM Architects. (2016). One World Trade Center. *ArchDaily*. Retrieved from https://www.archdaily.com/795277/one-world-trade-center-som

SOM Website. (2016). One World Trade Center Becomes Tallest LEED Building in the Western Hemisphere. Retrieved from https://www.som.com/news/one-world-trade-center-becomes-tallest-leed-building-in-the-western-hemisphere

Ulrich, R. S. (1984). View through a window may influence recovery from surgery. *Science, 224*(4647), 420–421.

Werbicki, R. (2019). A Sustainable Outlook in an Era of Uncertainty: A Case Study of Manitoba Hydro. Retrieved from http://hdl.handle.net/1993/33855

Wood, A. (2011). Tall Buildings: Search for a New Typology. Doctoral Dissertation, University of Nottingham.

Xia, J., Poon, D., & Mass, D. (2010). Case study: Shanghai Tower. *CTBUH Journal*, Issue II, 12–18.

9 Replacing Harmful Plastics with Biodegradable Alternatives

Innovations and Applications in Healthcare

Velur V. V. Reddy, Prasanthi Chidipudi, Sujatha Alla, and Nagesh Bheesetty

9.1 INTRODUCTION TO BIODEGRADABLE MATERIALS IN HEALTHCARE

Every year, the healthcare industry contributes significantly to the global plastic waste crisis, generating an estimated 1 million tons of plastic waste. This alarming statistic raises a critical question: Can biodegradable alternatives provide a solution to this escalating environmental challenge?

Biodegradable materials, derived from natural sources such as plants, animals, algae, and microorganisms, have emerged as a promising solution. Their ability to break down naturally over time makes them a sustainable alternative to the fossil-based plastics traditionally used in healthcare. The adoption of these materials is gaining momentum due to their environmental benefits and their ability to perform safely in medical applications without adverse human reactions.

In healthcare, biodegradable materials are being used across a wide array of applications including pharmaceuticals, wound management, organ implants, pacemakers, vacutainers, and sutures. These materials degrade naturally, minimizing their environmental impact while ensuring patient safety. By integrating biodegradable alternatives into healthcare products, the industry is working toward minimizing its carbon footprint and reducing the reliance on fossil fuels [1].

The increasing use of biodegradable materials in healthcare is driven by the urgent need to address the environmental consequences of traditional plastics. These non-biodegradable plastics, when improperly disposed of, accumulate in landfills and oceans, causing severe damage to wildlife and ecosystems. Moreover, the production of traditional plastics relies heavily on fossil fuels, contributing to greenhouse gas emissions and exacerbating climate change. In medical settings, the incineration of

 DOI: 10.1201/9781003513834-9

TABLE 9.1
Breakdown of Organic and Inorganic Matter of Biodegradable Plastics

Biodegradable Plastic	Organic Matter Produced	Biocompatibility
Polylactic acid (PLA) [50]	Lactic acid	Derived during PLA breakdown; further metabolized by microorganisms [50]
Polyhydroxyalkanoate (PHA) [51]	Short-chain fatty acids	Decomposes into monomers and fatty acids, serving as nutrients for soil microbes
Thermoplastic starch (TPS) [52]	Sugars and simple carbohydrates	Starch-based plastics degrade into simple sugars, consumed by microorganisms
General biodegradable plastics [53]	Humic substances	Stable organic compounds formed during breakdown, enriching the soil
	Cell biomass	Microbial biomass generated as microorganisms metabolize the material
	Alcohols and organic acids	Small amounts of byproducts like ethanol and acetic acid formed under specific conditions
	Lipids	Lipid-like organic compounds released during degradation

plastic waste releases harmful toxins and chemicals into the air, further degrading air quality and posing risks to surrounding communities and marine ecosystems [2].

Switching to biodegradable alternatives offers a powerful strategy to combat these environmental challenges. Materials like thermoplastic starch, polylactic acid (PLA), and polyhydroxyalkanoate (PHA) decompose faster and more naturally than conventional plastics. They are produced from renewable resources, making them an environmentally friendly choice. When these biodegradable materials break down, they convert into water, carbon dioxide, and organic matter, leaving minimal environmental impact. This shift not only promotes a circular economy, where resources are recycled and reused, but also paves the way for more sustainable medical practices [3]. The organic and inorganic matter that gets produced when a biomaterial broken down is listed in Table 9.1.

In recent years, significant advances in the development of biodegradable materials have made these alternatives more affordable and practical. Innovative bioplastics, such as PLA and PHA, are being increasingly used in various industries, including healthcare. Natural polymers like polysaccharides and proteins are also being explored for their potential applications in medical packaging and devices [4]. These innovations are helping industries transition away from conventional plastics, offering hope for a more sustainable future in healthcare.

9.2 CURRENT LANDSCAPE OF PLASTIC USE IN HEALTHCARE

The use of plastics in healthcare has become ubiquitous, with medical devices, packaging, and single-use items like syringes, gloves, and personal protective equipment (PPE) relying heavily on plastic materials. These plastics provide essential benefits such as durability, flexibility, and sterility, making them indispensable in modern medical settings. However, this reliance on plastic has led to significant environmental challenges, particularly in the wake of the COVID-19 pandemic, which saw a surge in the use of disposable medical items.

9.2.1 Common Types of Plastics Used in Medical Devices and Packaging

Several types of plastics dominate the healthcare industry due to their specific properties suited to medical applications. Polyethylene terephthalate (PET), polypropylene (PP), polyvinyl chloride (PVC), and polyurethane are widely used in everything from medical packaging to devices like catheters, tubing, and surgical instruments. These plastics are valued for their biocompatibility, resistance to chemicals, and ease of sterilization. However, their non-biodegradable nature has serious environmental consequences, contributing to the mounting plastic waste problem.

The pandemic exacerbated this issue, with disposable PPE such as face masks, gloves, and face shields leading to an unprecedented rise in healthcare-related plastic waste. This surge in single-use plastics highlights the ongoing dependency on materials that are difficult to recycle or dispose of sustainably. The usage of certain plasticizers like di-2-ethylhexyl phthalate (DEPH) in tubes has significant concern due to its potential health hazards, including carcinogenicity, endocrine dysfunction, and reproductive harm. This highlights the importance of safer alternatives [5].

9.2.2 Challenges Associated with Plastic Waste in Healthcare

Healthcare plastic waste presents unique challenges. A significant portion of this waste, including contaminated PPE and packaging materials, cannot be easily recycled due to the risk of infection or contamination. As a result, much of it ends up in landfills or is incinerated, contributing to environmental pollution. Incineration, while necessary for some medical waste to prevent the spread of infectious diseases, releases harmful chemicals and toxins into the air, negatively impacting both human health and ecosystems [6].

Additionally, certain plastics used in healthcare, such as those containing DEHP, a common plasticizer in medical tubing, pose direct health risks. DEHP has been linked to endocrine disruption, carcinogenicity, and reproductive harm, raising concerns about its continued use in medical products [7]. Although alternatives are available, the transition to safer materials has been slow due to cost and regulatory challenges.

The increased use of plastics in healthcare is also tied to pre-packaged supply kits, which are designed for convenience and sterility but result in large quantities of single-use plastic waste. This shift toward disposability has made it even more difficult for healthcare facilities to manage plastic waste sustainably.

9.2.3 Waste Management and Recycling Efforts

Efforts to manage healthcare plastic waste have focused on improving recycling processes and finding safer alternatives to harmful plastics. Technologies such as hydrogen peroxide and peracetic acid are being used to disinfect medical plastics, making them safer for recycling and reuse. However, the infrastructure to support widespread recycling of single-use medical plastics is often lacking, with few facilities equipped to handle the unique demands of healthcare waste.

Some hospitals and healthcare providers are starting to adopt more sustainable practices, such as segregating waste more efficiently and investing in closed-loop recycling systems that can turn medical plastics into new products. Additionally, the debate around DEHP in medical devices has prompted increased research into safer alternatives, though balancing safety, cost, and regulatory compliance remains a challenge.

9.3 ADVANCES IN BIODEGRADABLE POLYMERS

Despite these efforts, the sheer volume of plastic waste generated by healthcare systems continues to grow, making it imperative to find sustainable solutions. Reducing reliance on traditional plastics through the adoption of biodegradable alternatives represents a promising path forward, but it requires coordinated efforts from healthcare providers, policymakers, and industry leaders.

Switching to biodegradable bioplastics is an important step in decreasing plastic pollution around the world, which takes less time to degrade than regular plastics; see Figure 9.1. The key area of innovation is the creation of biodegradable elastomers, improved through chemical synthesis and processing technologies. These elastomers include special features like self-healing, which allows the material to repair itself after damage, antibacterial effects, preventing infections, and fluorescence that helps in medical imaging and diagnostics. These different types of elastomers are biodegradable polyesters and polyurethanes which are transforming biomedical devices and therapeutic strategies, making them more efficient, safer, and more adaptable to different medical needs.

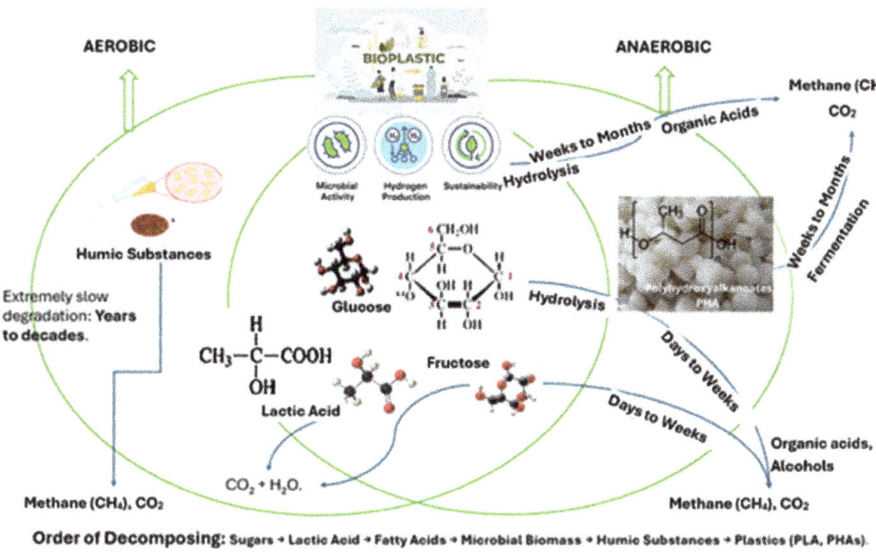

FIGURE 9.1 Degradation time rates of biodegradable plastics.

Another innovation is the use of polysaccharide-based polymers in the biomedical sector. These polysaccharides are natural polymers found in plants and organisms which are biocompatible. These polymers are flexible, renewable with strong mechanical properties. These polymers can be used to create scaffolds that support the growth of new tissues. A significant innovation is the development of U.S. Food and Drug Administration (FDA)-approved biodegradable esophagus stents [54]. These stents are used to treat esophageal strictures, to replace traditional stents. As these stents are biodegradable, and disintegrate by random hydrolysis in 12 weeks, they do not need to be removed and have drug-eluting features where they can release medication slowly to treat the condition more effectively [8].

9.3.1 Properties and Performance Comparison with Traditional Plastics

The specialty polymers used in healthcare offer many mechanical properties, such as toughness and flexibility, compared to traditional plastics. These advanced polymers are meticulously designed to meet the demands of medical applications, providing durability and reliability. Unlike traditional plastics, specialty polymers exhibit biocompatibility and reabsorbing capacity. This meticulous designing involves understanding and managing the effects of temperature, pH, and humidity of biodegradable plastics. The partial pressure of oxygen (PO_2) present in the bloodstream, is significantly lower than that found in the surrounding atmosphere, a phenomenon attributable to the body's intricate physiological mechanisms that meticulously regulate oxygen availability to satisfy metabolic requirements while simultaneously mitigating oxidative injury. The disparity in partial pressure is imperative for the effective oxygenation of tissues, which is fundamental for metabolic and cellular processes [65]. This gradient is of paramount importance for the effective transportation and utilization of oxygen within various tissues. Biodegradation processes occurring within the organism, particularly those involving mesenchymal stromal cells (MSCs) as well as anaerobic fermentation, are markedly influenced by this diminished PO_2. The duration necessary for biodegradation processes is contingent upon the specific biological milieu and prevailing environmental conditions.

For devices such as bioresorbable implants and drug delivery devices, controlled degradation rates are crucial to match the healing or treatment timeline. Similarly, material formulations may require additives or coatings to regulate environmental sensitivity. Irrespective of these challenges, their innovation and usage helped for the development of medical devices that offer improved quality and performance, effectively addressing the needs of the healthcare industry [9].

Table 9.2 shows the comparison between traditional plastics and biodegradable plastics, highlighting their pros and cons.

This table outlines key differences, highlighting that while biodegradable plastics are more environmentally friendly, they face challenges in cost and scalability compared to traditional plastics.

9.3.2 Design and Development of Biodegradable Polymers

The prospective trajectory of biodegradable healthcare materials is on the brink of substantial progress, propelled by groundbreaking advancements in material science

TABLE 9.2
Comparison Analysis of Traditional vs. Biodegradable Plastics

Feature	Traditional Plastics	Biodegradable Plastics
Material composition	Made from petroleum-based compounds (e.g., polyethylene, polypropylene)	Made from renewable resources (e.g., plant starch, PLA, PHA)
Degradation time	Can take hundreds of years to decompose	Degrades within months to years under specific conditions
Environmental impact	Significant pollution, contributes to landfill and ocean waste	Lower environmental impact, fewer microplastics
Production cost	Lower cost due to established processes and scale	Generally higher cost due to limited production scale and resources
Carbon footprint	High carbon footprint from fossil fuel extraction and processing	Lower carbon footprint, especially if sourced from plant-based materials
Recycling potential	Can be recycled but often not due to contamination or cost issues	Can be recycled but often not due to contamination or cost issues
Use in healthcare	Widely used in medical devices, packaging, PPE due to durability	Increasing use in medical packaging, wound care, and drug delivery systems
Biocompatibility	Often non-biodegradable, requires special disposal in healthcare	Biocompatible options available, reducing long-term patient risks
Durability	Very durable and resistant to wear and tear	Less durable, often designed to degrade after a specific use
End-of-life options	Landfill, incineration, or recycling (with limitations)	Composting, biodegrading under suitable conditions

and engineering disciplines. These materials are progressively being customized to fulfill the distinct requirements of medical applications, thereby providing superior biocompatibility, mechanical attributes, and operational capabilities. The incorporation of biodegradable materials within the healthcare sector not only mitigates ecological issues but also enhances patient outcomes through improved tissue integration and diminished cytotoxic effects.

The formulation of biodegradable polymers necessitates an extensive comprehension of their degradation mechanisms across various environmental contexts. This encompasses the meticulous selection of suitable feedstock materials and the refinement of production and recycling methodologies to augment biodegradability [11]. Biodegradable polymers can be derived from both natural and synthetic sources. Natural polymers offer high renewability and are easily degraded by microorganisms, making them suitable for medical applications [14].

9.3.3 Natural Biodegradable Materials

Derived from animal, plant, and microbial sources, these materials are gaining popularity due to their eco-friendliness and biocompatibility. They are used in various medical applications, including wound treatment and tissue engineering, without triggering immune responses [19].

9.3.3.1 Protein-Based Composites

Recent investigations have concentrated on the advancement of protein-based composites, exemplified by those originating from human serum albumin, intended for application in biodegradable sutures. The materials highlighted here prove to have superior biodegradability and biocompatibility, which are key for effective tissue engineering. These sutures possess mechanical traits like tensile strength and elongation that can be fine-tuned by integrating organic additives that decompose, which makes them fitting for numerous medical uses [39].

9.3.3.2 Polysaccharide-Based Polymers

There is a growing acknowledgment of biodegradable polymers that originate from polysaccharides, valued for their fundamental compatibility with biological entities and multifunctional capabilities. These substances are being employed in the domains of tissue engineering, pharmaceutical delivery systems, and as protective coatings for medical apparatus. Their capacity to construct intricate architectures and engage positively with biological tissues renders them highly suitable for applications within the realm of regenerative medicine, including the regeneration of cartilage, dermal tissues, and osseous structures. The use of these materials aligns well with the aims of fostering environmental responsibility, playing a role in curbing carbon footprints and advancing the United Nations' Sustainable Development Initiatives [40].

9.3.4 Synthetic Biodegradable Polymers

Synthetic polymers like polyesters and polyurethanes have been pivotal in creating biodegradable elastomers with properties such as self-healing, antibacterial, and shape-memory capabilities. These materials are engineered for specific biomedical applications, ensuring controlled biodegradability and functionality [16].

9.3.4.1 Synthetic Biodegradable Elastomers

Synthetic biodegradable elastomers, such as polyesters and polyurethanes, are being developed with advanced functionalities like self-healing, and antibacterial properties. These materials are crucial for creating biomedical devices with controllable properties, enhancing their applicability in various therapeutic strategies. Innovations in chemical synthesis and processing technologies are enabling the development of elastomers with tailored biodegradability and elasticity, expanding their use in the healthcare sector [41].

9.3.4.2 PLA in Medical Applications

The polymer PLA is recognized for its compatibility with biological systems and its ability to decompose, leading to its significant exploration for potential medical uses, including systems for drug delivery, wound healing, bone implants, and vascular grafts. Its capacity for degradation within the human body, yielding no detrimental byproducts, renders it exceptionally appropriate for these applications. Recent advancements encompass the modification of PLA through the incorporation of supplementary polymers to augment its properties, as well as the application of techniques such as cold plasma treatment to modify its surface for enhanced drug delivery efficacy. The technique of coaxial electrospinning offers an extra approach for producing various PLA-based goods aimed at specific healthcare applications [42].

9.3.4.3 Biodegradable Esophageal Stents

Innovative biodegradable substances, featuring synthetic polyester and magnesium-based alloys, are being designed for esophageal stents to lessen the problems tied to regular stents, like migration and restenosis. The ability of drug-eluting stents (DES) to effectively load and release drugs makes them a vital focus of study, yielding better options for managing esophageal strictures. Advances such as unidirectional drug release and anti-migration functionalities are currently under examination to enhance stent efficacy. The development of emergent technologies, featuring 3D printing and groundbreaking biodegradable materials such as hydrogels, is central to the improvement of advanced esophageal stents [43].

9.4 APPLICATIONS OF BIODEGRADABLE POLYMER

Constructed from synthetic and naturally derived biodegradable substrates, these devices are increasingly used across diverse medical fields, providing benefits such as reduced environmental impact and improved patient outcomes. The following sections explore the key aspects of biodegradable medical devices, including material innovations, applications, and future trends.

9.4.1 Biodegradable Alternatives for Medical Packaging

Biodegradable composites derived from sustainable biomaterials are emerging as innovative solutions for intelligent medical packaging. These materials, including starch, PLA, cellulose, and bio-composites, offer enhanced biodegradability, improved mechanical properties, and the potential for advanced functionalities like embedded nanosensors for monitoring product quality. Designed to decompose safely in the environment, they address the environmental challenges posed by traditional plastics while reducing pollution and medical waste [10,12].

Recent advancements have introduced unconventional sources, such as banana peels, combined with additives like glycerin and corn starch, to develop biodegradable materials with strong mechanical properties and effective degradation under composting conditions. For instance, researchers at the University of Cartagena created biodegradable packaging from banana peels, offering a renewable solution with significant potential for medical applications [13,15]. Similarly, companies like Teysha Technologies and Danimer Scientific have pioneered bioplastics from agricultural waste and PHA, respectively, to develop customizable, sustainable medical packaging with controlled degradation rates and excellent biocompatibility.

These materials show promise in applications such as sterile medical device packaging and pharmaceutical storage. For example, Apeel Sciences developed biodegradable coatings with antimicrobial properties to extend product shelf life, which are being adapted for medical packaging. However, scalability and economic feasibility remain significant barriers. Higher production costs, variability in biodegradability under different environmental conditions, and the lack of standardized biodegradability testing hinder broader adoption in healthcare [11,15].

To address these challenges, international standards by organizations like International Organization for Standardization (ISO) and the American Society for Testing and Materials (ASTM) are critical for ensuring reliable biodegradability under real-world conditions. Despite these hurdles, the growing global demand for sustainable packaging underscores the importance of continued innovation and economic incentives to advance biodegradable solutions in the medical sector.

9.4.2 Biodegradable Plastics in Pharmaceutical Applications

Biodegradable polymers have garnered considerable scholarly interest within the realm of pharmaceutical applications, especially in the context of drug delivery systems, attributable to their favorable biocompatibility, regulated degradation profiles, and potential to augment therapeutic effectiveness. These materials present an environmentally sustainable alternative to conventional non-biodegradable polymers, thereby addressing both ecological issues and the imperative for sophisticated drug delivery methodologies.

Biodegradable polymers function as vehicles for the administration of pharmaceuticals, offering a protective barrier that encapsulates therapeutic agents and guarantees a regulated release at the designated site of action. The substances produced during their decay are safe and can be removed from the organism safely, making them particularly fitting for integration into medicinal compositions [21]. Poly (butyl cyanoacrylate) (PBCA) is a notable example, used as a carrier matrix in drug delivery systems. Advances in polymer synthesis have allowed for the control of molecular weight and stability, crucial for pharmaceutical applications [22].

9.4.3 Biodegradable Medical Devices

Biodegradable medical devices represent a significant advancement in healthcare technology, offering sustainable and ecologically sound solutions for various medical applications. Designed to perform their intended functions and safely degrade within the biological environment, these devices eliminate the need for surgical removal and reduce long-term ecological impact. Their development relies on innovative materials and advanced fabrication methodologies for effective integration into healthcare practices.

Implantable Devices: Materials that break down naturally, including PLA, polyglycolic acid (PGA), and their various copolymers, find extensive application in orthopedic surgical implants and sutures. This collection of substances satisfies important benchmarks of non-harmfulness, performance, and biological harmony, thereby making them fit for temporary or semi-durable implantation [18].

Microsystems and Electronics: Advances in micro and nanofabrication have helped in the development of biodegradable implantable microsystems for monitoring, recording, and drug delivery. These devices are designed so as to lessen invasive damage while maximizing interaction with tissues [17].

Bio-based Polymers: Polymers such as PLA and polycaprolactone (PCL) are used in different medical devices, such as diagnostic tools, healthcare electronics, and medical tubing, due to their excellent biocompatibility and processability [20].

The integration of biodegradable materials in medical devices is expected to grow, with ongoing research focusing on enhancing material properties and expanding applications. Challenges remain in ensuring consistent performance and addressing regulatory hurdles for widespread adoption [16,17]. Although biodegradable medical devices present a plethora of benefits, there exist significant challenges associated with their mechanical characteristics and long-term durability. Ongoing investigation is imperative to refine these materials for more extensive applications, guaranteeing their compliance with the stringent requirements of the healthcare sector while upholding ecological sustainability.

9.5 APPLICATIONS IN BIOMEDICAL DEVICES

Synthetic biodegradable elastomers, like polyesters and polyurethanes, have notably revolutionized the domain of biomedical devices. These elements are precisely formulated to reveal both decomposability and elasticity, including functions like self-healing properties and anti-germ features, thereby enhancing their function in treatment devices [23]. Biodegradable polymers are also used in the fabrication of tablets, implants, and nanoparticles, providing versatility in drug delivery systems and tissue engineering [24].

9.5.1 Ocular Drug Delivery

In ocular drug delivery, biodegradable polymers overcome anatomical barriers, allowing for sustained drug release and improved bioavailability. They are used in formulations like nanoparticles and hydrogels, targeting diseases such as glaucoma and retinal disorders [25]. Although biodegradable plastics present significant advancements in pharmaceutical applications, obstacles persist in refining formulation strategies and complying with regulatory standards for clinical utilization. Ongoing research is imperative to confront these challenges and comprehensively harness the capabilities of biodegradable polymers in improving therapeutic outcomes.

9.5.2 Impact on Drug Stability and Efficacy

Polymers that can decompose, see Figure 9.2, particularly those created from polyesters including PLA and poly (lactic-co-glycolic acid) (PLGA), bring noteworthy benefits to the enhancement of pharmaceutical stability. These materials are extensively employed in drug delivery systems owing to their capacity to modulate drug release profiles and safeguard active pharmaceutical compounds from degradation. Biodegradable polyester matrices can be meticulously designed to establish a microenvironment conducive to drug stabilization. By fine-tuning how the polymer deteriorates, we can better manage the timing of the drug's release, thus supporting its stability over longer times [26]. Biodegradable polymers are not only used for drug delivery but also in other biomedical applications, such as wound healing

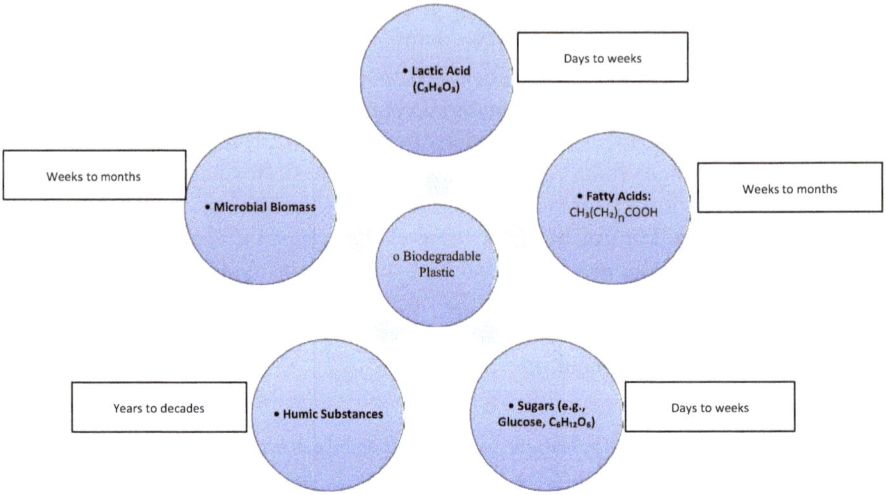

FIGURE 9.2 Decomposition process of bioplastics.

and cancer treatment. Their ability to degrade in response to specific stimuli, such as reactive oxygen species, allows for targeted drug release, which can enhance the stability and efficacy of the drug in the target area [27]. While biodegradable plastics offer numerous benefits for drug stability, challenges remain, such as ensuring uniform degradation rates and preventing premature drug release. Continued research into polymer engineering and stabilization techniques is essential to fully realize the potential of these materials in pharmaceutical applications.

9.5.3 Sustainability and Lifecycle Analysis of Biodegradable Plastics

The examination of the sustainability and lifecycle assessment of biodegradable plastics constitutes a complex subject that necessitates a comprehensive evaluation of their ecological ramifications from the stages of production to eventual disposal. Products like biodegradable plastics, which feature polybutylene adipate terephthalate (PBAT), polybutylene succinate (PBS), poly(3-hydroxybutyrate-co-3-hydroxyvalerate) (PHBV), and PLA, could provide environmental gains versus traditional plastic types; nevertheless, they bring forth particular challenges and considerations that must be taken into account across their entire lifecycle.

9.5.4 Material Properties and Production

Biodegradable materials, including PBAT, PBS, PHBV, and PLA, showcase remarkable characteristics in chemistry, heat tolerance, and mechanics that significantly shape their processing methods and applications. For example, PBAT and PBS demonstrate closed-cell structures, in contrast to the open-cell configuration of PHBV, which consequently impacts their prospective applications and ecological ramifications [28]. The production of biodegradable plastics can have a higher global warming potential (GWP) compared to fossil-based plastics. For example, the GWP for 1 kg of poly(3-hydroxybutyrate-co-4-hydroxybutyrate) (PHB) and PLA is 3.09 and 5.79 kg CO_2 equivalent, respectively [29].

9.5.5 End-of-Life Scenarios

Biodegradable plastics provide better end-of-life options, such as anaerobic digestion and incineration, that reduce their overall environmental impact when managed properly [29]. Mechanical recycling is a favorable end-of-life scenario for PHBV, as it retains material circularity and provides environmental credits by replacing recycles with virgin materials [30].

9.5.6 Environmental and Ecotoxicity Considerations

Despite the fact that biodegradable plastics decompose into water, carbon dioxide, and biomass, they could still possess additives that introduce ecotoxicological threats. As an illustration, phthalate esters (PAEs) have the ability to seep from these substances, possibly putting ecological systems at risk. Notwithstanding their inherent biodegradability, the inclusion of non-degradable additives necessitates a thorough examination of their environmental ramifications [31].

9.6 CHALLENGES AND LIMITATIONS

Biodegradable plastics are increasingly used for medical devices due to their sustainability benefits. However, challenges such as inferior barrier properties, low heat resistance, and high costs limit their widespread adoption. Strategies like blending and nanomaterial reinforcement are being explored to enhance their applicability and performance [32]. While biodegradable plastics offer potentially effective strategies for mitigating plastic pollution, their lifecycle assessments uncover intricate challenges that necessitate further examination. These challenges encompass aspects of production, degradation, market integration, and regulatory frameworks, thereby influencing their comprehensive sustainability and industrial feasibility.

9.6.1 Production and Material Challenges

The pursuit of sustainable feedstocks and efficient production processes is a significant challenge. Biodegradable plastics often require specific conditions for production and degradation, which are not always met, leading to inefficiencies and higher costs [33]. Biodegradable materials, such as those made from PLA or PHA, tend to be more expensive than traditional plastics due to the current scale of production. For large healthcare facilities, this can result in higher upfront costs for medical supplies and packaging. This economic barrier restricts their widespread adoption [34,35].

A range of policy measures could facilitate the adoption of these substances, underscoring the significance of regulatory frameworks, financial incentives, and cooperative efforts within the sector.

9.6.1.1 Regulatory Frameworks

The formulation of explicit protocols and benchmarks for the utilization of biodegradable substances in medical contexts can enhance their integration into practice. This encompasses the delineation of biocompatibility and biodegradability parameters that materials are required to satisfy in order to gain authorization for medical application. Advancing the efficiency of the approval process for biodegradable materials could facilitate innovation and curtail the period required for the debut of innovative products in the marketplace [59].

9.6.1.2 Financial Incentives

The implementation of fiscal incentives or subsidies for enterprises participating in the research and development of biodegradable materials possesses the ability to spur innovation and reduce the economic hurdles related to the transition from standard plastics [60]. The establishment of grants or funding initiatives tailored specifically for endeavors that seek to innovate or employ biodegradable materials within the healthcare sector may significantly bolster this transition [59]. Similarly, providing tax incentives to healthcare organizations that integrate biodegradable substances into their offerings can alleviate the economic strain associated with the shift toward sustainable options [61].

9.6.1.3 Government Grants and Funding

Governments possess the capacity to allocate financial grants aimed at facilitating research endeavors concerning biodegradable materials, with a particular emphasis on their advancement, empirical testing, and validation within the medical domain. The undertaking might demand the availability of financial backing to aid scholarly activities that examine biodegradable polymers, including PCL and PLGA [59].

9.6.2 Recycling and End-of-Life Management

The breakdown of these polymers is notably impacted by environmental variables, such as heat levels and the existence of microbes, and these variables may not uniformly occur in natural ecosystems, especially those in aquatic settings [36,37]. In some environments, biodegradable plastics do not fully degrade, leading to microplastic pollution, which poses a threat to aquatic ecosystems [36]. The insufficiency of efficient recycling pathways and infrastructure tailored for biodegradable plastics represents a significant concern. Existing recycling techniques are inadequately equipped to handle these materials, thereby requiring the innovation of novel technologies and methodologies [34,37]. Effective end-of-life management strategies, including chemical and biological recycling, are essential to enhance the sustainability of biodegradable plastics [34,37].

9.6.3 Supply Chain Limitations

The supply chain for biodegradable plastics is still developing. This presents challenges in ensuring a consistent and reliable supply of high-quality biodegradable materials for healthcare facilities. Hospitals need to work closely with suppliers to ensure that biodegradable products meet the necessary medical standards and regulatory requirements.

9.6.4 Market and Policy Barriers

There is a lack of consumer awareness and understanding of biodegradable plastics, which hampers market adoption. Additionally, the market is not yet competitive with conventional plastics due to these materials' higher costs and limited applications [33,35]. The absence of standardized policies and financial incentives for biodegradable plastics further complicates their adoption. Clear definitions and communication are needed to support their market integration [33,37].

9.6.5 Challenges with Sterilization

Standard sterilization methods pose significant challenges for biodegradable materials like PLA, PHA, and PCL due to their sensitivity to heat, moisture, and reactive agents. Autoclaving, which involves high temperatures (121°C–134°C) and moisture, can degrade these materials, leading to a loss of mechanical strength and alterations in their chemical composition. Similarly, chemical sterilization methods, such as using ethylene oxide or formaldehyde, can cause unwanted chemical reactions with biodegradable polymers, potentially altering their properties or leaving residues that compromise biocompatibility. Radiation sterilization, including gamma and electron beam methods, can further degrade polymer chains, reducing the strength and functionality of these materials. These limitations necessitate alternative sterilization techniques specifically suited for biodegradable medical devices.

Several alternative sterilization methods are well-suited for biodegradable medical devices, preserving material integrity while ensuring effective sterilization. Low-temperature gas plasma sterilization, using hydrogen peroxide vapor, operates below 50°C, is residue-free, and environmentally friendly but requires designs that allow effective plasma penetration. Supercritical CO_2 sterilization, combined with agents like peracetic acid, is ideal for heat- and moisture-sensitive materials, though it involves higher operational costs. Low-dose electron beam (E-beam) radiation offers fast, controlled sterilization with minimal material degradation but is limited to surface-level applications. Ultraviolet sterilization provides a quick, non-invasive solution for flat surfaces, while ozone sterilization is effective at 20°C–30°C with no toxic residue, requiring controlled environments. Lastly, peracetic acid immersion works at low temperatures and combats a wide range of microorganisms but requires thorough rinsing and is unsuitable for complex geometries. These methods provide viable alternatives to traditional sterilization for sensitive biodegradable devices (Table 9.3).

By selecting the most appropriate sterilization technique based on the material and application, it is possible to ensure both safety and performance of biodegradable medical devices.

TABLE 9.3
Summary Table of Sterilization Methods

Method	Temperature	Impact on Material	Applications
Gas plasma (H_2O_2)	<50°C	Minimal	Implants, sutures, drug delivery devices
Supercritical CO_2	30°C–50°C	Minimal	Heat- and moisture-sensitive materials
Low-dose E-beam radiation	Ambient	Low degradation risk	Thin films, surface sterilization
UV sterilization	Ambient	Surface sterilization only	Packaging, flat or exposed surfaces
Ozone sterilization	20°C–30°C	Minimal	Lightweight, porous devices
Peracetic acid immersion	<50°C	Residual rinsing required	Simple geometries, flat surfaces

9.6.6 Economic and Infrastructural Barriers

The synthesis of biodegradable polymers frequently incurs higher costs relative to traditional plastics, thereby constraining their market competitiveness. The successful biodegradation process necessitates the presence of specialized waste management systems, which are not universally accessible, consequently curtailing the practical advantages associated with biodegradable plastics [38]. The economic evaluation of biodegradable plastics in relation to conventional plastics represents a crucial determinant affecting their acceptance within the market. Typically, biodegradable plastics are associated with elevated costs stemming from the expenses related to raw materials, manufacturing methodologies, and constrained economies of scale. This financial divergence poses a significant obstacle to their extensive utilization, notwithstanding the ecological advantages they confer.

9.6.6.1 Raw Material and Production Costs

Biodegradable polymers, exemplified by those derived from algal substances, encompass intricate manufacturing procedures and necessitate specialized materials, thereby resulting in elevated expenditures. For example, the fabrication of films derived from seaweed necessitates supplementary constituents such as cellulose nanofibers, which augment the total financial outlay [55]. The fabrication of biodegradable plastics encompasses a more intricate series of methodologies, which may lead to heightened production expenses. For instance, the synthesis of PHB necessitates particular fermentation techniques that incur greater costs in comparison to the polymerization processes employed for traditional plastics [56]. The expenditure associated with the fabrication of biodegradable straws utilizing stereo-complexed poly (lactic acid) (SC-PLA) is comparatively modest, estimated at around 2.06 cents per straw; however, this cost is still elevated in relation to traditional plastic straws because of the distinct processing methodologies necessitated [57].

In the field of horticultural applications, it has been documented that biodegradable alternatives, including viscose polymer and jute fiber, exhibit a price increase of 49% compared to traditional options such as PP raffia and polyethylene mulching film. The elevated expenses are ascribed to the necessity for specialized manufacturing infrastructures and the prevailing absence of economies of scale within the biodegradable plastics sector [58].

9.6.6.2 Energy Consumption and Processability

The energy expenditure linked with the manufacturing and reprocessing of biodegradable plastics frequently surpasses that of petroleum-derived plastics. This phenomenon can be attributed to the supplementary processing stages required to guarantee biodegradability, which may elevate operational expenditures. The administration and reprocessing of biodegradable polymers additionally necessitate elevated energy investments, which further augment their total expenses in comparison to conventional plastics [66].

Although the progress observed in biodegradable healthcare materials is encouraging, significant obstacles persist, including the necessity for regulatory adherence and the realization of large-scale manufacturing. Furthermore, the equilibrium between biodegradability, mechanical performance, and cost-efficiency remains a pivotal domain of inquiry. Confronting these challenges will be imperative for the extensive integration of these pioneering materials within healthcare applications.

9.7 CASE STUDIES: SUCCESSFUL IMPLEMENTATION OF BIODEGRADABLE ALTERNATIVES

The transition of healthcare facilities from traditional plastics to biodegradable materials has been gaining traction as part of broader efforts to reduce environmental impacts, minimize healthcare waste, and promote sustainability. This in-depth analysis explores healthcare facilities that have adopted biodegradable materials, their challenges, and the benefits they have realized.

9.7.1 Sustainability Initiatives in Hospitals

Several hospitals and healthcare systems around the world are taking steps to implement biodegradable materials into their operations, particularly for disposable medical items such as syringes, gloves, surgical gowns, and packaging.

Case Study 9.1: Cleveland Clinic

Cleveland Clinic, a prominent healthcare institution in the United States, has integrated sustainable practices as part of its overall environmental strategy. One key component has been the transition to biodegradable packaging materials, particularly for food services within the hospital. The clinic replaced traditional plastic utensils and containers with compostable alternatives made from plant-based materials. This move reduced the amount of non-recyclable waste produced by the facility and led to significant cost savings in waste management.

Case Study 9.2: University Hospitals Birmingham

University Hospitals Birmingham in the UK has also implemented biodegradable materials into its healthcare waste strategy. The facility has adopted biodegradable packaging for certain pharmaceutical products and switched to biodegradable food service containers. The goal is to align with the UK's stringent environmental policies aimed at reducing single-use plastics. The switch to biodegradable alternatives has helped the hospital reduce its waste sent to landfills by over 20%.

9.7.2 Medical Device and Packaging Transitions

In healthcare, a significant amount of plastic waste stems from packaging and disposable devices such as gloves, syringes, and medical drapes. With increasing regulatory pressures and environmental targets, healthcare facilities are looking to biodegradable alternatives for these products.

Case Study 9.3: Karolinska University Hospital, Sweden

Karolinska University Hospital, a world leader in medical research and patient care, has shifted to biodegradable alternatives for many single-use medical devices. The hospital partnered with suppliers of biodegradable plastics for surgical drapes, gowns, and certain medical packaging, achieving a 10% reduction in its plastic waste output. The facility also runs pilot programs to test biodegradable medical products such as drug delivery systems and patient identification wristbands made from plant-based materials.

Case Study 9.4: Kaiser Permanente

Kaiser Permanente, one of the largest healthcare providers in the United States, has set ambitious sustainability goals, including transitioning to biodegradable plastics in various operational areas. They replaced traditional petroleum-based plastic food containers with compostable alternatives and introduced biodegradable packaging for pharmaceuticals. This initiative is part of their long-term goal to reduce waste and lower carbon emissions across their facilities.

9.7.3 Environmental and Economic Benefits

The benefits of transitioning to biodegradable materials in healthcare facilities are substantial, especially when viewed through the lens of long-term environmental sustainability and cost reduction in waste management.

Waste Reduction: Biodegradable materials help healthcare facilities reduce the amount of plastic waste sent to landfills or incinerators. This is particularly important in large facilities, which generate tons of waste each year. By using biodegradable materials, healthcare systems can significantly cut down on the environmental footprint associated with healthcare operations.

Compliance with Environmental Policies: Many healthcare facilities are adopting biodegradable materials to comply with stricter environmental regulations aimed at reducing single-use plastic waste. For example, the European Union has introduced policies that limit the use of certain plastics in packaging, and many U.S. states are following suit.

Public Perception and Sustainability Credentials: Transitioning to biodegradable materials can enhance a healthcare facility's reputation as an environmentally responsible organization. Hospitals that actively reduce their environmental impact are often viewed more favorably by patients and stakeholders who value sustainability. This can translate into increased patient trust and support from environmentally conscious consumers.

9.8 POLICY AND REGULATION FOR BIODEGRADABLE PLASTICS IN HEALTHCARE

The incorporation of biodegradable polymers within the healthcare sector represents a potentially effective strategy for mitigating environmental repercussions while simultaneously upholding the functionality of medical apparatus and products. This methodology is congruent with international sustainability objectives and responds to the urgent demand for environmentally sustainable alternatives within the medical industry. The advancement and governance of biodegradable polymers in healthcare encompass numerous critical dimensions, including material characteristics, market dynamics, and regulatory frameworks.

9.8.1 Regulatory Environment and Standards

The regulatory landscape for biodegradable plastics is crucial for their successful integration into healthcare. Standards and certifications ensure that these materials meet safety and performance criteria, facilitating their acceptance and use in medical applications [46]. Emphasizing regulatory approvals and environmental sustainability is essential for advancing the use of biodegradable polymers in healthcare, aligning with global sustainability goals and reducing carbon emissions [44].

9.8.2 Environmental and Socio-Economic Impacts

The implementation of biodegradable plastics within the healthcare sector has the potential to markedly diminish environmental contamination and carbon output. These substances are specifically engineered for degradation by microbial organisms, thereby reducing the longevity of plastic materials within ecological systems. This initiative is in harmony with international endeavors aimed at mitigating climate change and addressing the issue of microplastic pollution. The socio-economic ramifications of the shift toward biodegradable plastics encompass the prospective generation of employment opportunities within the bioplastics industry and the facilitation of a circular economic model. It is imperative for policymakers to weigh these advantages against the necessity for stringent standards and certifications to guarantee the safety and efficacy of the products [45].

While biodegradable plastics offer significant advantages, challenges remain in terms of scalability, cost, and regulatory compliance. Addressing these issues through coordinated policy efforts and technological advancements will be key to unlocking the full potential of biodegradable plastics in healthcare.

9.8.3 Economic and Market Considerations

The market for biodegradable polymers is experiencing substantial growth, propelled by the surging demand for sustainable commodities and the progressive bio-economic paradigm shift. Still, the market is open to the impacts of political and economic conditions, such as variations in GDP and petroleum pricing, which can alter both production abilities and levels of adoption [47]. Despite their potential, biodegradable plastics currently represent a small fraction of the global plastics market. Continued research and commercialization efforts are necessary to increase their market share and realize their environmental benefits [46].

9.8.4 Market Trends and Economic Analysis of Biodegradable Plastics in the Healthcare Industry

The biodegradable plastics market is experiencing significant growth, driven by increasing environmental concerns and regulatory pressures to reduce plastic waste. By 2030, the market is expected to reach USD 10 billion, indicating strong economic potential [48]. Biodegradable polymers, such as polysaccharides, are gaining traction due to their inherent biocompatibility and versatility in biomedical applications, including tissue engineering and drug delivery systems [41]. The packaging industry, a significant consumer of biodegradable plastics, is expected to grow at a compound annual growth rate (CAGR) of 9.7%, highlighting the broader market potential for these materials [49]. The global biodegradable plastics market is growing rapidly, with BASF, Corbion, and NatureWorks being some of the largest players. For example, the biodegradable packaging segment alone accounted for 53.9% of the total market share in 2023. BASF and Corbion hold significant portions of the biodegradable healthcare plastics market, as they are leaders in producing PLA and other biodegradable polymers used in medical applications. NatureWorks and TIPA have strong footholds in the market due to their focus on high-performance, sustainable packaging solutions (Table 9.4).

9.9 IMPACT ON PATIENT SAFETY AND CARE

The integration of biodegradable materials into healthcare has significant implications for both patient safety and care. These materials, designed to naturally break down within the body or environment, offer an innovative approach to

TABLE 9.4
Market Share of Biodegradable Manufacturing Companies

Company	Products	Market Presence/Share	Market Size (USD)
Arkema Group	Bio-based materials for medical packaging, wound care, and disposables	Key player in bio-based materials with significant market influence in healthcare plastics (Expert Market Research)	Tier 1 company in the global plant-based plastic industry with market revenue above USD 50 million
BASF SE	PLA, PBS for medical packaging, drug delivery, and disposable products	Leading producer with large market share in biodegradable plastics (Expert Market Research; Grand View Research)	Tier 1 company in the global plant-based plastic industry with market revenue above USD 50 million
Corbion	Lactic acid-based bioplastics for medical devices and drug delivery systems	A major player in healthcare bioplastics; leader in PLA derivatives (Expert Market Research; Mordor Intelligence)	Recognized as a key player in the bio-based chemicals market, contributing to a market projected to grow significantly
NatureWorks LLC	Ingeo biopolymer used in medical packaging, nonwoven fabrics for healthcare	Dominates in biodegradable healthcare packaging; significant market share (Grand View Research; Mordor Intelligence)	Leading player in the polylactic acid market, which is projected to grow from USD 1.0 billion in 2021 to USD 1.9 billion by 2026
Polymateria	Biodegradable solutions for healthcare packaging and personal hygiene products	Notable for advanced biodegradability; growing market presence (Emergen Research)	Identified among key players in the bioplastics market, expected to reach USD 20.48 billion by 2028
TIPA Corp Ltd	Biodegradable packaging for medical supplies, customizable compostable films	Strong presence in healthcare packaging with innovative solutions (Emergen Research)	Recognized in the bioplastics market, which is anticipated to grow at a rate of 17.1% to USD 20.48 billion by 2028

medical treatments, reducing the need for secondary surgeries to remove implants or devices. From biodegradable sutures and stents to drug delivery systems, these materials enhance patient outcomes by minimizing long-term complications and improving the biocompatibility of medical products. Additionally, the shift toward biodegradable materials in packaging and devices aligns with growing concerns about environmental sustainability, which increasingly influences patient perceptions of healthcare practices. However, ensuring that these materials meet rigorous safety standards and perform reliably under various conditions remains crucial for widespread adoption.

9.9.1 Evaluating the Safety and Effectiveness of Biodegradable Materials for Patients

Evaluating the safety and effectiveness of biodegradable materials in healthcare is a multifaceted process that requires a balance between medical innovation, patient safety, and regulatory oversight. Biodegradable materials, while offering numerous advantages, also present unique challenges that must be critically assessed to ensure they meet the stringent safety and performance requirements of medical applications.

9.9.2 Advantages of Biodegradable Materials for Patient Care

Biodegradable materials have the potential to revolutionize patient care by reducing the need for secondary surgeries and minimizing long-term complications. For instance, biodegradable sutures and stents naturally degrade within the body, eliminating the risks associated with permanent implants, such as infection, inflammation, or rejection. Moreover, biodegradable drug delivery systems can offer controlled release of medications, improving therapeutic outcomes by ensuring consistent dosing over time.

One key benefit of these materials is their biocompatibility. They are designed to interact harmoniously with biological systems, breaking down into non-toxic byproducts that the body can safely absorb or eliminate. This minimizes adverse reactions and contributes to overall patient safety. In applications such as wound healing and tissue engineering, biodegradable materials allow for natural tissue regeneration without the risk of immune responses or the need for further interventions.

9.9.3 Challenges in Safety Evaluation

Despite their potential, evaluating the safety of biodegradable materials is complex due to the variability in their degradation rates and byproducts. One major challenge lies in ensuring that these materials degrade in a controlled and predictable manner. Variations in individual patient physiology, such as differences in pH levels or enzyme activity, can influence how quickly or completely these materials degrade. Incomplete degradation could lead to complications such as localized inflammation, infection, or the formation of harmful byproducts, thus undermining patient safety.

Additionally, while these materials are designed to degrade, the degradation process itself must be rigorously monitored to ensure it does not compromise the device's structural integrity or function before it is meant to do so. For example, biodegradable stents must maintain their structural support long enough to allow proper healing before safely degrading. If the material degrades prematurely, it could result in device failure, potentially putting patients at risk.

9.9.4 Effectiveness across Different Medical Applications

The effectiveness of biodegradable materials varies significantly depending on their application. In some cases, such as biodegradable sutures, the material has been proven highly effective and has largely replaced traditional non-biodegradable alternatives. However, in more complex medical devices, such as biodegradable implants or drug delivery systems, challenges remain in ensuring consistent performance across different patients and conditions.

Clinical trials have shown mixed results for certain biodegradable medical devices. For example, biodegradable vascular stents have demonstrated promise in reducing the need for follow-up surgeries, but concerns remain about their long-term effectiveness and the possibility of restenosis (re-narrowing of the blood vessels). Similarly, while biodegradable polymers used in drug delivery can enhance patient outcomes, issues with the uniformity of drug release and the material's interaction with the body can affect overall efficacy.

9.9.5 Regulatory and Standardization Challenges

One of the biggest barriers to the widespread adoption of biodegradable materials in healthcare is the lack of standardized testing protocols and clear regulatory guidelines. The long-term safety of these materials, particularly in implantable devices, must be thoroughly established before they can become mainstream. Regulatory bodies such as the FDA and the European Medicines Agency (EMA) require extensive clinical data to demonstrate the safety, efficacy, and biodegradability of these materials under diverse conditions.

Furthermore, the challenge of ensuring uniform biodegradability across different environmental and biological conditions complicates the regulatory approval process. Manufacturers must not only demonstrate that their materials are safe and effective in controlled environments but also prove that they will perform reliably in the varied physiological conditions encountered in actual patients.

While biodegradable materials offer significant potential to enhance patient safety and care, especially by reducing the need for invasive procedures and improving the biocompatibility of medical devices, their safety and effectiveness require careful evaluation. The unpredictable nature of degradation, the variability in patient response, and the lack of standardized protocols are key areas that must be addressed through ongoing research and regulatory refinement. As technology advances and these challenges are resolved, biodegradable materials are poised to play an increasingly critical role in the future of patient care.

9.9.6 Patient Perceptions and Acceptance of Biodegradable Healthcare Products

The growing emphasis on sustainability and environmental responsibility in healthcare is influencing patient perceptions and acceptance of biodegradable healthcare products. As patients become more informed about the environmental impact of medical waste, particularly single-use plastics, their expectations for sustainable alternatives are rising. However, patient acceptance of biodegradable products depends on a combination of factors, including perceived safety, effectiveness, cost, and environmental benefits.

9.9.7 Environmental Awareness and Sustainability

In recent years, there has been a significant increase in patient awareness regarding the environmental consequences of healthcare practices, particularly the reliance on disposable plastic products. Many patients, especially those with a strong environmental consciousness, view biodegradable healthcare products as a positive innovation. Products such as biodegradable packaging, sutures, and medical devices are often seen as environmentally friendly alternatives that align with broader societal efforts to reduce plastic waste and pollution.

For example, patients who understand that biodegradable materials reduce the burden of medical waste on landfills and oceans are more likely to embrace these products. A growing number of consumers are now looking for sustainable options in all areas of their lives, including healthcare, which has prompted medical institutions to adopt greener practices to meet patient expectations.

9.9.8 Perceived Safety and Effectiveness

While environmental concerns are important, patient acceptance ultimately depends on their confidence in the safety and effectiveness of biodegradable products. Patients are generally willing to accept biodegradable materials if they are assured that these products are as safe and effective as traditional alternatives. Studies have shown that patients tend to trust healthcare providers' recommendations, especially when the benefits of biodegradable products, such as reduced surgical interventions for biodegradable implants or drug delivery systems, are clearly explained.

The dilemma inherent in balancing the minimization of plastic waste with the imperative of maintaining patient safety and dependability in medical devices constructed from biodegradable materials presents a multifaceted challenge. While biodegradable materials confer substantial ecological advantages by mitigating plastic waste, they are nonetheless required to adhere to rigorous safety and reliability criteria pertinent to medical applications.

9.9.8.1 Environmental Benefits

Substances that decompose over time, like PCL and PLGA, can greatly lessen the ecological consequences of medical waste through their natural breakdown, compared to regular plastics [59,63]. DNA-derived bioplastics present environmentally sustainable disposal alternatives and are sourced from renewable materials, thereby enhancing the principles of sustainability [62].

9.9.8.2 Patient Safety and Reliability

Biodegradable substances are required to uphold the essential attributes of strength, flexibility, and biocompatibility to guarantee the safety of patients. As a demonstration, PCL paired with PLGA has shown advantageous outcomes regarding their compatibility with living tissues and therapeutic efficacy [59,64]. The shift to biodegradable materials requires affecting challenges associated with material selection, testing, and regulatory approval to guarantee they meet the medical industry's stringent requirements [59]. However, a lack of understanding about biodegradable products can lead to hesitation. For example, patients may question whether a biodegradable medical device or implant will degrade too quickly, potentially compromising their treatment. Therefore, clear communication from healthcare providers about the reliability and safety of these materials is crucial in building patient trust and encouraging acceptance.

9.9.9 Cost Considerations

The cost of biodegradable healthcare products can also influence patient acceptance. In many cases, biodegradable alternatives are more expensive than conventional plastic products due to the higher cost of materials and manufacturing processes. This price difference may be a barrier for some patients, particularly those who do not prioritize environmental benefits or are more concerned about immediate costs. However, for environmentally conscious patients, the perceived long-term benefits of using sustainable materials may outweigh the higher initial costs.

To enhance acceptance, healthcare providers and insurers may need to explore cost-sharing models or subsidies that make biodegradable products more accessible to a broader range of patients. Additionally, as technology advances and biodegradable materials become more widely used, their costs are likely to decrease, making them more appealing to both patients and healthcare providers.

9.9.10 Cultural and Demographic Factors

Patient acceptance of biodegradable healthcare products can also vary based on cultural and demographic factors. Younger generations, who are generally more engaged with sustainability issues, tend to be more open to the use of eco-friendly products. This group is more likely to seek out healthcare providers that prioritize sustainability and offer biodegradable options. On the other hand, older patients or those less familiar with environmental issues may need more education and reassurance about the safety and efficacy of these materials.

Cultural factors also play a role in shaping perceptions. In regions where environmental conservation is a key public concern, patients are more likely to accept biodegradable healthcare products. Conversely, in areas where environmental issues are not a high priority, patient awareness and demand for such products may be lower.

9.9.11 Trust in Healthcare Providers

A key determinant of patient acceptance is the level of trust they place in their healthcare providers. When doctors and healthcare professionals advocate for the use of biodegradable products, explaining the benefits for both the environment and the patient's health, patients are more likely to accept these alternatives. Trust in the healthcare system and the information provided about new products plays a crucial role in patient decisions, making provider communication essential in promoting the use of biodegradable materials (Table 9.5).

TABLE 9.5
Impact of Biodegradables and Metrics

Category	Metrics to Evaluate	Considerations
Environmental impact	• Reduction in plastic waste volume • Biodegradability rate • Carbon footprint reduction	• Assess environmental pollution reduction benefits. • Analyze long-term sustainability in healthcare systems.
Patient safety	• Risk of material degradation during use • Biocompatibility (toxicity, inflammatory response) • Sterilization stability	• Evaluate risks of material failure during procedures. • Ensure compliance with FDA and ISO safety standards.
Device reliability	• Performance consistency • Durability under various conditions • Resistance to mechanical stress	• Compare biodegradable materials' lifecycle reliability to traditional plastics. • Test prototypes thoroughly.
Cost-effectiveness	• Production costs of biodegradable vs. traditional plastics • Manufacturing adaptation costs • Waste disposal savings	• Analyze long-term cost benefits. • Balance initial investments with operational cost savings.
Regulatory compliance	• Conformance to medical device standards (FDA, CE marking) • Environmental compliance (EPA, EU standards)	• Ensure materials meet strict medical-grade and environmental requirements. • Factor in compliance timelines.
Operational feasibility	• Compatibility with manufacturing processes • Integration into healthcare systems	• Assess logistical challenges in adoption. • Train healthcare staff for use and disposal.
Social and ethical considerations	• Public perception of biodegradable devices • Ethical balance between safety and sustainability	• Address public trust concerns. • Prioritize patient safety while meeting sustainability goals.

9.10 INTERDISCIPLINARY APPROACHES TO BIODEGRADABLE PLASTICS

The development and implementation of biodegradable plastics in healthcare require a robust interdisciplinary approach, integrating expertise from materials science, environmental science, healthcare, biology, and chemistry. This collaboration is essential for addressing the multifaceted challenges of creating sustainable, functional alternatives to traditional plastics that meet the stringent demands of medical applications.

Materials scientists play a pivotal role by designing innovative biodegradable polymers and composites with specific properties, such as controlled degradation rates, biocompatibility, and mechanical strength. These materials must be strong enough to meet the needs of medical devices while ensuring they degrade safely within the body or in the environment. At the same time, environmental scientists assess the lifecycle and ecological impact of these materials. Their research ensures that biodegradable plastics do not contribute to microplastic pollution or toxic byproducts and can be integrated into sustainable waste management systems.

Biologists and chemists contribute by exploring natural and renewable sources for biodegradable materials, such as plant-based polymers or proteins derived from animals. These natural materials are refined to ensure their safety and functionality in healthcare settings, including their ability to degrade without causing harm to human health or the environment. For example, polysaccharides and proteins are being developed for use in wound dressings, implants, and drug delivery systems, requiring collaboration across disciplines to ensure biocompatibility and efficacy.

Healthcare professionals offer crucial insights into the practical application of biodegradable materials in clinical settings. Their feedback helps guide the design and testing process, ensuring that the materials meet real-world healthcare requirements, such as sterility, ease of use, and patient safety. This collaboration between researchers and medical practitioners is critical for the successful adoption of biodegradable plastics, as it ensures that these materials are not only scientifically sound but also feasible and effective in everyday medical practice.

By integrating these multidisciplinary perspectives, the development of biodegradable plastics becomes more comprehensive and effective. Interdisciplinary collaboration accelerates innovation, translating laboratory discoveries into market-ready solutions that are both environmentally sustainable and clinically viable. This holistic approach is vital for overcoming the complex challenges associated with biodegradable materials, fostering advancements that improve patient care while reducing the environmental footprint of healthcare. Through the integration of materials science, environmental research, and healthcare expertise, the healthcare industry can adopt biodegradable plastics that meet regulatory standards, enhance patient safety, and contribute to a more sustainable future.

9.11 CONCLUSION

The transition to biodegradable materials in healthcare facilities is gaining momentum as part of the broader global movement toward sustainability. While challenges related to cost, regulatory approval, and supply chain limitations exist, the environmental and long-term economic benefits make this transition a critical focus for healthcare providers. Facilities like Cleveland Clinic, Karolinska University Hospital, and Kaiser Permanente are leading the way, demonstrating that the adoption of biodegradable alternatives in healthcare is both feasible and impactful. As technology advances and biodegradable materials become more widely available, more healthcare systems are likely to follow suit, making sustainability an integral part of healthcare operations.

REFERENCES

1. Hafiza, A. A., Khairunnisa-Atiqah, M. K., Mazlan, N. S. N., Salleh, K. M., & Zakaria, S. (2023). Biocompatible and biodegradable materials in medical applications. In: *Green Sustainable Process for Chemical and Environmental Engineering and Science* (pp. 331–358). Elsevier. doi:10.1016/B978-0-323-95169-2.00010-9.
2. Gopinath, P. M., Parvathi, V. D., Yoghalakshmi, N., Kumar, S. M., Athulya, P. A., Mukherjee, A., & Chandrasekaran, N. (2022). Plastic particles in medicine: A systematic review of exposure and effects to human health. *Chemosphere, 303*, 135227.
3. Flury, M., & Narayan, R. (2021). Biodegradable plastic as an integral part of the solution to plastic waste pollution of the environment. *Current Opinion in Green and Sustainable Chemistry, 30*, 100490.
4. Sen Gupta, R., Samantaray, P. K., & Bose, S. (2023). Going beyond cellulose and chitosan: Synthetic biodegradable membranes for drinking water, wastewater, and oil–water remediation. *ACS Omega, 8*(28), 24695–24717.
5. Wyssusek, K., Avudainayagam, M., Paramor, J., & Barner, L. (2024). Product stewardship in health care: The importance of minimising the environmental and health impacts of plastic products. *Journal of Perioperative Nursing, 37*(2), e27–e32.
6. Shenoy, S. R., Wagdarikar, M. J., & Desai, N. D. (2024). Polymers in medical devices and pharmaceutical packaging. In: *Polymers for Pharmaceutical and Biomedical Applications* (pp. 333–382). Elsevier. doi:10.1016/b978-0-323-95496-9.00009-0.
7. Kheirabadi, S., & Sheikhi, A. (2022). Recent advances and challenges in recycling and reusing biomedical materials. *Current Opinion in Green and Sustainable Chemistry, 38*, 100695.
8. Yang, Y., Yang, Y., Hou, Z., Wang, T., Wu, P., Shen, L., … & Sun, S. (2023). Comprehensive review of materials, applications, and future innovations in biodegradable esophageal stents. *Frontiers in Bioengineering and Biotechnology, 11*, 1327517.
9. Ashter, S. A. (2022). *Applications of Polymers and Plastics in Medical Devices: Design, Manufacture, and Performance*. William Andrew.
10. Alexandrova, L. V., Uspenskaya, M. V., & Ishevsky, A. L. (2023). Overview: Biodegradable packaging film materials. *Proceedings of the Voronezh State University of Engineering Technologies, 85*(2), 216–225. doi:10.20914/2310-1202-2023-2-216-225.
11. Emanuella, F., Fiandra, L., Shaw, M., Starck, C. J., McGurk, C., & Mahon, S. (2023). Designing biodegradable alternatives to commodity polymers. *Chemical Society Reviews*. doi:10.1039/d3cs00556a.
12. Bharadwaj, S., Dhand, V., & Kalyana Lakshm, Y. (2022). Biodegradable composite for smart packaging applications. In: Inamuddin, T. A. (Ed.), *Biodegradable Materials and their Applications*. Wiley. doi:10.1002/9781119905301.ch21.
13. Estefanía, L., Alison, A., Yesly, I., Aline, P., Adriana, P., Pamela, V., & Aracely, S. (2022). Biodegradable packaging made from banana peels. *Alimentos Ciencia e Ingeniería*. doi:10.31243/aci.v29i2.1843.
14. Bruna, A., Araujo, L., de Silva, F., Kênia, K., Freitas, S., Vanessa, R., …, de Medeiros, M. (2021). A aplicação de polímeros biodegradáveis como uma alternativa sustentável. *Research, Society and Development*. doi:10.33448/RSD-V10I9.18248.
15. Danijela, Š., Senka, P., Nevena, H., & Jovana, U. (2020). Degradable packaging materials: Sources, application and decomposition routes. doi:10.5937/JPEA25-30971.
16. Shuo, C., Yihan, W., Lei, Y., Chengzhen, C., Shichun, C., Zhao, W., …, Jiajia, X. (2023). Biodegradable elastomers for biomedical applications. *Progress in Polymer Science*. doi:10.1016/j.progpolymsci.2023.101763.
17. Park, J., & Jürgen, B. (2022). Biodegradable implantable microsystems. doi:10.1109/IEDM45625.2022.10019376.

18. Suzuki, S., & Ikada, Y. (2022). Medical applications. In: *Poly (Lactic Acid) Synthesis, Structures, Properties, Processing, Applications, and End of Life* (pp. 581–604) Wiley. doi:10.1002/9781119767480.ch25.
19. Hafiza, A. A., Khairunnisa-Atiqah, M. K., Mazlan, N. S. N., Salleh, K. M., & Zakaria, S. (2023). Biocompatible and biodegradable materials in medical applications. In: *Green Sustainable Process for Chemical and Environmental Engineering and Science* (pp. 331–358). Elsevier. doi:10.1016/b978-0-323-95169-2.00010-9.
20. Syed, A. A. (2021). Applications of biobased polymers in medical devices. doi:10.1016/b978-0-12-820980-6.00011-4.
21. Nandini, G., Chandrani, S., & Sampa, S. (2022). Biodegradable polymers: Carriers for drug delivery. *Materials Horizons*. doi:10.1007/978-981-99-3307-5_7.
22. Benjamin-Luca, K., Claudia, L., Samuel, O., & Kyeremateng, G. F. (2022). Synthesis and characterization of biodegradable poly(butyl cyanoacrylate) for drug delivery applications. *Polymers*. doi:10.3390/polym14050998.
23. Shuo, C., Yihan, W., Lei, Y., Chengzhen, C., Shichun, C., Zhao, W., …, Zhengwei, Y. (2023). Biodegradable elastomers for biomedical applications. *Progress in Polymer Science*, doi:10.1016/j.progpolymsci.2023.101763.
24. Sudarshan, S., Chuda, C., Bhupendra, G., Prajapati, A., & Chandel, S. (2023). Editorial: Biodegradable polymeric materials in tissue engineering and their application in drug delivery. *Frontiers in Bioengineering and Biotechnology*. doi:10.3389/fbioe.2023.1296119.
25. Ta-Hsin, T., Yu-Chien, T., Hsin-Pei, L., Yi-Hao, C., & Lu, D. (2023). Biodegradable polymer-based drug-delivery systems for ocular diseases. *International Journal of Molecular Sciences*. doi:10.3390/ijms241612976.
26. Nisar Ul, K., Dhawal, C., Dhawal, C., Coralie Adele, R., Monica, R. S., & Yoon, Y. (2021). Engineering microenvironment of biodegradable polyester systems for drug stability and release control. *Therapeutic Delivery*. doi:10.4155/TDE-2020-0113.
27. Zehao, J. (2022). Application of degradable polymers for the treatment of wounds and tumors. *Highlights in Science, Engineering and Technology*. doi:10.54097/hset.v26i.3987.
28. Guilherme, M. R. L., Adrivit, M., Francesco, P., & Ranjita, K. B. (2024). Characterization of biodegradable polymers for porous structure: Further steps toward sustainable plastics. *Polymers*. doi:10.3390/polym16081147.
29. Danbee, P., & Wangyun, W. (2024). Unveiling the environmental gains of biodegradable plastics in the waste treatment phase: A cradle-to-grave life cycle assessment. *Chemical Engineering Journal*. doi:10.1016/j.cej.2024.150540.
30. Trang, T. N., Lieselot, B., Valérie, G., Lucile, C., Maria, R., Mariana, M., & Jo, D. (2024). Environmental sustainability assessment of biodegradable bio-based poly(3-hydroxybutyrate-co-3-hydroxyvalerate) from agro-residues: Production and end-of-life scenarios. *Journal of Environmental Management*. doi:10.1016/j.jenvman.2024.120522.
31. Min, A. J., Minkyung, L., Seonghyn, C., Seul, A. P., Huijeong, P., Hyeon-Jong, J., …, Hyo, J. K. (2024). Ecotoxicity assessment of additives in commercial biodegradable plastic products: Implications for sustainability and environmental risk. *Science of the Total Environment*. doi:10.1016/j.scitotenv.2024.172903.
32. Juan, C., Rui, G., Yong, Z., & Qinbao, L. (2024). Applications of biodegradable materials in food packaging: A review. *Alexandria Engineering Journal*. doi:10.1016/j.aej.2024.01.080.
33. Tim, B., & Manfred, Z. (2024). Key challenges in the advancement and industrialization of biobased and biodegradable plastics: A value chain overarching perspective. *Frontiers in Bioengineering and Biotechnology*. doi:10.3389/fbioe.2024.1406278.
34. YingChao, L., Shuai, W., Song, Q., Zhijie, L., Yujing, W., & Yulong, Z. (2024). Depolymerization and re/upcycling of biodegradable PLA plastics. *ACS Omega*. doi:10.1021/acsomega.3c08674.

35. Puck, B. L. G. R., van Sonja, D., Ruud, B., & Conny, B. (2024). Bio-based plastics in product design: The state of the art and challenges to overcome. *Sustainability.* doi:10.3390/su16083295.
36. Jennifer, J. S., Nur, A., Amirul, A.-A. A., Wei, W., Sevakumaran, V., & Kesaven, B. (2024). Exploring the advantages and limitations of degradation for various biodegradable micro-bioplastic in aquatic environments. *Journal of Environmental Management.* doi:10.1016/j.jenvman.2024.121777.
37. Lara, S.-A., & Auxiliadora Prieto, M. (2024). Can bioplastics always offer a truly sustainable alternative to fossil-based plastics? *Microbial Biotechnology.* doi:10.1111/1751-7915.14458.
38. Ikponmwosa, A., Uwaga, M. A., & Eseoghene, K. (2024). Impact of biodegradable plastics on U.S. environmental conservation: A comprehensive review, exploring the effectiveness, challenges, and broader implications of bioplastics in waste management and eco-preservation. *Engineering Science & Technology Journal.* doi:10.51594/estj.v5i7.1309.
39. Nasar, M., Moeaz, W., & Sayed, A. M. A (2024). Biodegradable suture development-based albumin composites for tissue engineering applications. *Dental Science Reports.* doi:10.1038/s41598-024-58194-5.
40. Jian-Hua, Z., Haiying, W., Hui, Z., Penghao, H., Lei, L., & Haibing, H. (2023). Recent advances in biodegradable electronics- from fundament to the next-generation multi-functional, medical and environmental device. *Sustainable Materials and Technologies.* doi:10.1016/j.susmat.2022.e00530.
41. Zia, U. A. (2024). The role of polysaccharide-based biodegradable soft polymers in the healthcare sector. *Advanced Industrial and Engineering Polymer Research.* doi:10.1016/j.aiepr.2024.05.001.
42. Junhua, Z. (2023). Exploring the utilization of polylactic acid-based materials in medicine: Contemporary innovations and trends. doi:10.54254/2753-8818/23/20231021.
43. Yaochen, Y., Yuanyuan, Y., Zhipeng, H., Tingting, W., Peng, W., Lufan, S., …, Siyu, S. (2023). Comprehensive review of materials, applications, and future innovations in biodegradable esophageal stents. *Frontiers in Bioengineering and Biotechnology.* doi:10.3389/fbioe.2023.1327517.
44. Zia, U. A. (2024). The role of polysaccharide-based biodegradable soft polymers in the healthcare sector. *Advanced Industrial and Engineering Polymer Research.* doi:10.1016/j.aiepr.2024.05.001.
45. Taofeeq, D. M., Gusman, N., Fatimah, M., Fazeeda, B. M., Mohd, H. A., & Airin, A. G. (2021). Expanding policy for biodegradable plastic products and market dynamics of bio-based plastics: Challenges and opportunities. *Sustainability.* doi:10.3390/SU13116170.
46. Eva, G., Sánchez, R., Emiliano, M. A., & Joxemari, S. F. (2017). *Polímeros Biodegradables Con Moléculas Biológicamente Activas Para la Prevención de Infecciones en Dispositivos Biomédicos.* UPV/EHU.
47. Anju, S., Prajitha, N., Sukanya, V. S., & Mohanan, P. V. (2020). Complicity of degradable polymers in health-care applications. *Materials Today Chemistry.* doi:10.1016/J.MTCHEM.2019.100236.
48. Ensieh, S. H., Saoirse, D., Priyanka, G., & Ravinder, D. (2021). Biodegradable materials for sustainable health monitoring devices. doi:10.1021/ACSABM.0C01139.
49. Sushil, K. V., Arbind, P. S., & Vimal, K. (2024). State of art review on sustainable biodegradable polymers with a market overview for sustainability packaging. *Materials Today Sustainability.* doi:10.1016/j.mtsust.2024.100776.
50. Ma, Y., Guo, X., Du, M., Kang, S., Dong, W., Nicolosi, V., … & Qiu, B. (2024). Beyond biodegradation: Upcycling of polylactic acid plastic waste into amino acids via cascade catalysis under mild conditions. *Green Chemistry, 26*(7), 3995–4004.

51. Ali, M. I., Perveen, Q., Ahmad, B., Javed, I., Razi-Ul-Hussnain, R., Andleeb, S., … & Hameed, A. (2009). Studies on biodegradation of cellulose blended polyvinyl chloride films. *International Journal of Agriculture and Biology*, *11*(5), 577–580.
52. Dake, M. (2015). Biodegradable polymers: Renewable nature, life cycle, and applications. In: *Microbial Factories: Biodiversity, Biopolymers, Bioactive Molecules* (Vol. 2, pp. 29–56). Springer.
53. Senko, O., Maslova, O., Stepanov, N., Aslanli, A., Lyagin, I., & Efremenko, E. (2024). Role of humic substances in the (bio) degradation of synthetic polymers under environmental conditions. *Microorganisms*, *12*(10), 2024.
54. Richardson, T., Naidoo, G., Rupasinghe, N., Smart, H., & Bhattacharya, S. (2018). Biodegradable stents in resistant peptic oesophageal stricture: Is it the right way to go? *Clinical Medicine Insights: Gastroenterology*, *11*, 1179552218819492.
55. Yahaya, W. A. W., Azman, N. A. M., Adam, F., Subramaniam, S. D., Abd Hamid, K. H., & Almajano, M. P. (2023). Exploring the potential of seaweed derivatives for the development of biodegradable plastics: A comparative study. *Polymers*, *15*(13), 2884.
56. Sakamoto, Y. (2012). Life cycle assessment of biodegradable plastics. *Journal of Shanghai Jiaotong University (Science)*, *17*, 327–329.
57. Li, R., Feng, Y., Gong, R. H., & Soutis, C. (2023). A biodegradable stereo-complexed poly (lactic acid) drinking straw of high heat resistance and performance. *Materials*, *16*(6), 2438.
58. Thrän, J., Garcia-Garcia, G., Parra-López, C., Ufarte, A., García-García, C., Parra, S., & Sayadi-Gmada, S. (2024). Environmental and economic assessment of biodegradable and compostable alternatives for plastic materials in greenhouses. *Waste Management*, *175*, 92–100.
59. Moshkbid, E., Cree, D. E., Bradford, L., & Zhang, W. (2024). Biodegradable alternatives to plastic in medical equipment: Current state, challenges, and the future. *Journal of Composites Science*, *8*(9), 342.
60. Weerarathna, I. N., Kumar, P., Luharia, A., & Mishra, G. (2025). Sustainable biomaterials for pharmaceutical and medical applications. *Multidisciplinary Reviews*, *8*(5), 2025141–2025141.
61. Mishra, P., Kumar, S., Maurya, A. K., Tiwari, P., Tirkey, S., & Sharma, S. (2024). Bio-based materials in drug delivery. In: *Sustainable Bio-Based Composites: Biomedical and Engineering Applications* (Vol. 20, p. 79). doi:10.1515/9783111321530.
62. Ji, Y., Kim, T., Han, D., & Lee, J. B. (2024). Self-healing and thermal responsive DNA bioplastics for on-demand degradable medical devices. *ACS Materials Letters*, *6*(4), 1277–1287.
63. Soman, R., Mangla, D., & Annu. (2024). Bioplastics in medical devices. In: *Biopolymers for Biomedical Applications* (pp. 417–437). doi:10.1002/9781119865452.ch16
64. Sushma, M. V., kadam, A., Kumar, D., & Mutreja, I. (2023). Biodegradable polymers. In: *Biomaterials and Biopolymers* (pp. 33–54). Springer.
65. Sharma, S., Hashmi, M. F. (2022). Partial pressure of oxygen. In: StatPearls [Internet]. Treasure Island (FL): StatPearls Publishing. PMID: 29630271.
66. Stachowiak, T., & Łukasik, K. (2021). The management of polymer and biodegradable composite waste in relation to petroleum-based thermoplastic polymer waste-in terms of energy consumption and processability. Sustainability (Switzerland), 13(7). https://doi.org/10.3390/su13073701.

10 Circular Sustainable Electronics from Design and Manufacturing to Business Models

Fatemeh Abedi, Ulla A. Saari, Maria Smolander, Liisa Hakola, Tilak Lakshmana, and Thomas M. Kraft

10.1 INTRODUCTION

The healthcare sector is one of the fastest growing industries worldwide and faces significant challenges. A major concern is the large volume of hospital waste produced by the increasing global population. This issue leads to significant environmental, social, and economic challenges (Kenny and Priyadarshini, 2021; MacNeill et al., 2020). To tackle these problems, it is important to focus on how healthcare systems, especially electronic medical devices, are designed and managed. These devices are key to diagnosing, treating, and preventing diseases. They are carefully made to be highly effective, safe, and hygienic, while also aiming to be environmentally friendly and cost-effective (Guzzo et al., 2020).

A major barrier to recycling electronic medical devices and healthcare waste is the regulatory framework, which often classifies significant portions of hospital waste as non-recyclable (Hoveling et al., 2024). Furthermore, the healthcare sector's prioritization of safety and hygiene has led to widespread use of single-use devices, complicating efforts to implement sustainable recycling processes (Leung et al., 2019; Rizan et al., 2020).

Recycling within the healthcare sector is generally limited to non-clinical and uncontaminated materials, such as paper, plastic, and decontaminated glassware, along with certain types of medical and pharmaceutical packaging. However, the potential for recycling a broader range of healthcare waste exists in hospitals, primary care centers, and private clinics. This potential is often prevented by legal and logistical barriers (Kenny and Priyadarshini, 2021).

Adding to these challenges are the rapid technological advancements and the growing complexity of materials used in medical devices. These factors make it difficult to establish standardized recycling processes, as many components are not designed for reuse or repurposing (Kenny and Priyadarshini, 2021; MacNeill et al.,

DOI: 10.1201/9781003513834-10

2020). This issue underscores the urgent need for sustainable waste management strategies tailored to healthcare electronics (Płotka-Wasylka et al., 2022).

To overcome these obstacles, applying circular economy principles to the healthcare sector presents a promising pathway forward. By integrating circular approaches with innovative business models, the so-called Circular Business Models (CBMs) (Geissdoerfer et al., 2018; Płotka-Wasylka et al., 2022), the industry can make progress toward reducing waste and promoting sustainability. In addition, as technology continues to evolve, these strategies must align with updated regulations for medical devices to maintain compliance and effectiveness (Rizos and Bryhn, 2022).

Circular economy is a prominent topic in scientific research, engaging researchers, entrepreneurs, and government officials to develop alternatives to traditional linear production methods (Sehnem et al., 2022). It aims to create economic, social, and environmental value throughout the entire system. Integrating circular economy principles with business model innovation has led to the development of CBMs. These models are designed to enhance resource efficiency and reduce environmental impact by optimizing resource loops, minimizing waste and emissions within organizational value networks (Bocken et al., 2016; Geissdoerfer et al., 2018). CBMs enable companies to create economic value by utilizing materials, products, and components in multiple use cycles (Lüdeke-Freund et al., 2019). CBMs aim to reorganize value creation and supply chains to promote sustainable production and consumption (Hofmann, 2019). Research by Mukoro et al. (2022) indicates that circular economy principles can be incorporated into company operations through the business models (Mukoro et al., 2022).

The European Commission's shift toward a circular economy involves strategies such as enhancing recycling, preventing the loss of valuable materials, creating jobs, driving economic growth, and reducing greenhouse gas emissions and environmental impacts (Bocken et al., 2016; Directorate-General for Communication, European Commission, 2020). This transition is driven by the new Circular Economy Action Plan (CEAP), adopted in 2020, which advances the foundational efforts of the first CEAP introduced in 2015 (Digital EU Commission, 2024). The initial action plan included comprehensive measures aimed at accelerating Europe's transition toward a circular economy by focusing on the entire product life cycle, from production and consumption to waste management and the market for secondary raw materials. These plans aim to facilitate Europe's transition to a circular economy, ultimately promoting sustainable economic growth and creating new employment opportunities.

This transition highlights how innovative business models and eco-design principles can guide Europe toward a zero-waste future. Eco-design takes a holistic approach to the entire product life cycle, focusing on minimizing the environmental impacts (Mendoza et al., 2017). Therefore, by considering different factors such as materials, processes, logistics, and recyclability, the environmental impact of a product can be improved (Milousi and Souliotis, 2023). Hence, the adoption of eco-design and circular economy principles is crucial for driving sustainability in electronics used within the healthcare sector (Sanyé-Mengual et al., 2014).

Previous studies have explored various aspects of sustainability in electronics, emphasizing recycling, waste reduction, and energy efficiency (Lee et al., 2012; O'Connor et al., 2016). However, the challenges in implementing circular economy principles specifically in the healthcare sector have not been fully addressed. Fernandes et al. (2023) conducted a thorough review of methods and solutions for tracing the value chain of electric and electronic equipment. Their study also examines technologies that could support and advance the circular economy model within this value chain (Fernandes et al., 2023). In addition, other studies conducted by Hapuwatte and Jawahir (2021) show that designing products with circular design principles involves creating goods intended for reuse, refurbishment, remanufacturing, or recycling, while minimizing waste and reducing environmental impact (Hapuwatte and Jawahir, 2021). By adopting a circular design approach, manufacturers aim to capture value throughout the entire product life cycle. In addition to studies conducted in healthcare (Guzzo et al., 2020; Rizan et al., 2020), the study done by Mendoza et al. (2019) explores cleaner production methods for disposable baby diapers, focusing on the economic and environmental benefits of using optimized absorbent cores and innovative bonding technologies (Mendoza et al., 2019). Evaluating these methods across various production scales highlights significant potential for cost reductions and enhanced eco-efficiency within the diaper industry.

Integrating circular economy principles into the electronics sector involves considering various elements. For instance, a study by Bocken et al. (2016) shows the need to expand research frameworks to include aspects such as supply chain management, developing technologies, and robust infrastructural support. Furthermore, it also points to the lack of methods for assessing the sustainability impacts of circular products and business models across environmental, social, and economic dimensions (Bocken et al., 2016). In addition, the current literature on customer satisfaction identifies a gap in reliable metrics for assessing customer satisfaction with the sustainability of the products they purchase and use (Globocnik and Holzmann, 2024).

The study conducted by Koide et al. (2023) outlines an analysis of consumer preferences for CBMs such as reuse, refurbishment, and subscription services. It also suggests that future studies explore consumer behavior toward reparability. However, recycling strategies need to be considered to ensure the circular economy approach addresses both product life cycle extension and material recovery (Koide et al., 2023). This multi-viewpoint approach is important as it highlights the various challenges and solutions in adopting circular economy principles.

There is also a lack of studies on integrating circular economy principles within healthcare electronics, particularly in smart hygiene products. Although various studies have explored the circular economy and CBMs, few address the challenges and requirements of the healthcare sector, where hygiene, safety, and product lifespan are critical (MacNeill et al., 2020; Mendoza et al., 2019).

This chapter aims to investigate how circular economy principles can be integrated into healthcare product design, particularly smart hygiene products, from the perspectives of the customer, technology developers, as well as sales and marketing. These perspectives provide valuable insights for researchers and industry professionals aiming to promote sustainable practices within the healthcare industry. The data for this study was collected during a focus group workshop on circular electronics at the IEEE FLEPS 2024 conference, hosted by the Technical Research Centre of Finland Ltd (VTT) and Tampere University, Finland. The workshop brought together a diverse group of experts from the academia, research institutes, and industry.

They explored integrating circular economy principles into electronics, focusing on smart hygiene products in healthcare environments. The primary objectives of the workshop were to identify the most prevalent barriers within the circular product value chain, pinpoint critical aspects of product circularity, and explore potential CBMs applicable to the electronics sector. This research aims to investigate how circular economy principles can be integrated into the design of healthcare electronics, particularly smart hygiene products, by focusing on the customer, technology developers, as well as sales and marketing perspectives. The findings are summarized in a framework for both academics and practitioners for enhancing sustainability in healthcare product design, addressing existing gaps, and contributing to the development of CBMs in this sector.

This study addresses the following research questions (RQs):

- **RQ1**: How can reusable electronics and detachable components enhance sustainability while ensuring hygiene and care efficiency in the healthcare industry? (Customer perspective)
- **RQ2**: What key technological development would enable the extension of product life cycles and enhance the recyclability of electronic components in smart hygiene products? (Technology development perspective)
- **RQ3**: What needs to be incorporated into sales and marketing strategies to meet consumer expectations and promote a sustainable electronics industry? (Sales perspective)

This study is structured into several sections. Following this introduction, Section 10.2 explores the background literature. Section 10.3 outlines the research methodology. Section 10.4 presents the results. Finally, Section 10.5 discusses the findings, draws conclusions, and proposes areas for future research.

10.2 LITERATURE REVIEW

Section 10.2.1 presents the background on the CBM concept. Section 10.2.2 provides an overview of customer needs and requirements within the healthcare industry. Section 10.2.3 focuses on sustainable technology development for a circular economy, and Section 10.2.4 addresses different aspects that need to be considered in the sales and marketing strategies.

10.2.1 Circular Business Models

Circular economy aims to minimize resource input, waste, emissions, and energy leaks by optimizing material and energy loops through digitalization, servitization, and sustainable practices like long-lasting product design, maintenance, repair, reuse, remanufacturing, refurbishing, and recycling (Geissdoerfer et al., 2023). Research on the circular economy has shifted from focusing on technological aspects, such as recycling methods, to examining business models. This change aims to better analyze the factors that influence the adoption of existing circular technologies (Antikainen and Valkokari, 2016; Geissdoerfer et al., 2023; Guldmann and Huulgaard, 2020).

Scholarly interest in CBMs has increased from 2015 onward, as evidenced by the growing number of publications that provide thorough reviews and detailed insights into this field (Geissdoerfer et al., 2023). CBM definitions utilize the value creation framework, which includes the elements of value proposition, value creation and delivery, and value capture in the context of the circular economy. These components are aligned with the principles and strategies of the circular economy (Galvão et al., 2020; Mentink, 2014; Nußholz, 2018).

The definition of CBMs varies across different sources. For instance, Mentink (2014) defined a CBM as the rationale of how an organization creates, delivers, and captures value with and within closed material loops. Bocken et al. (2016) and their colleagues present CBM strategies suitable for transitioning to a circular economy, based on the taxonomy of slowing, closing, and narrowing resource loops (Bocken et al., 2016). Furthermore, Zucchella and Previtali (2019) emphasize that the primary goal of the business model is to incorporate circular economy principles into the design or redesign of business processes and partnerships (Zucchella and Previtali, 2019).

In the healthcare sector, CBMs provide financial benefits that could motivate healthcare providers to transition to sustainable practices. The study conducted by Guzzo et al. (2020) discusses how CBMs in the medical device industry enable cost savings through product life extension and resource efficiency. For example, implementing take-back schemes and refurbishing programs for electronic medical equipment not only reduces environmental impact but also reduces procurement costs for healthcare facilities. Moreover, their research showed that hospitals can achieve operational cost reductions of approximately 28% by adopting circular practices, such as leasing medical devices instead of purchasing new ones (Guzzo et al., 2020).

The refurbished medical device market is projected to grow significantly, driven by increasing public and private investments in developing countries. The market size, estimated at $9.9 billion in 2022, is expected to increase to $22.2 billion by 2032, with a compound annual growth rate (CAGR) of 11.6% from 2023 to 2032. North America and Europe are established markets, with North America holding a leading 28.24% share in 2021 ("Global refurbished medical equipment market," 2023; Pinheiro et al., 2024). Major medical equipment manufacturers, such as Siemens and Philips, have set up facilities specifically for refurbishing equipment and reselling it with warranties under distinct brand names. This approach has been especially effective for high-cost, complex devices like magnetic resonance imaging (MRI) machines, X-ray systems, patient monitors, and anesthesia machines, which can be refurbished and sold at 60%–70% of their original price (Kane et al., 2018).

Hospitals are adopting the reprocessing of single-use devices as a strategic response to rising costs and limited budgets, aiming to reduce both expenses and waste. By considering single-use devices as reusable resources rather than disposable items, hospitals can implement a circular model that provides both financial and environmental benefits. In 2023, reprocessed single-use devices enabled hospitals to save over $465 million, reduce waste by 23 million pounds, and lower greenhouse gas emissions. Expanding reprocessing practices across additional facilities could lead to savings and aligns with the growing "right to repair" movement, which supports hospitals' sustainable management of their equipment. This approach strengthens the argument for CBMs in healthcare, offering a cost-effective and environmentally responsible solution (Association of Medical Device Reprocessors, 2024).

10.2.2 Customer Value Creation in the Circular Economy

The main aim of a company is to create value for its customers, leading to the generation of profit (Kumar and Reinartz, 2016; Van Boerdonk et al., 2021). When businesses align with customer values that shape satisfaction and loyalty, they build trust and strengthen relationships. Customer satisfaction influences both purchasing decisions and subsequent buying behavior (Chen, 2010; Pinkse and Bohnsack, 2021; Van Boerdonk et al., 2021). This is the case also for products that are the result of sustainable product innovations (Pinkse and Bohnsack, 2021) and in the context of healthcare products designed for the circular economy (Van Boerdonk et al., 2021).

The existing research on customer satisfaction highlights a lack of dependable metrics for evaluating how satisfied customers are with the sustainability of the products they buy and use (Globocnik and Holzmann, 2024). Previous research has explored various aspects of customer satisfaction (Danaher and Haddrell, 1996) and its components. These components include satisfaction with specific functions (Tandon et al., 2016), usability (Bai et al., 2008), design (Homburg et al., 2015), and service quality (Rajeswari et al., 2017).

Companies need to also understand their customers' business models. They should consider value propositions as performance targets and effectively communicate their products and services. Mishra et al. (2018) highlighted the importance of diverse business models in delivering customer value within a circular economy. Therefore, improving customer service, particularly through services such as maintenance and return agreements, can enhance the service quality (Mishra et al., 2018; Van Boerdonk et al., 2021). Customers also benefit from enhanced reliability, improved service levels, and reduced risk of defects or maintenance issues as well as increased flexibility (Bocken et al., 2018; Pascual et al., 2016).

10.2.3 Sustainable Technology Development for a Circular Economy

Consumer interest in sustainable products is growing, especially in those with reduced content of toxic substances, improved durability, and increased potential for reuse (Essoussi and Linton, 2010; Van Boerdonk et al., 2021). This interest emphasizes the importance of technological innovations in facilitating the transition toward a circular economy within the electronics industry, particularly for smart hygiene products in healthcare applications. The integration of circular economy principles into product design and manufacturing necessitates advancements in materials science, product architecture, and digital technologies. These advancements aim to enhance product longevity, enable reuse, and recycling processes, which helps minimize environmental impact (Bocken et al., 2016; Geissdoerfer et al., 2017).

Design for disassembly, modularity, and reusability are key strategies for extending product lifespans and facilitating end-of-life processing. These strategies focus on designing products so that components can be separated and recovered, reducing the complexity and cost of recycling (Charter and Gray, 2008). Furthermore, designing for sterilization ensures that reusable components maintain their integrity and functionality after multiple sterilization cycles (Garvey, 2023). Modularity allows for individual components to be independently replaced, upgraded, or repaired without the need to discard the entire product, thus conserving resources and reducing waste (den Hollander et al., 2017). In the case of smart hygiene products, implementing modular designs where electronic components, such as sensors and communication modules, are detachable can enhance circularity.

Advancements in materials science are vital for developing sustainable electronics that align with circular economy principles. The use of bio-based and biodegradable materials in electronic components facilitates reducing the environmental impacts associated with electronic waste (e-waste) (Irimia-Vladu, 2013; Jaiswal et al., 2023). For example, printing-based manufacturing methods enable the use of a wide variety of several environmentally friendly substrates like paper, bioplastics (e.g. polyethylene terephthalate (PET)), or veneer in combination with conductive inks like silver or even more preferably carbon or copper for the production of disposable sensors and circuits. These devices can minimize environmental impact at the end of their life cycle in comparison to conventionally fabricated electronic devices (Naji Nassajfar et al., 2023).

Smart diapers, embedded with sensors and connected technologies, offer real-time monitoring of the user's condition, enhancing comfort and care for infants and the elderly (Baek, 2023). In other words, sensor technology supports smart hygiene products by enabling the real-time monitoring of physiological parameters. The development of flexible, stretchable, and skin-mountable sensors provides high sensitivity and user comfort (Amjadi et al., 2015). Hence, these wearable sensors can monitor a range of biomarkers, including moisture levels, temperature, and biochemical indicators, which are crucial for patient care within healthcare facilities. While technological advancements offer different benefits, incorporating circular economy principles into electronic product design faces different challenges including the following:

- **Hygiene Standards and Performance**: In healthcare products, reusable electronic components are designed to maintain reliable performance across multiple use cycles while meeting high hygiene and safety standards to prevent contamination. This requires that materials and components are not only durable but also capable of withstanding repeated sterilization processes without degradation (Garvey, 2023).
- **Material Compatibility**: Combining biodegradable materials with electronic components is challenging due to differences in material properties like thermal and mechanical stability. Therefore, it is imperative that biodegradable components do not compromise the functionality of electronic devices to promote sustainable product design (Irimia-Vladu, 2013).

The Internet of Things (IoT) is an advanced technological framework where physical and virtual objects with unique identifiers (IDs) are connected through a global network. These objects interact within the network, offering and receiving services as part of business processes, while addressing security and privacy concerns (Kiritsis, 2011). IoT systems and solutions are designed for various purposes, including wearable devices and sensors that are integrated into our living environments (Hyysalo et al., 2022). Smart healthcare leverages advanced technologies like IoT, Internet of Medical Things (IoMT), artificial intelligence (AI), big data, and cloud computing to enhance the availability, convenience, efficiency, and personalization of digitalized healthcare services (Baek, 2023; Hyysalo et al., 2022; Tian et al., 2019). However, this study does not explore the various technology models in detail.

Wearable healthcare technologies have evolved from being tools for medical professionals to becoming available for everyday use for consumers to enhance their personal well-being (Hyysalo et al., 2022). Digitalization and the IoT enhance the functionality and sustainability of smart hygiene products by enabling connectivity and data exchange. IoT technologies facilitate remote monitoring, analysis of the data, and integration with healthcare information systems, improving patient care and operational efficiency (Atzori et al., 2010; Baek, 2023; Walden et al., 2021). This is also helping the healthcare personnel whose workload is increasing as the numbers of elderly are growing in the developed countries (World Health Organization, 2016).

10.2.4 Sales and Marketing of Circular Economy Products

Sales strategies play a crucial role in the adoption of circular economy products in the healthcare sector, where product effectiveness, safety, and regulatory compliance are critical (Kane et al., 2018). Transitioning to CBMs requires innovative sales approaches that align with sustainability principles while addressing the specific needs and high-quality standards of stakeholders such as healthcare providers, patients, and regulatory authorities (Hofmann, 2019). However, to the best of the authors' knowledge, there is a lack of studies specifically addressing sales and marketing strategies for circular economy products in the healthcare sector. This gap highlights the need for further research to develop effective approaches that can facilitate the adoption of circular products in this industry.

Baek (2023) emphasizes the importance of educating consumers about the benefits of smart diapers, including health monitoring and environmental advantages when integrated into a circular economy. Tunn et al. (2019) suggest that marketing messages can be designed to provide educational information about products. From these studies, it becomes evident that incorporating educational aspects into marketing strategies is crucial for promoting smart diapers. This ensures that consumers are aware of both their personal health benefits and their positive environmental impact (Tunn et al., 2019).

Developing customer-centric value propositions is key to promoting circular products (Lee, 2017; Muchenje et al., 2023). In the healthcare sector, addressing the needs of multiple stakeholders including healthcare managers, nurses, patients, and their relatives in value propositions enhances their effectiveness (Pereno and Eriksson, 2020). Incorporating feedback such as surveys and polls enables companies to understand real customer needs and tailor their products accordingly (Frishammar and Parida, 2019). Engaging customers in the product development process enhances satisfaction and loyalty, leading to increased sales (Globocnik and Holzmann, 2024). For instance, understanding the specific requirements of nurses and caregivers can facilitate product improvements that make smart hygiene products user-friendly and effective. Therefore, marketing strategy focuses on the added value provided by smart features and sustainability. This emphasizes how the product contributes to health monitoring while also reducing environmental impact, affecting its competitiveness in the market (Chamberlin and Boks, 2018). Moreover, Life Cycle Assessment (LCA) can identify hotspots in the product life cycle where improvements are most needed, informing not only product development but also targeted marketing messages. Integrating LCA insights into marketing efforts helps companies meet regulatory requirements and address consumer expectations for sustainability (Chamberlin and Boks, 2018).

Several aspects related to CBMs and their application in the healthcare sector have been identified from the literature review, focusing on customer needs, technology development, and marketing strategies. Nevertheless, there is still a gap in the development of reliable metrics to assess customer satisfaction with the sustainability features of products (Globocnik and Holzmann, 2024). Moreover, there is a lack of research on the incorporation of customer-centric approaches in the development of sustainable technologies for the healthcare sector. This gap highlights the need for research to incorporate consumer perspectives into the design and functionality of smart hygiene products, aligning with the objectives of circular economy principles. Therefore, exploring and addressing consumer needs in this context is vital for driving the adoption of sustainable technologies and achieving environmental and economic benefits within the healthcare industry (Van Boerdonk et al., 2021). Various CBM strategies such as slowing, closing, and narrowing resource loops have been explored (Bocken et al., 2016; Moreno et al., 2016), but their application in the healthcare sector is limited by specific customer needs and regulations. Sales and marketing strategies in this context demonstrate a gap, requiring further research and the development of frameworks for implementation.

10.3 METHODS AND DATA COLLECTION

Focus group research is a qualitative methodology for collecting expert data, providing either primary evidence or supplementary information (Gill et al., 2008). In this study, we applied focus group methods during the IEEE FLEPS 2024 workshop on Circular and Sustainable Electronics. This workshop was organized as part of an EU project, the Sustronics project, and aims to support future product development and policymaking in sustainable electronics. We gathered participants from diverse backgrounds to share and discuss their experiences relevant to our research topic. In addition, the Impact Canvas (IC) tool is employed to analyze the RQs and assess the most critical aspects of product circularity in electronics within smart hygiene products from three different viewpoints: Customer, Technology-developer, and Sales (Saari et al., 2017). The following paragraphs provide further details on the IC tool and its implementation.

In healthcare research, methods like interviews and focus groups are often utilized (Gill et al., 2008). The focus group method was introduced by sociologists Robert Merton and Paul Lazarsfeld in the 1940s (Caretta and Vacchelli, 2015). This method is utilized for sociological research and later expanded to market research to explore consumer attitudes toward products (Gill et al., 2008). Focus groups are useful for gathering collective opinions and exploring participants' experiences and perspectives (Gill et al., 2008; Traynor, 2015). However, it is important to acknowledge that the focus group method introduces potential biases due to participant subjectivity, which may limit the generalizability of our findings.

Workshops in participatory action research democratize the research process by involving participants in formulating objectives and contributing to findings (Caretta and Vacchelli, 2015). In the workshop session, a moderator is required to introduce the topic, explain the research objectives, and clarify what participants can expect. This allows participants to share their knowledge, questions, concerns, and ideas about the specific topic under discussion (Gill et al., 2008; Traynor, 2015). In general, workshop activities such as brainstorming, role-playing, creating collages, sorting pictures, and ranking are supported by materials like pictures, flipcharts, posters, and project plans (Caretta and Vacchelli, 2015).

The IC tool is designed to support researchers and pre-start-up teams in the early stages of idea development and testing. It addresses critical areas necessary for shaping business concepts with social impact. In addition, the IC tool consists of seven different content elements that represent the key areas that need to be developed: vision, customer, solution, competition, resources, actions, and team (Saari et al., 2018, 2017). Each section provides guiding questions to help users explore and refine their ideas (see Figure 10.1) (Saari et al., 2017). In IEEE FLEPS 2024 workshop, three specific elements of the IC tool were focused on: (i) customer, (ii) solution (technology developer), and (iii) competition (sales and marketing), as these elements are relevant to CBMs and represent critical considerations when designing CBMs for novel products. Figure 10.1 shows the layout of the IC tool used in the workshop.

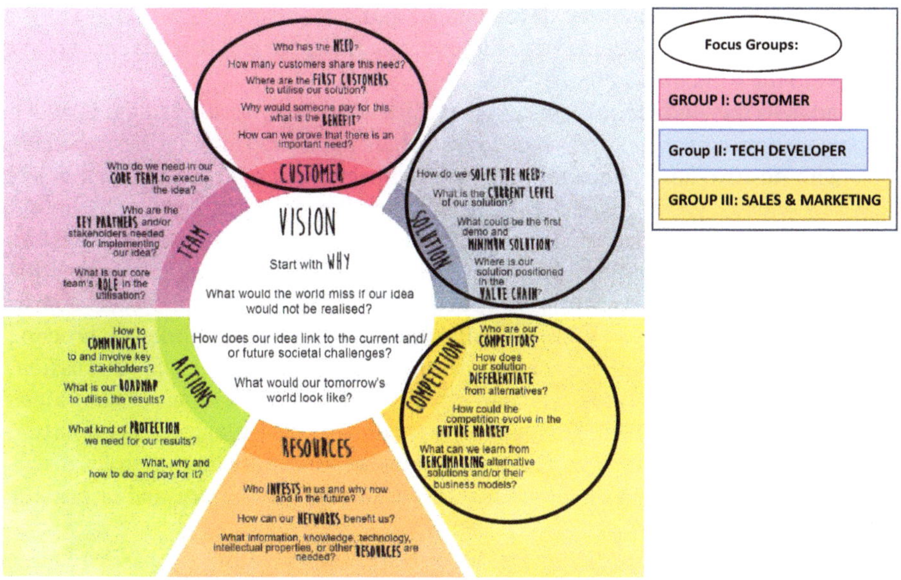

FIGURE 10.1 The Impact Canvas tool layout (Saari et al. 2017).

This study is conducted in three steps: (i) Data collection using the IC tool via the focused group at the IEEE FLEPS 2024 workshop, (ii) Data analysis, incorporating data gathered from Post-it notes, and (iii) Formulation of conclusions and recommendations based on the findings. The following paragraphs provide an in-depth explanation of the process.

The workshop focused on advancing the design, manufacturing, and commercialization of circular and sustainable electronics in line with European environmental agendas. The discussions were organized based on three key perspectives:

1. **Customer**: Focusing on user needs, user-centric designs that prioritize ease of use, reliability, and the sustainability of smart hygiene products.
2. **Technology Developer**: Exploring innovative technologies that can enhance the use, extend the lifespan, and enhance the recyclability of electronic components used in healthcare products.
3. **Sales and Marketing**: Developing marketing strategies for circular electronics that align with consumer expectations and promote industry sustainability standards.

The focus group for the IEEE FLEPS 2024 workshop consisted of 16 participants with diverse backgrounds in circular and sustainable electronics. Among the participants from different European and international countries, four were academics from universities. Five participants were research and development (R&D) personnel from research and technology organizations (RTOs). The remaining seven were industry experts representing different companies. The participants specialized in areas including product design, business development, and technological innovations in circular healthcare products. This mix allowed us to explore a wide range of insights on customer needs, technology development, and sales strategies for circular electronics in healthcare, balancing both theoretical knowledge and practical experience relevant to the workshop's objectives.

To address the guiding question at the FLEPS workshop, we utilized the IC tool to investigate how it enables experienced researchers to develop circular business solutions with positive environmental and social impacts. Our analysis concentrates on the tool's selected guiding content elements: Customer, Solution, and Competition.

In the workshop, the participants were divided into three working groups and each of the three groups was guided by a moderator who played a crucial role in detailing the procedures for various exercises and activities that the participants were required to perform collaboratively. Figure 10.2 illustrates the flow of the workshop process.

The workshop included focused brainstorming sessions and group discussions, each serving distinct purposes. The participants in the brainstorming sessions aimed to generate comprehensive ideas and solutions addressing challenges and opportunities in circular product design for smart hygiene products, while the group discussions were crucial for refining these ideas, assessing their feasibility, and prioritizing practical steps.

First, the workshop facilitator introduced the IC tool to all the participants in the workshop. Then, participants used Post-it notes to share their ideas within three focus groups: Group I (Customer), Group II (Technology developers), and Group III

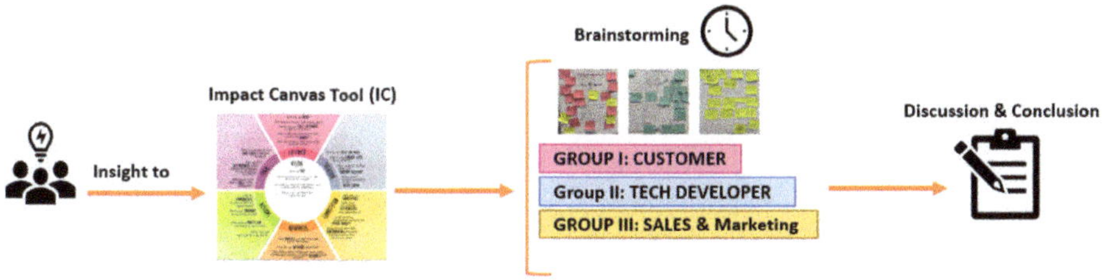

FIGURE 10.2 Workshop process flow.

(Sales and marketing). The main tasks during these sessions involved identifying major barriers in product circularity, exploring potential technical and CBM solutions, and developing recommendations for integrating circular economy principles in healthcare electronics.

The collaborative effort followed a rotating iterative process, involving three distinct groups in brainstorming sessions. For instance, one group concentrated on the customer perspective. Meanwhile, they actively engaged in discussions about sales strategies and technological developments, contributing their ideas to both areas.

Each brainstorming session lasted approximately 15-minutes and there were three different rounds, and each expert participated in three workgroups which resulted in the end to a total of 45 minutes input per expert. Afterward, participants consolidated the key points from their Post-it note discussions into three summarized tables (Tables 10.1–10.3). At the end of the workshop, the lead representatives from each group presented these summaries to all the participants in the workshop.

10.4 RESULTS

The results from the focus group workshop highlighted several important factors for the business viability of smart hygiene products. The evaluation of technology readiness and market readiness has become a crucial aspect in assessing the market viability of smart hygiene products. This approach is based on insights gathered from a focus group workshop, where participants emphasized the importance of assessing both the technical maturity and market potential of a product. Therefore, evaluating both aspects is necessary to align with customer expectations and promote sustainability initiatives. Understanding these findings requires insight into technology readiness and market readiness, as these were important themes discussed in the workshop.

Technology readiness refers to the product's technical maturity, including aspects like validation and interoperability. It ensures that the technology meets functional requirements and integrates with existing systems (Ardilio et al., 2015). On the other hand, market readiness focuses on market acceptance and innovation, demonstrating that the product addresses customer needs and aligns with market demands (Kwon and Son, 2018).

Figure 10.3 outlines how technology readiness and market readiness serve as key components in ensuring the business viability of smart hygiene products. It emphasizes the importance of product validation and interoperability to achieve innovation and market acceptance.

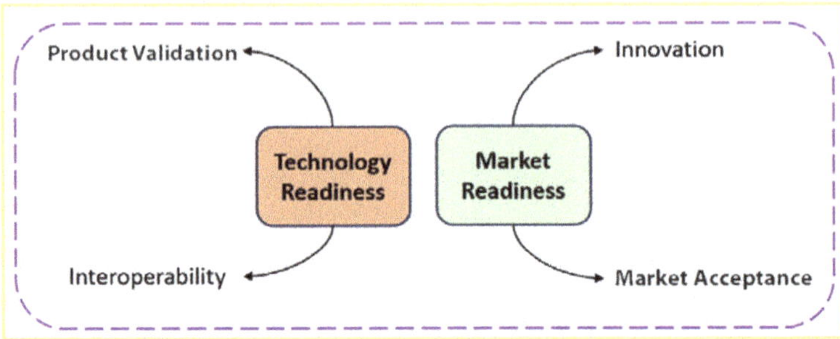

FIGURE 10.3 Business viability through technology and market readiness.

Since sustainability and circularity have become critical factors, customer insights play an important role in guiding product development to meet these demands. According to the workshop results, technology developers should prioritize these insights to address both technical and sustainability requirements, making the product ready for the market.

10.4.1 Customer Needs and Circularity Aspects in Healthcare Industry for Smart Hygiene Product

This section explores customer needs and the circularity of smart hygiene products in the healthcare industry based on the results from the focus workgroup discussions. It highlights efficiency, reliability, and user-friendliness, while promoting sustainability through modular designs and reusable components.

10.4.1.1 Customer Perspective

Group I, consisting of various professionals in the electronics industry, focused on identifying the needs and potential circular solutions for health monitoring products used in elderly care facilities.

The primary needs identified by the group include:

- **Efficiency and Simplicity**: It is important to prioritize efficiency and simplicity of the product due to the lack of nurses for caring, ensuring quality care without staff burnout.
- **Reliable Health Monitoring**: It is crucial to monitor vital health indicators such as glucose levels, infection markers, and the hygiene status of the diaper.
- **User-Friendliness**: There is a need for smart hygiene product that are easy to handle, with a simple process in their use and disposal, requiring only a minimal number of steps.

In the workshop for the CBM part, the important aspect is the consideration of circularity and the extension of product lifespan, especially for temporary-use products like smart diapers and medical devices for short-term health monitoring such as electrocardiogram (ECG) devices. According to the participants' views, incorporating modular and detachable electronic components can facilitate extending the lifetime of these devices. This enables components to be utilized in various contexts and devices which helps minimize waste. Furthermore, the advantages of circular products within the healthcare sector are varied. These can enhance patient care by providing more durable and reliable equipment, reducing the risk of infections, and improving overall care quality. Hence, circular products can help reduce the workload of healthcare providers by minimizing maintenance and repair requirements. As sustainability is important in today's world, the environmental benefits of circular products, such as reduced waste and resource consumption, further incentivize healthcare facilities to invest in these innovative solutions.

Table 10.1 shows an overview of customer needs, health monitoring requirements, and circularity strategies discussed at the workshop. It categorizes the distinct requirements of different customer groups such as healthcare managers of elderly homes, nurses, patients, elderly, babies, and caretakers. The requirements of these groups emphasize the importance of optimizing nursing resources, maintaining quality care, and balancing budgets. Specific health monitoring needs focus on

TABLE 10.1
Customer Perspective

Group I (Customer)	Requirements	Circularity and Sustainability Features
Healthcare managers, nursing staff, private and public healthcare sector	• Optimizing nursing time • Ensuring care quality • Budget management • Efficiency in care procedure	• Reusable electronics where applicable • Close recycling facilities
Patient and user	• Effective health monitoring (e.g., diaper status, glucose level, viral infections) • Enhance patient care and hygiene • Prevent skin diseases • Better hygiene (Reduce smell)	• Detachable and disinfectable components • Reuse and reset of electronic modules
Babies, elderly, caretakers	• Quality of life • Maintaining data integrity • Quick response to alarms • Efficiency • User-friendly product design • Low cost • Indication and timing for changing hygiene products	• Easy recycling and disposal processes
Caretakers, nursing homes	• Easy to use • Low cost • Uncomplicated recycling • No skin irritation • Indication and timing for changing hygiene products	• Close recycling facilities • Easy disposal

continuous updates on vital health indicators such as diaper status, glucose levels, and signs of viral infections. The table also outlines the integration of circular economy principles for smart hygiene products through features like reusable electronics and easily detachable components, highlighting the workshop's commitment to sustainability.

In addition, during the workshop different factors such as ease of use, cost-effectiveness, and recycling processes, highlighting how these aspects enhance user experience and support environmental goals, were discussed. This part of the workshop concentrated on understanding customer goals by examining the interaction between stakeholder needs and the circular economy strategies explored. This will aid in future product development and service improvements in the healthcare sector.

10.4.1.2 Technology Developers

Group II focused on the technology aspects of smart hygiene products with circular economy principles, as illustrated in Table 10.2. A major focus was on addressing the life cycle of both the product's materials and its electronic components to develop a sustainable CBM. To address the need for product circularity, especially concerning the materials and electronic components in smart hygiene products, the group highlighted the significance of designing products with consideration for their end of life and reusability.

Participants in Group II proposed solutions for the disposal of electronic components, which are essential for the functionality of smart hygiene products but difficult to discard. They emphasized that these components should be designed to be easily separable from the disposable or potentially biodegradable parts to facilitate different end-of-life scenarios like reuse or repurposing. For example, sensors used for monitoring health parameters could be designed modularly to allow their transfer to a new product after the initial product's end of life. This reusability not only aligns with circular economy principles but is also critical for reducing e-waste.

Further discussion highlighted that once these components are separated, they can either be reused, refurbished for extended use, or recycled. While reusability was

TABLE 10.2
Technology Developers' Perspective

Group II (Technology Developers)	
Focus Area	**Key Points**
Complex product composition	Plastics, bio-waste, biodegradable, electronics
Reusable parts	In clothes, easy sensor separation for recycling
Environmental impact of sensors	E-waste, biodegradability
Upgradability of sensors	Sensor programming for different patients
Microfluidics for sample transfer	Sensors outside, channels on paper
Diagnostic sensor	Sensor indicating absence of output
Digitalization benefits	Achieving sustainability benefits
Market demand vs. technology	Technology driven by market needs
Separation of components	Electronics: Bio-waste collection, reusable electronics

emphasized by participants as an important approach, it was not considered the only relevant R-strategy. The participants recognized reusability, recycling, refurbishing, and repurposing as important strategies within a CBM. For instance, metals within electronics could be reused, which requires a carefully managed collection and recycling process integrated into the company's value chain (Van Yken et al., 2021). This step is crucial and rated as medium to high in importance. Therefore, it supports sustainability goals and provides economic returns through material recovery.

Group II focused on the environmental impact by exploring innovative technological approaches. They suggested microfluidics for efficient sample transfer and enhanced sensor separability to facilitate recycling.

10.4.1.3 Sales and Marketing

The last group, Group III, shared their ideas on sales and marketing for creating market readiness for a new sustainable circular solution on sensor-equipped diapers tailored for both infants and elderly users.

Table 10.3 summarizes the main points discussed in the workgroups concerning sales and marketing strategies for different customer segments and features of products related to elderly and baby care.

From the sales perspective, the key stakeholders are the future potential users, caretakers, medical professionals, and regulatory bodies, who are also integral to the product's development and deployment. Engaging these groups requires establishing effective communication, ongoing feedback processes, and partnerships with

TABLE 10.3
Sales and Marketing Perspectives

Group III (Sales and Marketing)

Focus Area	Key Points
Product features	• Easy to use, handle, and dispose • No extra costs or special disposal processes
Efficiency	Time and resource management, motivating nurses
Value propositions based on user needs	• Babies at home: quality of life, response to alarms. • Elderly at home: data for mobile nursing personnel and data for relatives.
Feedback	Use question polls for real needs
Costs	Clear cost model and value propositions
Industry standards	Standardization of diaper industry
Sensor technology	Sensors for timely response, simplicity, and enhanced sensitivity
Marketing and awareness	Informing public about product availability, enhanced functionality like global positioning system (GPS) and emergency alerts, potential adaptations for other uses like sound and wound monitoring.
Product development	Home smart diapers for infants, potential future adaptations for wound monitoring.

healthcare facilities and regulatory bodies to ensure that the product meets market and compliance standards.

According to the workshop findings, it is important for smart hygiene products to offer user-friendly operation, easy handling, and straightforward disposal without incurring additional costs or requiring complex procedures. Emphasizing benefits such as enhanced efficiency, reduced workload for nursing staff, and improved patient care can encourage healthcare providers to adopt these products. Hence, to achieve widespread deployment in the healthcare sector, it is crucial to standardize industry practices and enhance sensor technology for improved performance. Furthermore, developing a clear cost model incorporating reimbursement mechanisms ensures affordability and minimizes financial barriers for institutions adopting these solutions. By addressing these key areas, institutions can overcome financial challenges and facilitate broader adoption, securing both the economic and technical foundations necessary for successful implementation.

10.5 DISCUSSION AND CONCLUSION

The IEEE FLEPS 2024 workshop brought together a multidisciplinary group of 16 participants, including researchers from the academia, research institutes, industry, product developers, business developers, and researchers specializing in the circular economy, who came together to share their innovative ideas on the design and manufacturing of circular and sustainable electronics. Through focused brainstorming sessions and group discussions, the workshop identified key barriers, critical aspects of product circularity, and potential CBM designs for the electronics sector.

The focus of the workshop was then shifted to the healthcare sector, guided by a use case (smart hygiene products such as diapers) from the Sustronics project as a European Union initiative aimed at transforming the electronics industry by promoting sustainable materials, eco-friendly design, energy-efficient manufacturing, and CBMs.

Participants explored how circular design principles could be effectively applied to healthcare, emphasizing the need for practical and user-friendly solutions tailored to the unique demands of this environment.

The workshop participants highlighted in the workgroup discussions the critical role of addressing customer needs in the healthcare sector. It emphasized the necessity for smart hygiene products to be efficient, reliable, and user-friendly. In addition, the ease of use and simple processes for disposal came up. Moreover, the discussions highlighted the integration of circular economy principles into product design to extend product lifetime, reduce waste, and enhance environmental benefits.

One limitation of this study is its small sample size, comprising 16 participants from academia ($n=4$), research institutes ($n=5$), and industry ($n=7$). This limited sample size, combined with the specific expertise of the participants, may have influenced the scope of the discussions. Integrating circularity and sustainability into healthcare, particularly for customers (Group I), indicates a shift toward a more sustainable paradigm. The adoption of reusable electronic devices, along with the development of local recycling facilities, reduces environmental impact and enhances resource efficiency in the healthcare sector (MacNeill et al., 2020).

This aligns with the circular economy's goals of extending product life cycles, reducing waste, and minimizing greenhouse gas emissions. Despite challenges such as ensuring the safety of single-use devices and addressing regulatory barriers related to disposables, adopting circular strategies is crucial for creating resilient and environmentally responsible healthcare systems (Hoveling et al., 2024; Leung et al., 2019; MacNeill et al., 2020). Healthcare managers and staff play important roles in driving this transition.

When considering the role of customers such as caretakers, nursing homes in the circular economy, it is important to expand their involvement beyond the recycling phase. While recycling is a crucial element of a CBM, engaging customers throughout the entire product life cycle is vital. By encouraging practices such as extended use and remanufacturing, customers can help prolong the product's lifespan and reduce its environmental impact. For instance, extended use involves designing products that are durable, easy to maintain, and adaptable to changing needs (Bocken et al., 2016; Geissdoerfer et al., 2018). Incorporating these phases into the customer perspective allows businesses to increase engagement in sustainable practices and enhance their commitment to the principles of circularity.

From the perspective of technology developers, the importance of addressing the life cycle impacts of electronic components and materials was emphasized. The participants recommended to design electronic components, used in medical devices, that should be easily separable, reusable, or recyclable, aiming to minimize the environmental footprint while maintaining functionality.

As an example, the reuse of medical devices within a circular economy framework requires strict compliance with regulatory frameworks to guarantee patient safety (Garvey, 2023). Although implantable devices cannot be reused due to the inherent risks, reusable medical devices can be safely reprocessed by following the guidelines outlined in the International Standard Organization (ISO) 17664-1:2021 ("ISO-11.080.01-Sterilization and disinfection in general," 2023), which specifies procedures for cleaning, disinfection, and sterilization in clinical settings (Stuckey and Benowitz, 2020).

To facilitate the development of CBMs in the medical device industry, regulatory adjustments could focus on enhancing standardization for device design to support easier disassembly and reprocessing, without compromising functionality or safety (Hoveling et al., 2024; Joseph et al., 2021). Moreover, encouraging durability, adaptability, and modularity in medical device design would further align with circular principles, enabling extended use and remanufacturing while complying with stringent safety standards. By incorporating these practices, the medical device industry can address life cycle challenges similar to those highlighted by technology developers.

From a participant's perspective, the recovery phase has not been addressed. However, as Kumar et al. (2022) outlined, the recovery of valuable metals can reduce the reliance on virgin materials in production, leading to resource conservation and economic benefits. Integrating recovery strategies into the life cycle approach recommended for both electronic components and medical devices could bridge current gaps, ensuring a more comprehensive adoption of circular economy principles across industries.

The results from the discussions regarding the sales and marketing of more sustainable and circular electronics in the healthcare sector highlighted the importance of aligning market readiness strategies with the demands of various stakeholders, including caregivers and medical professionals. The objective should be to develop products that comply with regulatory requirements and meet the needs of end-users and caregivers, balancing cost efficiency with quality care outcomes. The workshop participants were primarily product developers and business-oriented professionals. However, the findings might lack a perspective on consumer-facing challenges and regulatory complexities often faced in the broader adoption of circular healthcare products.

In the "Marketing and Awareness" focus area, participants from Sales and Marketing (Group III) emphasized the importance of informing the public about product availability to enhance market penetration. They proposed incorporating advanced functionalities, such as global positioning system (GPS) tracking and emergency alert features. In addition, they suggested potential adaptations for broader applications, such as sound and wound monitoring. However, they also discussed limitations that need addressing. For instance, GPS technology exhibits reduced accuracy indoors, which could compromise its effectiveness in certain environments. Moreover, privacy concerns were raised regarding compliance with regulations like the General Data Protection Regulation (GDPR). These concerns highlight the importance of future research focusing on mitigating technological limitations and ensuring robust data protection measures are in place to maintain user trust and regulatory compliance.

From a CBM perspective, the value proposition centers on manufacturers leveraging the residual value of products. This is achieved by providing customers with affordable, "new" products through remanufacturing, reuse, repair, recycling, and other strategies that extend product lifespans (Bocken et al., 2016). The value proposition highlights high-quality, durable products designed for longevity. This approach enables manufacturers to provide durable products with supportive services (Bocken et al., 2016).

Furthermore, the value proposition for sales and marketing perspectives (Group III) highlights specific benefits for both babies and the elderly. For babies, it focuses on improving quality of life through alert responses that enhance comfort and safety. For the elderly, it underlines advantages for mobile nursing personnel, where real-time data access facilitates prompt and personalized care, improving efficiency. Sales efforts can leverage feedback and collaborations with care facilities to build trust and loyalty, showcasing these sustainable and practical benefits.

The optimization of CBMs for cost, efficiency, and sustainability in the manufacturing and sale of smart hygiene products is crucial. A key strategy for enhancing sustainability in electronic product development is the integration of modularity into design practices (Kane et al., 2018). Modularity involves manufacturing products with easily separable components, which facilitates the reuse and refurbishment of electronic parts. This approach reduces production costs and environmental waste by extending the lifespan of electronic components (Das et al., 2022).

The workshop findings emphasize that enhancing manufacturing processes with energy-efficient technologies can result in cost reductions. This strategy not only decreases operational expenses but also advances sustainability goals by reducing energy consumption and emissions. These improvements provide benefits to both economic and environmental aspects. Furthermore, Bocken et al. (2016) outline the role of sustainability in business models. For example, they discuss how companies like Miele apply strategies such as designing for durability and reducing resource use, showing how business model innovation can be linked to sustainable practices (Bocken et al., 2016). For sales strategies, companies are required to use transparent communication about the environmental and economic benefits of these products to gain consumer acceptance and drive market growth. By focusing on the long-term cost savings offered by reusable and durable components, companies can engage both budget-conscious and environmentally conscious customers. Future research on smart hygiene products should prioritize new technologies like biodegradable materials and advanced recycling methods to enhance sustainability while maintaining affordability and functionality. These strategies will support circular economy and meet the healthcare sector's need for cost-effective, high-performance products.

Participants also suggested that the product could be developed further to enhance its diagnostic features and expand into other applications, such as wound monitoring, drawing on successful business models from similar health technology products. Moreover, they highlighted the benefits of reusable or environmentally friendly products, offering insights into sustainable practices and consumer preferences that could influence ongoing product innovation and marketing strategies.

This study focuses on three elements of the IC Tool: customer, solution, and competition, chosen for their relevance to CBMs in healthcare electronics. The other elements, including vision, resources, actions, and team, were not studied in this analysis. In addition, the participant backgrounds in product development limited discussion on end-of-life processing. Further research could incorporate all IC Tool elements and broader expertise to achieve a thorough understanding of CBM integration.

This research presents perspectives that can support the advancement of policy development in sustainable electronics. Identifying specific challenges and opportunities from customer, technology developer, as well as sales and marketing perspectives enables policymakers to develop targeted regulations and incentives that facilitate the adoption of circular economy principles in the electronics sector. For example, policies could encourage R&D in biodegradable materials and advanced recycling methods. They could establish design standards for product modularity and recyclability while offering financial incentives for companies that adopt sustainable practices, such as utilizing reusable electronic components in healthcare products. Furthermore, transparency in cost models and value propositions can enable policymakers to design frameworks that balance economic viability with environmental sustainability. Therefore, promoting collaboration among stakeholders and adopting circular economy principles are essential for transitioning toward a more sustainable and economically viable electronics industry.

10.5.1 Funding

The work was carried out as part of Sustronics project that is co-funded by the European Union under grant agreement 101112109. Views and opinions expressed are however those of the author(s) only and do not necessarily reflect those of the

European Union or the Chips Joint Undertaking. Neither the European Union nor the granting authority can be held responsible for them. This project is supported by the Chips Joint Undertaking and its members under grant agreement 1021112109 including top up funding by the Netherlands, Austria, Germany, Spain, Finland, France, Latvia, Poland, and Sweden. The project also receives funding from the Swiss State Secretariat for Education, Research and Innovation (SERI). VTT and Tampere University have received top-up funding from Business Finland under grant agreements 7926/31/2922 and 8306/31/2022, respectively.

REFERENCES

Amjadi, M., Kyung, K.-U., Park, I., Sitti, M., 2015. Stretchable, skin-mountable, and wearable strain sensors and their potential applications: A review. *Advanced Functional Materials* 26. https://doi.org/10.1002/adfm.201504755.

Antikainen, M., Valkokari, K., 2016. A framework for sustainable circular business model innovation. *Technology Innovation Management Review* 6(7), 5–12.

Ardilio, A Seidenstricker S Schmitz (2015). Measuring and assessing application-specific technology readiness. International Journal on Advanced Science Engineering Information Technology 5(6): 475-480.

Association of Medical Device Reprocessors, 2024. AMDR|Association of Medical Device Reprocessors. https://amdr.org/portfolio-items/reducing-costs-by-reprocessing/ (accessed 11 August 24).

Atzori, L., Iera, A., Morabito, G., 2010. The internet of things: A survey. *Computer Networks* 54, 2787–2805. https://doi.org/10.1016/j.comnet.2010.05.010.

Baek, J., 2023. Smart predictive analytics care monitoring model based on multi sensor IoT system: Management of diaper and attitude for the bedridden elderly. *Sensors International* 4, 100213. https://doi.org/10.1016/j.sintl.2022.100213.

Bai, B., Law, R., Wen, I., 2008. The impact of website quality on customer satisfaction and purchase intentions: Evidence from Chinese online visitors. *International Journal of Hospitality Management* (Special Issue on Hospitality Management in China) 27, 391–402. https://doi.org/10.1016/j.ijhm.2007.10.008.

Bocken, N.M.P., De Pauw, I., Bakker, C., Van Der Grinten, B., 2016. Product design and business model strategies for a circular economy. *Journal of Industrial and Production Engineering* 33, 308–320. https://doi.org/10.1080/21681015.2016.1172124.

Bocken, N.M.P., Mugge, R., Bom, C.A., Lemstra, H.-J., 2018. Pay-per-use business models as a driver for sustainable consumption: Evidence from the case of HOMIE. *Journal of Cleaner Production* 198, 498–510. https://doi.org/10.1016/j.jclepro.2018.07.043.

Caretta, M.A., Vacchelli, E., 2015. Re-thinking the boundaries of the focus group: A reflexive analysis on the use and legitimacy of group methodologies in qualitative research. *Sociological Research* 20. https://doi.org/10.5153/sro.3812.

Chamberlin, L., Boks, C., 2018. Marketing approaches for a circular economy: Using design frameworks to interpret online communications. *Sustainability* 10, 2070. https://doi.org/10.3390/su10062070.

Charter, M., Gray, C., 2008. Remanufacturing and product design. *International Journal of Product Development* 6, 375. https://doi.org/10.1504/IJPD.2008.020406.

Chen, W., 2010. An exploratory research on adoption of mobile commerce technology in the supply chain, in: Zhao, X., Zhu, G., Flynn, B. (Eds.), *Capital University of Economics & Business. Presented at the Proceedings of the Fourth International Conference on Operations and Supply Chain Management (ICOSCM 2010)*, China, June 26–30, pp. 90–95.

Danaher, P.J., Haddrell, V., 1996. A comparison of question scales used for measuring customer satisfaction. *International Journal of Service Industry Management* 7, 4–26. https://doi.org/10.1108/09564239610129922.

Das, A., Konietzko, J., Bocken, N., 2022. How do companies measure and forecast environmental impacts when experimenting with circular business models? *Sustainable Production and Consumption* 29, 273–285. https://doi.org/10.1016/j.spc.2021.10.009.

den Hollander, M.C., Bakker, C.A., Hultink, E.J., 2017. Product design in a circular economy: Development of a typology of key concepts and terms. *Journal of Industrial Ecology* 21, 517–525. https://doi.org/10.1111/jiec.12610.

Digital_EU_Commission1.pdf., 2024. n.d. 2030 Digital Decade: Report on the State of the Digital Decade 2024. doi:10.2759/122170 KK-02-24-716-EN-C. https://digital-strategy.ec.europa.eu/en/library/report-state-digital-decade-2024

Directorate-General for Communication, European Commission, 2020. *Circular Economy Action Plan: For a Cleaner and More Competitive Europe*. Publications Office of the European Union, Brussels, Belgium.

Essoussi, L.H., Linton, J.D., 2010. New or recycled products: How much are consumers willing to pay? *Journal of Consumer Marketing* 27, 458–468. https://doi.org/10.1108/07363761011063358.

Fernandes, L., Rosado da Cruz, A.M., Cruz, E.F., Lopes, S.I., 2023. A review on adopting blockchain and IoT technologies for fostering the circular economy in the electrical and electronic equipment value chain. *Sustainability* 15, 4574. https://doi.org/10.3390/su15054574.

Frishammar, J., Parida, V., 2019. Circular business model transformation: A roadmap for incumbent firms. *California Management Review* 61, 5–29. https://doi.org/10.1177/0008125618811926.

Galvão, G.D.A., Homrich, A.S., Geissdoerfer, M., Evans, S., Ferrer, P.S.S., Carvalho, M.M., 2020. Towards a value stream perspective of circular business models. *Resources, Conservation and Recycling* 162, 105060. https://doi.org/10.1016/j.resconrec.2020.105060.

Garvey, M., 2023. Medical device-associated healthcare infections: Sterilization and the potential of novel biological approaches to ensure patient safety. *International Journal of Molecular Sciences* 25, 201. https://doi.org/10.3390/ijms25010201.

Geissdoerfer, M., Morioka, S.N., De Carvalho, M.M., Evans, S., 2018. Business models and supply chains for the circular economy. *Journal of Cleaner Production* 190, 712–721. https://doi.org/10.1016/j.jclepro.2018.04.159.

Geissdoerfer, M., Santa-Maria, T., Kirchherr, J., Pelzeter, C., 2023. Drivers and barriers for circular business model innovation. *Business Strategy and the Environment* 32, 3814–3832. https://doi.org/10.1002/bse.3339.

Geissdoerfer, M., Savaget, P., Bocken, N.M.P., Hultink, E.J., 2017. The circular economy: A new sustainability paradigm? *Journal of Cleaner Production* 143, 757–768. https://doi.org/10.1016/j.jclepro.2016.12.048.

Gill, P., Stewart, K., Treasure, E., Chadwick, B., 2008. Methods of data collection in qualitative research: Interviews and focus groups. *British Dental Journal* 204, 291–295. https://doi.org/10.1038/bdj.2008.192.

Global Refurbished Medical Equipment Market, 2023. Data Bridge Market Research. Global Refurbished Medical Equipment Market - Industry Trends and Forecast 2030. https://www.databridgemarketresearch.com/reports/global-refurbished-medical-equipment-market (accessed 11 August 24).

Globocnik, D., Holzmann, P., 2024. Sustainability-related product satisfaction – Development and application of a multi-dimensional measurement instrument. *Journal of Cleaner Production* 448, 141567. https://doi.org/10.1016/j.jclepro.2024.141567.

Guldmann, E., Huulgaard, R.D., 2020. Barriers to circular business model innovation: A multiple-case study. *Journal of Cleaner Production* 243, 118160. https://doi.org/10.1016/j.jclepro.2019.118160.

Guzzo, D., Carvalho, M.M., Balkenende, R., Mascarenhas, J., 2020. Circular business models in the medical device industry: Paths towards sustainable healthcare. *Resources, Conservation and Recycling* 160, 104904. https://doi.org/10.1016/j.resconrec.2020.104904.

Hapuwatte, B.M., Jawahir, I.S., 2021. Closed-loop sustainable product design for circular economy. *Journal of Industrial Ecology* 25, 1430–1446. https://doi.org/10.1111/jiec.13154.

Hofmann, F., 2019. Circular business models: Business approach as driver or obstructer of sustainability transitions? *Journal of Cleaner Production* 224, 361–374. https://doi.org/10.1016/j.jclepro.2019.03.115.

Homburg, C., Schwemmle, M., Kuehnl, C., 2015. New product design: Concept, measurement, and consequences. *Journal of Marketing* 79(3). https://doi.org/10.1509/jm.14.0199.

Hoveling, T., Svindland Nijdam, A., Monincx, M., Faludi, J., Bakker, C., 2024. Circular economy for medical devices: Barriers, opportunities and best practices from a design perspective. *Resources, Conservation and Recycling* 208, 107719. https://doi.org/10.1016/j.resconrec.2024.107719.

Hyysalo, J., Dasanayake, S., Hannu, J., Schuss, C., Rajanen, M., Leppänen, T., Doermann, D., Sauvola, J., 2022. Smart mask: Wearable IoT solution for improved protection and personal health. *Internet of Things* 18, 100511. https://doi.org/10.1016/j.iot.2022.100511.

Irimia-Vladu, M., 2013. "Green" electronics: Biodegradable and biocompatible materials and devices for sustainable future. *Chemical Society Reviews* 43, 588–610. https://doi.org/10.1039/C3CS60235D.

ISO-11.080.01, 2023. Sterilization and Disinfection in General. https://www.iso.org/ics/11.080.01/x/ (accessed 16 November 24).

Jaiswal, A.K., Kumar, V., Jansson, E., Huttunen, O., Yamamoto, A., Vikman, M., Khakalo, A., Hiltunen, J., Behfar, M.H., 2023. Biodegradable cellulose nanocomposite substrate for recyclable flexible printed electronics. *Advanced Electronic Materials* 9, 2201094. https://doi.org/10.1002/aelm.202201094.

Joseph, B., James, J., Kalarikkal, N., Thomas, S., 2021. Recycling of medical plastics. *Advanced Industrial and Engineering Polymer Research* 4, 199–208. https://doi.org/10.1016/j.aiepr.2021.06.003.

Kane, G.M., Bakker, C.A., Balkenende, A.R., 2018. Towards design strategies for circular medical products. *Resources, Conservation and Recycling* 135, 38–47. https://doi.org/10.1016/j.resconrec.2017.07.030.

Kenny, C., Priyadarshini, A., 2021. Review of current healthcare waste management methods and their effect on global health. *Healthcare* 9, 284. https://doi.org/10.3390/healthcare9030284.

Kiritsis, D., 2011. Closed-loop PLM for intelligent products in the era of the Internet of things. *Computer-Aided Design* 43, 479–501. https://doi.org/10.1016/j.cad.2010.03.002.

Koide, R., Yamamoto, H., Kimita, K., Nishino, N., Murakami, S., 2023. Circular business cannibalization: A hierarchical Bayes conjoint analysis on reuse, refurbishment, and subscription of home appliances. *Journal of Cleaner Production* 422. https://doi.org/10.1016/j.jclepro.2023.138580.

Kumar, A., Gaur, D., Liu, Y., Sharma, D., 2022. Sustainable waste electrical and electronic equipment management guide in emerging economies context: A structural model approach. *Journal of Cleaner Production* 336, 130391. https://doi.org/10.1016/j.jclepro.2022.130391.

Kumar, V., Reinartz, W., 2016. Creating enduring customer value. *Journal of Marketing* 80, 36–68. https://doi.org/10.1509/jm.15.0414.

Kown, Y-I Son J-K (2018). A case study on the promising product selection indicators for small and medium-sized enterprises (SMES). Journal of Open Innovation: Technology, Market, and Complexity. 4, 56, doi:10.3390/joitmc4040056

Lee, H.M., Sundin, E., Nasr, N., 2012. Review of end-of-life management issues in sustainable electronic products, in: Seliger, G. (Ed.), *Sustainable Manufacturing: Shaping Global Value Creation*, Springer, Berlin, Heidelberg, pp. 119–124. https://doi.org/10.1007/978-3-642-27290-5_18.

Lee, Y.-C., 2017. Corporate sustainable development and marketing communications on social media: Fortune 500 enterprises. *Business Strategy and the Environment* 26, 569–583. https://doi.org/10.1002/bse.1936.

Leung, L.W., Evranos, B., Grimster, A., Li, A., Norman, M., Bajpai, A., Zuberi, Z., Sohal, M., Gallagher, M.M., 2019. Remanufactured circular mapping catheters: Safety, effectiveness and cost. *Journal of Interventional Cardiac Electrophysiology* 56, 205–211. https://doi.org/10.1007/s10840-018-0497-x.

Lüdeke-Freund, F., Gold, S., Bocken, N.M.P., 2019. A review and typology of circular economy business model patterns. *Journal of Industrial Ecology* 23, 36–61. https://doi.org/10.1111/jiec.12763.

MacNeill, A.J., Hopf, H., Khanuja, A., Alizamir, S., Bilec, M., Eckelman, M.J., Hernandez, L., McGain, F., Simonsen, K., Thiel, C., Young, S., Lagasse, R., Sherman, J.D., 2020. Transforming the medical device industry: Road map to a circular economy. *Health Affairs* 39, 2088–2097. https://doi.org/10.1377/hlthaff.2020.01118.

Mendoza, J.M.F., D'Aponte, F., Gualtieri, D., Azapagic, A., 2019. Disposable baby diapers: Life cycle costs, eco-efficiency and circular economy. *Journal of Cleaner Production* 211, 455–467. https://doi.org/10.1016/j.jclepro.2018.11.146.

Mendoza, J.M.F., Sharmina, M., Gallego-Schmid, A., Heyes, G., Azapagic, A., 2017. Integrating backcasting and eco-design for the circular economy: The BECE framework. *Journal of Industrial Ecology* 21, 526–544. https://doi.org/10.1111/jiec.12590.

Mentink, B., 2014. Circular business model innovation: A process framework and a tool for business model innovation in a circular economy. Thesis for Master of Science. https://doi.org/10.13140/RG.2.2.10776.70404.

Milousi, M., Souliotis, M., 2023. A circular economy approach to residential solar thermal systems. *Renewable Energy* 207, 242–252. https://doi.org/10.1016/j.renene.2023.02.109.

Mishra, J.L., Hopkinson, P.G., Tidridge, G., 2018. Value creation from circular economy-led closed loop supply chains: A case study of fast-moving consumer goods. *Production Planning & Control* 29, 509–521. https://doi.org/10.1080/09537287.2018.1449245.

Moreno, M., De los Rios, C., Rowe, Z., Charnley, F., 2016. A conceptual framework for circular design. *Sustainability* 8, 937. https://doi.org/10.3390/su8090937.

Muchenje, C., Tapera, M., Mugoni, E., Katsvairo, H., 2023. Green marketing strategies and consumer behavior: Insights for achieving sustainable marketing success, in: *Sustainable Marketing, Branding, and Reputation Management: Strategies for a Greener Future,* IGI Global, pp. 465–484. https://doi.org/10.4018/979-8-3693-0019-0.ch024.

Mukoro, V., Sharmina, M., Gallego-Schmid, A., 2022. A framework for environmental evaluation of business models: A test case of solar energy in Kenya. *Sustainable Production and Consumption* 34, 202–218. https://doi.org/10.1016/j.spc.2022.09.007.

Naji Nassajfar, M., Välimäki, M., Hakola, L., Eiroma, K., Immonen, K., Abdulkareem, M., Horttanainen, M., 2023. The effect of conductive ink alternation on the sustainability and functioning of printed electronics. *Flexible and Printed Electronics* 8. https://doi.org/10.1088/2058-8585/acd650.

Nußholz, J.L.K., 2018. A circular business model mapping tool for creating value from prolonged product lifetime and closed material loops. *Journal of Cleaner Production* 197, 185–194. https://doi.org/10.1016/j.jclepro.2018.06.112.

O'Connor, M.P., Zimmerman, J.B., Anastas, P.T., Plata, D.L., 2016. A strategy for material supply chain sustainability: Enabling a circular economy in the electronics industry through green engineering. *ACS Sustainable Chemistry & Engineering Journal* 4, 5879–5888. https://doi.org/10.1021/acssuschemeng.6b01954.

Pascual, R., Santelices, G., Liao, H., Maturana, S., 2016. Channel coordination on fixed-term maintenance outsourcing contracts. *IIE Transactions (Institute of Industrial Engineers)* 48, 651–660. https://doi.org/10.1080/0740817X.2015.1122255.

Pereno, A., Eriksson, D., 2020. A multi-stakeholder perspective on sustainable healthcare: From 2030 onwards. *Futures* 122, 102605. https://doi.org/10.1016/j.futures.2020.102605.

Pinheiro, A.M., Chettri, B., Mehra, A., Deepti, I., Ravi, R., 2024. Regulatory landscape, risks, and solutions for refurbished medical devices: A comparative analysis in the US, EU, Malaysia, and Ghana. *Expert Review of Medical Devices* 21, 819–828. https://doi.org/10.1080/17434440.2024.2390581.

Pinkse, J., Bohnsack, R., 2021. Sustainable product innovation and changing consumer behavior: Sustainability affordances as triggers of adoption and usage. *Business Strategy and the Environment* 30, 3120–3130. https://doi.org/10.1002/bse.2793.

Płotka-Wasylka, J., Makoś-Chełstowska, P., Kurowska-Susdorf, A., Treviño, M.J.S., Guzmán, S.Z., Mostafa, H., Cordella, M., 2022. End-of-life management of single-use baby diapers: Analysis of technical, health and environment aspects. *Science of the Total Environment* 836, 155339. https://doi.org/10.1016/j.scitotenv.2022.155339.

Rajeswari, S., Srinivasulu, Y., Thiyagarajan, S., 2017. Relationship among service quality, customer satisfaction and customer loyalty: With special reference to wireline telecom sector (DSL service). *Global Business Review* 18, 1041–1058. https://doi.org/10.1177/0972150917692405.

Rizan, C., Mortimer, F., Stancliffe, R., Bhutta, M.F., 2020. Plastics in healthcare: Time for a re-evaluation. *Journal of the Royal Society of Medicine* 113, 49–53. https://doi.org/10.1177/0141076819890554.

Rizos, V., Bryhn, J., 2022. Implementation of circular economy approaches in the electrical and electronic equipment (EEE) sector: Barriers, enablers and policy insights. *Journal of Cleaner Production* 338, 130617. https://doi.org/10.1016/j.jclepro.2022.130617.

Saari, U., Aarikka-Stenroos, L., Köppä, L., Langwaldt, J., Boedeker, S., Mäkinen, S., 2018. Sustainable business model ideation and development of early ideas for sustainable business models: Analyzing a new tool facilitating the ideation process, in: *Sustainable Business Models,* Palgrave Macmillan, pp. 119–150. https://doi.org/10.1007/978-3-319-93275-0_5.

Saari, U.A., Aarikka-Stenroos, L., Boedeker, S., Köppä, L., Langwaldt, J., 2017. Assessing the usefulness of an early idea development tool among experienced researchers. *CERN IdeaSquare Journal of Experimental Innovation* 1, 3. https://doi.org/10.23726/cij.2017.476.

Sanyé-Mengual, E., Pérez-López, P., González-García, S., Lozano, R.G., Feijoo, G., Moreira, M.T., Gabarrell, X., Rieradevall, J., 2014. Eco-designing the use phase of products in sustainable manufacturing. *Journal of Industrial Ecology* 18, 545–557. https://doi.org/10.1111/jiec.12161.

Sehnem, S., de Queiroz, A.A.F.S.L., Pereira, S.C.F., dos Santos Correia, G., Kuzma, E., 2022. Circular economy and innovation: A look from the perspective of organizational capabilities. *Business Strategy and the Environment* 31, 236–250. https://doi.org/10.1002/bse.2884.

Stuckey, M.J., Benowitz, I., 2020. Reprocessing, CDC, and IPs. *Prevention Strategies* 12(3), 34–37.

Tandon, U., Kiran, R., N Sah, A., 2016. Customer satisfaction using website functionality, perceived usability and perceived usefulness towards online shopping in India. https://doi.org/10.1177/0266666915621106.

Tian, S., Yang, W., Grange, J.M.L., Wang, P., Huang, W., Ye, Z., 2019. Smart healthcare: Making medical care more intelligent. *Global Health Journal* 3, 62–65. https://doi.org/10.1016/j.glohj.2019.07.001.

Traynor, M., 2015. Focus group research. *Nursing Standard* 29, 37, 44–48. https://doi.org/10.7748/ns.29.37.44.e8822.

Tunn, V.S.C., Bocken, N.M.P., van den Hende, E.A., Schoormans, J.P.L., 2019. Business models for sustainable consumption in the circular economy: An expert study. *Journal of Cleaner Production* 212, 324–333. https://doi.org/10.1016/j.jclepro.2018.11.290.

Van Boerdonk, P.J.M., Krikke, H.R., Lambrechts, W., 2021. New business models in circular economy: A multiple case study into touch points creating customer values in health care. *Journal of Cleaner Production* 282, 125375. https://doi.org/10.1016/j.jclepro.2020.125375.

Van Yken, J., Boxall, N., Cheng, K.Y., Nikoloski, A., Moheimani, N., Kaksonen, A., 2021. E-waste recycling and resource recovery: A review on technologies, barriers and enablers with a focus on Oceania. *Metals* 11, 1313. https://doi.org/10.3390/met11081313.

Walden, J., Steinbrecher, A., Marinkovic, M., 2021. Digital product passports as enabler of the circular economy. *Chemie-Ingenieur-Technik* 93, 1717–1727. https://doi.org/10.1002/cite.202100121.

World Health Organization, 2016. *Global Strategy on Human Resources for Health: Workforce 2030*. World Health Organization, Geneva.

Zucchella, A., Previtali, P., 2019. Circular business models for sustainable development: A "waste is food" restorative ecosystem. *Business Strategy and the Environment* 28, 274–285. https://doi.org/10.1002/bse.2216.

11 Analyzing the Healthcare Performances of EU Countries via Decision Method

Fazıl Gökgöz and Engin Yalçın

NOMENCLATURE

AHP	Analytic hierarchy process
ASEAN	Association of Southeast Asian Nations
CODAS	Combinative distance-based assessment
COPRAS	Complex proportional assessment
CRS	Constant return to scale
DEA	Data envelopment analysis
DMU	Decision-making unit
DOBI	Dombi Bonferroni
EDAS	Evaluation based on distance from average solution
EU	European Union
GAIA	Geometrical analysis for interactive aid
MABAC	Multi-attributive border approximation area comparison
MARCOS	Measurement of alternatives and ranking according to compromise solution
MCDM	Multi-criteria decision-making
MPI	Malmquist productivity index
OECD	Organisation for Economic Co-operation and Development
PROMETHEE	Preference ranking organization method for enrichment evaluation
RAFSI	Ranking of alternatives through functional mapping of criterion sub-intervals into a single interval
SFA	Stochastic frontier analysis
TOPSIS	Technique for order of preference by similarity to ideal solution
VIKOR	VlseKriterijumska Optimizacija I Kompromisno Resenje

11.1 INTRODUCTION

The main goals of health systems are to satisfy public needs and to promote healthcare by reducing economic differences. If the healthcare system fails to meet societal demands and meet the expected outcomes, it may not uphold the whole society's

 DOI: 10.1201/9781003513834-11

state of health (Top et al. 2020). The performance assessment approaches comparing health systems in different countries are used as a measure for viewing the health systems in other countries as well as controlling and assessing the performance of health systems evolution and sustainability (Gavurova et al. 2021). Healthcare is essential not only to ensure safety but also for the economic stability of the European Union (EU) by making it one of the main pillars that aim to boost the performance of healthcare and provide citizens with high-quality preventive care. In this regard, the EU is expected to address this issue of inequality with respect to healthcare standards within its members. Instead, they will assist the particular states currently flagging behind as regards limited access to such healthcare products as services. Healthcare is necessary for both individual well-being and economic development, serving as an instrumental driver of economic growth through its beneficial impact on public health. A well-functioning healthcare system improves life expectancy, productivity levels in the workforce, and overall well-being, leading to a stronger and more productive labor market. The comparison of healthcare in nations is very useful because it provides opportunities to observe a country's performance in comparison to others and justification of precautions (Mitropoulos 2021).

Healthcare has long been at the forefront of the EU, simultaneously protecting citizens' health and bolstering economic stability and growth. The healthcare systems within the EU are built to deliver quality care and enhance the health of its citizens while stressing universal access and equitability. The EU's fourth initiative for health-related activities is called EU4Health. It is the most ambitious European Health Program to date, having been adopted in the wake of the COVID-19 pandemic. It provides substantial financial support for the resilience and recovery of European healthcare systems after the pandemic, as well as for the EU's preparedness to face major cross-border health threats like widespread communicable disease outbreaks (Casanova et al. 2023). The EU focuses on aligning across its member states toward reducing health disparities between them, with a specific emphasis on ensuring equal access to healthcare services for vulnerable populations. Besides, because healthcare leads to better worker productivity, a healthier population means higher productivity and economic growth. Well-functioning health systems prevent the economic and financial cost of health (EU Commission 2024).

Assessment of healthcare performance is a tough and complicated deed, which incorporates several conflicting criteria. Hence, making decisions in the healthcare industry becomes much more difficult. Given the significance of evaluating the performance of healthcare systems, it is essential to evaluate several competing criteria in the framework. Multi-criteria decision-making (MCDM) can be a useful strategy for making judgments that evaluate the performance of many nations with respect to several criteria by producing compromised solutions for each chosen option (Torkayesh et al. 2021).

Among the many available MCDM methods, the PROMETHEE technique is based on a number of important advantages: PROMETHEE is a simple technique; this enables it to be applied in many areas. The method allows flexibility regarding how preferences may be modeled because it allows a different preference function for each criterion, which also permits more precise consideration of the alternatives. Besides, PROMETHEE offers a partial ranking of alternatives, known as

PROMETHEE I, and a complete ranking of alternatives, known as PROMETHEE II, thus providing overall analysis for better decision-making. It integrates with the Geometrical Analysis for Interactive Aid (GAIA) plane to support visualization by underlining the identification of conflicts and synergies among criteria. Another important reason is that it has already been applied to various fields by proving its capability to handle complex decision-making problems. In contrast to other MCDM techniques, PROMETHEE represents a more understandable method that includes less computational burden (Markovic Brankovic et al. 2018).

MCDM approaches have gained ground in healthcare performance evaluation recently. For the ranking, MABAC, COPRAS, MAIRCA, VIKOR, RAFSI, and MARCOS have been used. According to MABAC, it gives strong stability in decision-making (Liang et al. 2019), while COPRAS weighs both the ideal and anti-ideal effects (Goswami et al. 2021). MAIRCA ranks all alternatives based on a reference point (Tepe et al. 2024), while VIKOR is used to find compromised solutions, which makes it very suitable for trade-off scenarios (Radulescu and Radulescu 2024). The RAFSI method improves the robustness of decision-making based on some combined ranking strategies (Komasi et al. 2025) and the MARCOS technique adapts well to the dynamic nature of decision environments because it takes into consideration ideal and anti-ideal solutions (Younis et al. 2025). PROMETHEE has been selected for this study, due to the outranking concept and ability to combine qualitative and quantitative criteria by providing preference flows. The PROMETHEE method has its well-founded preference structure, the flexibility of this method, and ability to provide clear rankings (Chen et al. 2018). While some other methods such as MABAC, COPRAS, and MAIRCA present results with a basis on weighted summation or directly normalized weights, PROMETHEE evaluates based on paired comparisons that would be suitable to assessments in the frame of healthcare performance. It is highly adaptable, taking into consideration that for each criterion different preference functions may be defined and ensure gradual or threshold-based effects. The PROMETHEE method balances rigorous mathematics with interpretability by offering insightful perspectives to the decision-makers, also through visualization devices such as the GAIA planes and net flow rankings. While methods such as VIKOR focus on a compromise solution PROMETHEE represents a rather simple yet powerful ranking system to discriminate between the best and the worst performances (Senvar et al. 2014). Its ability to handle maximization and minimization criteria provides additional strength and makes it more applicable to EU healthcare performance. With these benefits, PROMETHEE provides a strong methodology in healthcare performance analysis and thus can be considered superior to other MCDM methods. Compared to previous studies, the research aims to contribute to the significance of healthcare performance evaluation by integrating PROMETHEE and DOBI techniques.

Authorities are obliged to deal with the hazards to public health that come from COVID-19 and widespread outbreaks (Kargi et al. 2023). The COVID-19 pandemic has actually placed an unprecedented burden on healthcare systems in EU countries, thus making the evaluation of healthcare performance an urgent task. In this regard, we use PROMETHEE, which is a very effective MCDM approach that has been capable of providing a nuanced ranking regarding healthcare performance. While the existing literature on measuring healthcare performance has generally focused on either Data Envelopment Analysis (DEA) or Stochastic Frontier Analysis (SFA) methods, these approaches are regarded as presumptive and lacking in encapsulating the full complexity of multidimensional healthcare performance within a comparative framework. Although the number of related studies on healthcare performance is increasing, few studies have analyzed the effects of COVID-19 by using the MCDM approach. This chapter aims to contribute to the existing literature through the application of PROMETHEE and DOBI methods in analyzing the performance of healthcare systems in the EU during and after the pandemic. We pinpoint performance disparities over the investigated period.

The rest of our chapter is organized as follows. Section 11.2 summarizes healthcare performance studies. Section 11.3 reports the empirical method. Section 11.4 presents the analysis results. Section 11.5 details the conclusion and policy implications.

11.2 LITERATURE REVIEW

We explain the advantages of the PROMETHEE technique, which underlines its power compared to other MCDM methods. PROMETHEE has some advantages because of its simplicity and strength in ranking alternatives based on multiple conflicting criteria. Unlike methods such as analytic hierarchy process (AHP), which demand long pairwise comparisons, PROMETHEE depends on preference functions, which present a structured way for the decision-maker to express the level of preference on each criterion. This reduces cognitive load and limits inconsistencies in decisions. The major strength of PROMETHEE includes the use of both qualitative and quantitative data without complex normalization procedures, which is unlike in methods such as TOPSIS, where there is vector normalization. This is helpful in handling the variation of problems that have significant data variation. Furthermore, PROMETHEE allows decision-makers to define different types of preference functions by rendering them flexible in modeling the decision preferences of a decision-maker in comparison with rigid methods such as ELECTRE, which is largely based on threshold-based outranking relationships.

One of the other significant advantages is that it can provide either partial or complete rankings of the alternatives. A partial ranking provided by PROMETHEE I can be incomparable when alternatives become too close to be preferred. On the other hand, a whole ranking by PROMETHEE II, considering net flow values, reveals the ranked order. Such a double-ranking system provides more insights into decision problems than single-ranking methods. Moreover, PROMETHEE is empowered by the GAIA plane, which is a representation of the decision alternatives and criteria in graphical form. Such a graphical analysis tool allows decision-makers to observe the trade-offs between conflicting criteria and thus obtain a deeper understanding of the positioning of the alternatives. Such visualization capabilities are less developed in other MCDM techniques, hence making PROMETHEE preferable in decision-making situations where interpretability is crucial (Ozkaya and Demirhan 2023; Ranjan et al. 2016). Its adaptability to complex decision environments, besides the ability to integrate weights assigned by experts or through objective weighting methods, provides further credibility for it as a robust MCDM approach. Compared with AHP, which is more sensitive to rank reversals and requires consistency checks (Tu and Wu 2023), the PROMETHEE method is a more stable decision support system.

The literature has extensively addressed the examination of health systems performance by various decision analysis techniques. Some of them are summarized below.

Selamzade et al. (2023) use DEA and MCDM methods to evaluate health efficiency in Organisation for Economic Co-operation and Development (OECD) nations during COVID-19. The calculations are based on CRS and super-efficiency. The rankings are carried out via the MCDM techniques such as TOPSIS, EDAS, and CODAS methods. The number of doctors, nurses, and beds constituted the inputs whereas the health expenditure, the number of tests conducted, cases, and deaths are regarded as outputs. The study concludes that New Zealand is the most efficient country. The study stresses the necessity of low-capacity countries to tailor health policies that focus on increasing test capacity and reducing cases.

Gavurova et al. (2021) aim to assess and contrast the performance of the OECD's health systems by Dynamic Network DEA. The analysis focuses on how efficiently whole health systems, as well as healthcare and medical treatment, perform. The average efficiency is ranged between 84% and 88%. Efficiency in this case generally measures how effectively inputs are converted into desired outputs. A score of 84%–88% means that, on average, the decision-making units (DMUs) are operating at 84%–88% of their optimal potential. The efficiency score is comparable to the performance of countries in the sector being examined. It indicates how close the countries are to the frontier, where efficiency is the performance of the best-performing unit(s) based on the criteria. This non-parametric approach constructs an efficiency frontier and measures each DMU's distance from it, with a value between 0 and 1. With performance increases in healthcare, the Malmquist productivity index (MPI) outcomes demonstrate that the OECD countries have become more efficient over time.

Mitropoulos (2021) bases the study on a two-stage network DEA model, which is used to evaluate the healthcare systems in the EU countries. In the first stage, production efficiency is determined while the second stage focuses on service quality. The study has revealed trade-offs between production and quality, where some countries are willing to throw one away to make the other better. Even though there was a considerable increase in efficiency, during times of unemployment, the rate of technological development went down. The study draws attention to the balance between the savings and qualitative and social equity of health services.

Singh et al. (2021) assess the efficiency and productivity of the national healthcare systems in the ASEAN area by DEA and MPI. Both models incorporate life expectancy at birth and the death rate from diseases to evaluate the technical efficiency of the national healthcare system throughout the area. Resource use discrepancies, policies, and health systems contribute to the efficiency gaps among the ASEAN countries. Healthcare efficiency can be achieved by applying the most recent technologies and optimal use of resources. They conclude that policymakers should focus on resource efficiency and foster technological advancements in healthcare.

Top et al. (2020) analyze the healthcare systems of African countries using the DEA approach. Their findings show that 58% of the countries are efficient while socioeconomic factors and unequal resource distribution can be regarded as the main causes of efficiency variations. African healthcare systems and scale inefficiency are found to be significant. African nations find it very challenging to provide for the basic requirements of their people, including food, housing, security, and health. Health systems in African nations suffer from their undeveloped and financially distressed economies.

The research considered here emphasizes the use of MCDM methods for measuring healthcare performance in the EU countries. Various methods such as MCDM, static and dynamic models of DEA have been utilized to measure general system performance along with individual components of healthcare such as resource planning, service, and technological innovation. Findings indicate that the rate of efficiency highly varies depending on economic conditions, policy environments, and healthcare facilities. Evidence derived from other studies indicates the place of crises, such as pandemics, as forces behind healthcare efficiency and calls for policy intervention of an adaptive nature to enhance the ability for testing and make better use of existing resources. There are other studies focusing on trends in long-term efficiency, which show that healthcare infrastructure investment, staffing allocation, and technology developments have an important contribution to making the system better. One common feature throughout the literature is the need for policymakers to maximize resource utilization while promoting fair access to quality healthcare services. Overall, the results emphasize the key role of efficiency-based policy reform responsive to the unique needs and problems of various healthcare systems.

11.3 METHODS

11.3.1 MCDM Methods

The decision-making process needs to be consulted before any decisions are taken. Decision-making is a pivotal process where a complex set of factors are taken into account, in order to reach a certain goal. This process may entail some assumptions that are impacted by several circumstances. One of the most precise approaches to decision-making is MCDM (Taherdoost and Madanchian 2023). The process of MCDM may be viewed as dynamic and complicated (Opricovic and Tzeng 2004). The primary aim is how to evaluate a set of possibilities according to many criteria. Many modern researchers have considered MCDM framework as an effective way of decision-making. MCDM is the process of making decisions when confronted with several, conflicting variables (Zavadskas et al. 2014). Furthermore, there is a wide range of applications for MCDM techniques in many fields. These methods have demonstrated their effectiveness in handling difficult decision-making issues in a variety of fields, including engineering, business and management, environmental decision-making, healthcare, and public policy (Sahoo and Goswami 2023). Several techniques have been developed to evaluate alternatives based on several criteria. The PROMETHEE technique is one of those methods used in different fields.

11.3.1.1 The Shannon Entropy Method

In this study, the Shannon entropy is used to help facilitate the decision-making. The weights of criteria are determined by using the objective weighing technique known as entropy (Kousar et al. 2025). In 1948, Shannon developed a theory based on probability that is often known as the information theory (Žižović and Albijanić 2025). This method is adaptable and suitable for a range of intricate decision-making situations (Biswas et al. 2025). The Shannon entropy, which enables objective weighting structure, is a method for making decisions using several features. This method is widely used in many scientific fields. The concept of Shannon's entropy is essential to information theory and serves as a general measure of uncertainty. Thus, the metric of entropy can be used to illustrate the unpredictable nature of attributes (Del and Tabrizi 2020).

First, the normalization is calculated as follows (Yang et al. 2018):

$$p_{ij} = \frac{x_{ij}}{\sum_{i=1}^{m} x_{ij}} \tag{11.1}$$

where p_{ij} signifies normalized decision values.

The entropy value calculation is presented below.

$$E_j = -(\ln m)^{-1} \sum_{i=1}^{m} p_{ij} \ln\ p_{ij} \tag{11.2}$$

where E_j denotes the entropy values.

The weight obtained via the entropy method is presented as follows:

$$\frac{w_j = \left(1 - E_j\right)}{\left(n - \sum_{j=1}^{n} E_j\right)} \tag{11.3}$$

where w_j signifies criteria weight.

11.3.1.2 The PROMETHEE Method

Brans et al. (1986) developed the PROMETHEE technique as a novel MCDM methodology to make partial and ultimate rankings of alternatives. Pairwise comparisons of the options depending on each criterion form the basis of the PROMETHEE approach. Its user-friendly outranking mechanism is its primary benefit. Since it can effectively outrank competitors and comes in numerous variants, the PROMETHEE method is used extensively in several fields. PROMETHEE I allows a partial rating of choices, whereas PROMETHEE II allows a complete rating. PROMETHEE I is employed for limited performance, whereas PROMETHEE II utilizes a full rating of alternatives (Abdullah et al. 2019). The steps of the PROMETHEE technique are summarized below (Makan and Fadili 2020):

Step 1: Comparing pairs in order to identify deviations

$$d_j(a,b) = g_j(a) - g_j\ (b) \tag{11.4}$$

where $d_j(a,b)$ denotes the disparity between a and b's assessments on each criterion.

Step 2: Selecting and utilizing preference functions

$$P_j(a,b) = F_j d_j(a,b) \tag{11.5}$$

where $P_j(a,b)$ denotes the alternative preference of a in relation to alternative b on each criterion

Step 3: Calculation of the Global Preference Index

$$\forall\ a,b \in A,\ \pi(a,b) = \sum_{j=1}^{k} P_{j\ (a,b)\cdot w_j} \tag{11.6}$$

where $\pi(a,b)$ signifies the weighted sum $p(a,b)$ for each criterion, w_j denotes the weight corresponding to jth criterion.

Step 4: Utilizing the PROMETHEE I partial ranking to calculate the ranking flows

$$\phi^{+}(a) = \frac{1}{n-1}\sum_{x \varepsilon A} \pi(a,x) \tag{11.7}$$

$$\phi^{-}(a) = \frac{1}{n-1}\sum_{x \varepsilon A} \pi(x,a) \tag{11.8}$$

where $\phi^{+}(a)$ and $\phi^{-}(a)$ denote the positive and negative ranking flow of every unit respectively.

Step 5: Computing the PROMETHEE II total ranking

$$\Phi(a) = \phi^{+}(a) - \phi^{-}(a) \tag{11.9}$$

For each option, $\Phi(a)$ signifies the net ranking flow.

11.3.1.3 The Dombi Bonferroni (DOBI) Method

The DOBI technique is a novel MCDM method developed to rank alternatives. The DOBI technique is the first hybrid MCDM approach that uses an algorithm and an inverse sorting algorithm in conjunction with enhanced DOBI hybrid functions (Ecer and Pamucar 2022). The steps are summarized below (Nila and Roy 2023):

Step 1: The elements of decision matrix is normalized below

$$\beta_{ij} = \begin{cases} \dfrac{\alpha_{ij}}{\alpha_j^{+}}, & \text{if } i \text{ is benefit criterion} \\[2ex] -\dfrac{\alpha_{ij}}{\alpha_j^{+}} + \max_{1 \le i \le m}\left(\dfrac{\alpha_{ij}}{\alpha_j^{+}}\right) + \min_{1 \le i \le m}\left(\dfrac{\alpha_{ij}}{\alpha_j^{+}}\right), & \text{if } i \text{ is cost criterion} \end{cases} \tag{11.10}$$

where $\alpha_j^+ = \max_{1 \le i \le m}\left(\alpha_{ij}\right)$

Step 2: The Calculation of Weighted Significance

$$\zeta_i^{(1)\psi_1,\psi_2,\zeta} = \frac{\sum_{j=1}^{n} \beta_{ij}}{1+\left\{\left[\frac{1}{\left(\omega_i\omega_j\right)+(\psi_1+\psi_2} \sum_{\substack{i,j=1\\ i\neq j}}^{n} \frac{1-\omega_i}{\frac{1}{\omega_1\left(\frac{1-f(\beta_i)}{f(\beta_i)}\right)^{\xi}+\omega_2\left(\frac{1-f(\beta_i)}{f(\beta_i)}\right)^{\xi}}}\right]^{1/\xi}\right\}} \tag{11.11}$$

$$\zeta_i^{(2)\psi_1,\psi_2,\zeta} = \sum_{j=1}^{n} \beta_{ij} - \frac{\sum_{j=1}^{n} \beta_{ij}}{1+\left\{\left[\frac{1}{\left(\omega_i\omega_j\right)+(\psi_1+\psi_2} \sum_{\substack{i,j=1\\ i\neq j}}^{n} \frac{1-\omega_i}{\frac{1}{\omega_1\left(\frac{f(\beta_i)}{1-f(\beta_i)}\right)^{\xi}+\omega_2\left(\frac{f(\beta_i)}{1-f(\beta_i)}\right)^{\xi}}}\right]^{1/\xi}\right\}} \tag{11.12}$$

Step 3: The DOBI Function Integrated Value

$$\Re_i = \frac{\zeta_i^{(1)\psi_1,\psi_2,\zeta} + \zeta_i^{(2)\psi_1,\psi_2,\zeta}}{1+\left\{\left[\frac{1}{2}\left(\frac{1-\zeta_i^{(1)\psi_1,\psi_2,\zeta}}{\zeta_i^{(1)\psi_1,\psi_2,\zeta}}\right)^{\delta}+\frac{1}{2}\left(\frac{1-\zeta_i^{(2)\psi_1,\psi_2,\zeta}}{\zeta_i^{(2)\psi_1,\psi_2,\zeta}}\right)^{\delta}\right]\right\}} \tag{11.13}$$

ψ_1 and ψ_2 signify Bonferroni function's stabilization indicators while ξ denotes Dombi norm's stability factor.

Step 4: The alternatives are ranked based on $\Re_i$ values.

11.4 DATA AND VARIABLES

In this study, the healthcare performance in the EU countries is evaluated by using the PROMETHEE technique, which is one of the most frequently used MCDM approaches. The performance criteria are selected based on data availability and

TABLE 11.1

The Descriptive Statistics of Decision Variables

Decision Variables	Minimum	Average	Maximum	Standard Deviation
Healthcare expenditure	1,624	72,230	477,695	122,576
Total beds	267	523	807	172
Health personnel	1,336	40,126	191,020	52,164
Life expectancy at birth	68	80	80	434

Source: Authors' calculations.

current studies in healthcare studies. The selection of decision variables took place based on their being widely used key indicators in healthcare performance literature. Healthcare expenditure, total hospital beds as well as health personnel and life expectancy at birth were selected, as they are considered basic elements of healthcare performance. Healthcare expenditure can possibly reflect the financial input into and, by that, access to and quality of health services available. The total number of beds should inform about the hospital infrastructure available in terms of patient care capacity, while health personnel means the availability of a workforce that would directly translate into service delivery. Life expectancy at birth is an important health outcome indicator that reflects the overall efficiency of a healthcare system in a country. The use of these variables is well established in efficiency studies and performance measurement in healthcare, as was demonstrated by past research in health economics and health policy literature. To further justify our selection, we reviewed empirical studies that use similar indicators in other studies (Mitropoulos 2021; Top et al. 2020; Selamzade 2023). Ensuring compatibility with other existing methodologies strengthens the validity and comparability of our findings in the wider context of healthcare performance. The dataset used in this study is the most recent complete dataset available at the time of analysis.

First, we present the descriptive statistics of our variables in Table 11.1.

As Table 11.1 indicates healthcare expenditure shows the widest range, indicating significant disparities in financial resources allocated to healthcare among the countries. The average expenditure stands with a high standard deviation, reflecting large deviations from the average. There is a moderate variation in the total number of beds, which indicates the inequality of hospitals' capacity between the countries but a more plausible extent than the healthcare expenditure. The high standard deviation of health personnel points to the fact that there are serious inequalities in workforce availability, which have a crucial role in healthcare access and quality. The life expectancy at birth exhibits less fluctuation in comparison to the others. An average life expectancy of 80 years and a standard deviation of 4.3 show that despite regional differences most of the countries have similar levels of health and are the results of cooperation in terms of healthcare. These statistics provide the foundation for understanding the healthcare structure across the EU region.

TABLE 11.2
The Weights Attributed to Criteria by the Shannon Entropy Method

Criteria	Weights
Healthcare expenditure	0.263
Total beds	0.243
Health personnel	0.250
Life expectancy at birth	0.242

Source: Authors' calculations.

The homogeneity of the DMUs would, in the study, involve picking countries with similarities in their respective health systems. On this premise, all EU members selected nearly resemble each other based on existing characteristics related to healthcare structure and economic regime conditions. To further enhance comparability, we use standardized indicators, which are harmonized across all countries for healthcare expenditure, patient outcomes, and resource utilization and normalized for different population sizes, economic conditions, and healthcare infrastructures.

In our study, we ensure the homogeneity of the DMUs by carefully selecting EU countries that exhibit comparable healthcare characteristics. The selected are chosen because they represent fundamental aspects of healthcare system performance and are available across all EU countries. Although there is some deviation in healthcare expenditure, health personnel, and total beds, the values of the standard deviation indicate that the countries under analysis have relatively similar healthcare characteristics in relation to population size and health infrastructure. Besides, life expectancy has a very low variance, which implies that DMUs are homogeneous indicators. This ensures that the homogeneity of the DMUs is clearly addressed by highlighting that the selected countries share common characteristics in the context of their healthcare systems, which is crucial for valid analysis.

Before ranking the countries, it is necessary to attribute criteria weights. To this end, we use the Shannon entropy method. The criteria weights are presented in Table 11.2.

Table 11.3 reports the analysis results of the healthcare performance in EU countries over the 2021–2022 period.

PROMETHEE I provides partial rankings among one another using positive and negative flow values. It informs how much a country outranks or is outranked by the others. PROMETHEE II is the one that combines these flows into a net flow score, which thereby provides a full ranking of the countries. One of the primary criteria used in the PROMETHEE method to measure alternatives is to compare their positive and negative flows, which express how well or insufficiently an alternative perform is compared to others. The higher the $\Phi+$ value of a country, for example, in the case of Germany, the more frequent its positive comparisons in regard to other countries. Germany leads in both 2021 and 2022 in a consistent manner, displaying a strong performance, with a net flow increase. In 2021, Austria, Belgium, and Italy

TABLE 11.3

The Healthcare Performance of the EU Countries via the PROMETHEE I and II Methods

	PROMETHEE I 2021		PROMETHEE II 2021	Ranking	PROMETHEE I 2022		PROMETHEE II 2022	Ranking
EU Countries	Positive Flow	Negative Flow	Net Flow		Positive Flow	Negative Flow	Net Flow	
Germany	7.266	4.636	2.630	1	8.690	2.362	6.630	1
Austria	3.501	1.216	2.284	2	3.182	1.485	5.860	5
Belgium	2.863	1.620	1.243	3	2.665	1.779	3.391	6
Italy	4.426	3.227	1.919	4	5.521	0.849	−0.028	2
Czechia	2.848	1.799	1.049	5	2.284	2.311	1.697	7
Spain	3.878	3.020	0.857	6	4.488	2.380	0.886	4
France	4.159	3.328	0.831	7	6.709	2.129	2.108	3
Poland	2.996	2.388	0.608	8	2.653	2.683	−0.030	8
Malta	2.694	2.264	0.429	9	1.891	3.017	−0.631	10
Bulgaria	3.467	3.382	0.084	10	2.694	4.032	−1.126	12
Romania	2.979	2.990	−0.011	11	2.338	3.539	−1.201	11
Slovenia	2.167	2.444	−0.276	12	1.420	3.276	−2.157	9
Hungary	2.377	2.786	−0.408	13	1.690	3.405	−1.366	14
Croatia	2.107	2.526	−0.418	14	1.358	3.228	−1.715	16
Ireland	2.537	2.994	−0.456	15	2.043	3.409	−1.727	13
Netherlands	2.424	3.566	−1.415	16	2.644	3.147	−1.338	15
Lithuania	1.646	3.627	−1.981	17	0.911	4.294	−3.383	17
Estonia	1.298	3.690	−2.392	18	0.550	4.384	−3.834	18
Latvia	1.307	4.783	−3.475	19	0.563	5.435	−4.872	19

Source: Calculated by the authors.

are also in the top ranks. Besides, Italy showed a better position by moving to second place despite its slightly negative net flow. France made remarkable advancement, going up from seventh place in 2021 to third in 2022, thus showing better performance through the evaluation criteria. Latvia is at the bottom end of the ranking throughout the analysis period. Estonia along with Lithuania faced performance difficulties, as they are unable to move off the bottom of the ranking. These countries had negative flows, which means there are significant performance problems in their healthcare system. On the other hand, the fluctuating positions of some countries such as Spain and Italy point out that these countries may have an unstable reaction toward evaluation criteria or concurrent adverse effects. The negative flow $\left(\phi^{-}\right)$ reflects the degree of a country being outranked by all other countries with regard to all of the criteria involving healthcare efficiency. The higher the negative flow is, the greater the evidence of a country that is consistently inferior compared to all the other countries, reflecting health resource wasting, higher cost, or poor patient outcomes. In the context of EU healthcare systems, countries with highly negative flows

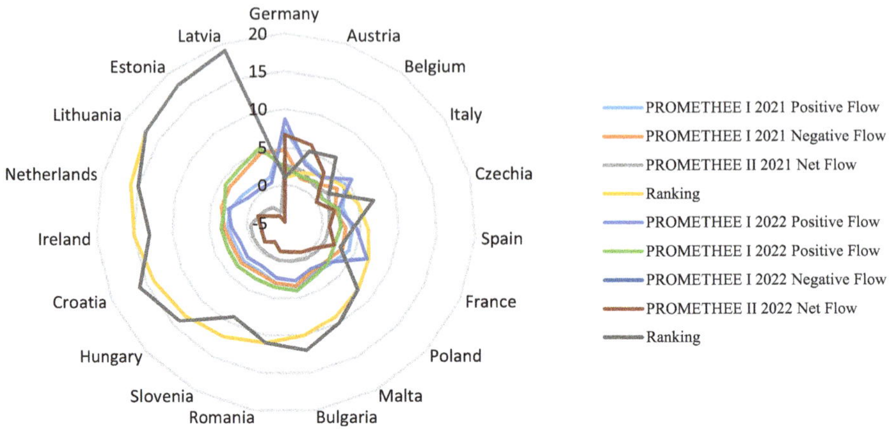

FIGURE 11.1 The rankings of EU countries in terms of healthcare performance between 2021 and 2022.

may face resilience issues regarding the COVID-19 pandemic: through hospital overcrowding, poor medical workforce availability, or simply bad public health policy. Less negatively flowing countries are less dominated, meaning that they perform comparatively well even when they are not ranked at the top overall. This, in turn, will determine that the countries requiring policy efforts for performance measurement of healthcare in future studies are clearly demarcated. The comparison of the PROMETHEE rankings of 2021 and 2022 illustrates the impact of the COVID-19 pandemic on the performance of EU nations, with various recovery trajectories for member states. Countries such as Germany, France, and Spain recorded significant improvement in the values of their net flow, reflecting that strong healthcare investment, effective economic stimulus policies, and adaptive recovery policies enabled them to be resilient following the pandemic. In addition, low-ranked nations with persistently low rankings such as Latvia, Estonia, and Lithuania showed an increased decline in their efficiency scores, highlighting structural deficiency in the healthcare system, economic resilience, and policy implementation. These results suggest that countries with well-designed and well-funded recovery plans were better able to regain stability, while those with slow responses remained behind during the post-pandemic period. The results highlight the essential policy intervention, healthcare preparedness, and funding support mechanisms in influencing national performance.

In this part, the ranking distribution of the EU countries is illustrated to present the performance in Figure 11.1.

Figure 11.1 shows a comparison among various countries in the EU, using both the PROMETHEE I and PROMETHEE II methods for 2021 and 2022. The ranking varies regarding the positive, negative, and net flow values of these countries. The PROMETHEE I method is used to segregate the positive and negative flows in order to evaluate the strengths and weaknesses of countries. By contrast, PROMETHEE II integrates these flows into one net flow score and hence allows ranking. The flow structure of the high-ranking countries is the one that exhibits a high positive and a low negative flow. The magnitude of the favorable flow reveals to what extent a country is better than countries in the analyzed aspects. Thus, it reveals the strong points of that country. Figure 11.1 indicates that some countries, such as Germany, Austria, and Belgium, are rather consistent in larger positive flow values and comparatively smaller negative flows; it would have tended to indicate better performance in these nations, possibly a result of more established economic policy and infrastructure investment. The mixture of their high positive and low negative flow reinforces their success in dealing with the problems of the healthcare system. Such results indicate the necessity of both the proper use of advantages and effective control of weak points for a robust rating.

A low negative flow signifies limited areas of underperformance relative to other countries, indicating fewer weaknesses. On the other end of the ranking, Latvia, Estonia, and Lithuania have lower rankings because of their negative flow. The lower net flow values indicate that negative features such as economic constraints, policy inefficiencies, or structural limitations may have dominated their positive contributions. A noteworthy fact is that ranking in general has considerably been turning to the positive side, which reflects the steps of improvement in the performance of the EU countries. Policy reforms, the development of sustainable infrastructure, or the enhancement of the governance framework might account for these advancements in EU countries.

We compare our PROMETHEE results with one of the novel MCDM methods, the DOBI technique, to validate the findings (Table 11.4).

TABLE 11.4

The Healthcare Performance of the EU Countries via the DOBI Method

EU Countries	DOBI Score 2021	Ranking 2021	DOBI Score 2022	Ranking 2022
Germany	0.882	1	0.908	1
France	0.638	2	0.672	2
Italy	0.518	3	0.456	4
Spain	0.474	4	0.420	6
Austria	0.466	5	0.475	3
Belgium	0.436	6	0.437	5
Czechia	0.398	7	0.377	9
Netherlands	0.389	8	0.390	8
Malta	0.385	9	0.391	7
Bulgaria	0.382	10	0.367	11
Ireland	0.381	11	0.370	10
Poland	0.380	12	0.333	14
Romania	0.362	13	0.343	12
Slovenia	0.349	14	0.334	13
Hungary	0.335	15	0.332	15
Croatia	0.323	16	0.314	16
Lithuania	0.258	17	0.273	17
Estonia	0.218	18	0.217	18
Latvia	0.197	19	0.200	19

Source: Authors' calculations.

The PROMETHEE and DOBI ranking comparison over the period 2021–2022, despite differences in methodology, reveals a high stability in terms of categorizing the best as well as worst-performing EU countries. Germany is the best-performing country in each year and according to both methodologies, which testifies to its stable economic structure, quality of policy-making, and healthcare performance. Similarly, Austria and Belgium rank consistently high in the leading countries in both PROMETHEE and DOBI rankings, which means that these countries exhibit resilience, sound management of resources, and sustainable performance improvements over time. At the bottom end of the rankings, Latvia, Lithuania, and Estonia are both ranked as the worst-performing countries in both DOBI and PROMETHEE techniques, indicating deeper structural performance shortages, economic limitations, and less robust institutional capacities that these countries find hard to surmount to achieve higher performance. Both methods rank the same countries similarly indicates that the shortcomings in their performance may indicate that problems need to be addressed through policy efforts. The middle-rank stability of nations such as Spain, Czechia, and Poland also supports the reliability of the performance rankings.

11.5 DISCUSSION

The PROMETHEE and DOBI approaches aim to enlighten the EU healthcare by presenting a sectoral overview. Traditional approaches such as DEA usually assume homogeneous DMUs and are founded on a measure of efficiency, not accounting for preference structures among the alternatives under consideration. By comparison, the PROMETHEE approach supports pairwise comparison as well as allowing for flexible ranking. This method allows decision-makers to rank EU countries concerning healthcare performance. Furthermore, the DOBI approach compares the PROMETHEE rankings to strength through ideal and anti-ideal reference points. The research proposes a hybrid MCDM model synthesizing PROMETHEE preference modeling with the reference-based stability of DOBI to overcome several weaknesses of earlier methods. More detailed decision-making is facilitated as the model compares the PROMETHEE and DOBI approaches. In applying this model to the healthcare systems in the EU, the research is able to deliver thoughtful policy recommendations to policymakers so that the stakeholders can trace inefficiency, unify resource application, and advance the performance of the healthcare system. The PROMETHEE and DOBI approaches are a new method of measuring healthcare efficiency by providing policymakers with a holistic means to assess performance.

The rankings between our methods and those of Kwilinski and Vysochyna (2024) and Medeiros and Schwierz (2015) highlight some significant similarities between countries. Germany, Austria, France, Italy, and Belgium were consistently ranked high-performing countries on both approaches by demonstrating outstanding performance in healthcare. Kwilinski and Vysochyna (2024) conclude that the highest healthcare finance efficiency value is found in Italy, which is one of the best-performing countries in our analysis as well. Further, Medeiros and Schwierz (2015) found comparable outcomes with our findings when calculating the financial efficiency of healthcare in EU nations. In particular, the authors conclude that the Czech Republic,

Lithuania, and Slovakia had the lowest performance indicators, while Belgium, France, Italy, Sweden, and the Netherlands had the highest.

Policymakers can utilize the PROMETHEE and DOBI methods to render healthcare more efficient in utilizing resources. The disparities in EU countries' healthcare personnel distribution indicate that policies enabling equal access to healthcare personnel and services are necessary. Moreover, investments in preventative healthcare can be given priority to realize cost savings in the long term, as well as improved patient outcomes. Tracking data can also be used to make adaptive policy adjustments to maintain the healthcare systems robust and resilient to emerging challenges. Healthcare expenditures also need to be made transparent for enhanced accountability and against wastage of resources. Policymakers can enhance the performance of healthcare systems and address these drawbacks more effectively by taking these steps.

11.6 CONCLUSION AND POLICY IMPLICATIONS

Performance measurement of healthcare carried out through MCDM methodology is crucial because it permits a comprehensive evaluation of multiple conflicting factors. The MCDM framework facilitates a better decision-making process for all stakeholders. The study focuses on PROMETHEE and DOBI techniques, which provides a structured way of evaluating several indicators simultaneously. Traditional performance measurement methods generally fail to incorporate the trade-offs among these elements, whereas MCDM makes it possible for a more integrated ranking process. MCDM methods enable one to establish which countries are performing best on different healthcare priorities. This is particularly useful for policymakers and stakeholders who need detailed insight into EU healthcare. This study focuses on integrated MCDM methods such as PROMETHEE and DOBI, which have rarely been applied together in this area. Unlike other decision techniques, the PROMETHEE method supports flexible preference modeling with the potential for trade-offs between key healthcare indicators. Concurrently, the DOBI method enhances decision-making through the incorporation of multi-objective optimization. The hybrid method provides a more substantial ranking. Moreover, the extension of the framework to European health systems provides a comparative analysis of performance among countries. The integration of PROMETHEE and DOBI increases the validity of healthcare performance evaluation. This research brings significant insight into healthcare performance measurement by integrating PROMETHEE with DOBI, with a holistic decision-making process. The findings inform the key variations in the healthcare performance of EU countries. Based on this methodology, the study establishes a solid framework by facilitating decisions on enhancing healthcare performance.

The study presents the main tendencies, which are the consistently high-performing countries such as Germany, and areas for improvement in the underperforming countries such as Latvia, Estonia, and Lithuania by evaluating positive and negative flows. The performance levels that the study presents not only represent the status of the EU countries but also shed light on the precautions underperforming EU countries need to take. Developing EU countries such as Spain and Poland, which display moderate performance, experienced some gaps in healthcare management. For instance, efficient expenditure management offsets Spain's relatively lower number of hospital beds and average healthcare staff, resulting in high life expectancy. This situation reveals how resource allocation is more planned and focuses more on the strategic part that can help improve the overall performance. These results highlight the importance of investment in the healthcare sector, which includes infrastructure, as well as workforce and services. This study enables policymakers to discover strengths and weaknesses in their healthcare systems and to adopt strategies for enhancement.

According to our PROMETHEE analysis, Germany, France, and Austria are the countries consistently at the top of the ranking with robust healthcare infrastructure and resource utilization. Gavurova et al. (2021) obtain similar results, simultaneously they focus on the fact that medical care efficiency is high in Germany, the steady progress with preventive care and medical outcomes is witnessed in France, while Austria remains stable in both public health and medical care. Mitropoulos (2021) obtains similar outcomes too. For instance, Germany and Austria reach efficiency through promoting the proper use of resources in addition to the treatment of service quality. On the other hand, Spain and Poland should focus on bed numbers and healthcare expenditure. In the case of low-performing countries such as Latvia and Lithuania, which were always at the bottom of our work as well as in Mitropoulos (2021), the findings suggest that there are inefficiencies within the system. Mitropoulos (2021) also identifies that the economic crisis played a critical role in aggravating inefficiencies. These countries are challenged with the struggle between output and quality, which causes unmet medical needs and declining patient safety. High-performing countries can address gaps in preventive care and public health initiatives to sustain their leadership, while underperforming nations require systematic reforms to link production efficiency with quality improvements.

Detailed policy implications are essential to address the challenges and improve healthcare performance in EU countries. Germany, France, and other high-performing countries may maintain their performance by investing in digital health technologies, including diagnostic tools and advanced platforms by improving the delivery of service, and decreasing inequality in the region (Stoumpos et al. 2023). EU members can focus on the implementation of several strategies such as the efficient management of resources, deployment of technological innovations, cooperation among the regions, and the adoption of sustainable policies to increase the performance of their health systems and improve health outcomes. For instance, Germany can maintain its high performance by allocating resources equally. Varabyova et al. (2017) compare the efficiency of Germany and Italy's hospital systems. Germany is considerably found more efficient than Italy in terms of hospital efficiency. In addition, France is also found to be among the leading countries according to our results, with high healthcare performance. Its ranking indicates effective health policies, well-established infrastructure, and an adequate workforce, which leads to improved overall performance. Cost-effective solutions to maintain its performance should be implemented (Dincă et al. 2020).

Workforce and infrastructure deficit solutions are most important for developing countries such as Spain and Poland. Spain possesses a strong primary healthcare system. Nevertheless, there are certain deficits to be addressed (González-de-Julián et al. 2024). Spain must improve their hospitals and the bed capacity (Rechel et al. 2016). Poland could balance investments in urban and rural healthcare infrastructure (Miszczynska and Miszczyński 2022). Both nations could expand their outpatient care facilities to lessen the burden of healthcare. Countries that do not perform well, for example, Latvia, Estonia, and Lithuania, require immediate attention and precautionary measures. The healthcare system should as a priority enhance preventive care, such as healthcare workforce development and the promotion of primary care services to achieve better performance. Such countries can also implement public-private partnerships to improve hospital infrastructure and implement public health programs to improve healthcare. Apart from this, employee retention programs such as competitive compensation and training sessions can help to minimize healthcare workforce shortages. EU-wide policies should be strengthened in order to enable the exchange of knowledge and resources among member states (Willis-Shattuck et al. 2008). EU countries can address their problems and collectively advance through a more effective healthcare system by adopting these precautions.

Despite the methodological strength, some weaknesses exist. The application of the PROMETHEE methodology is reliant upon the selection and weighting of healthcare indicators that, even if strictly adhered to, can have some degree of subjectivity. The analysis is also not controlled for exogenous factors that could affect a country's performance beyond the selected indicators.

In conclusion, MCDM methods have been utilized to measure healthcare performance, such as the PROMETHEE and DOBI methods. MCDM methods allow for an overall evaluation of the healthcare system that can be used to rank the best-performing countries by considering several different dimensions. Policymakers and practitioners could utilize MCDM as a decision support tool to identify the best-performing countries in the EU, thereby improving the healthcare system over the long term. Directions of future research may target several priority topics. Firstly, the addition of time-series or panel data would uncover the long-term dynamics by providing an improved view of long-term patterns of performance. Second, future research could explore hybridizing PROMETHEE and DOBI with other decision techniques to facilitate decision-making in healthcare management. Third, broadening the analysis to non-EU healthcare systems, especially developing countries, would form a more universal healthcare performance measurement. In addition, incorporating patient outcomes such as quality of care, access, and patient satisfaction as well as traditional efficiency measures would further strengthen the evaluation framework.

REFERENCES

Abdullah, L., Chan, W., & Afshari, A. (2019). Application of PROMETHEE method for green supplier selection: A comparative result based on preference functions. *Journal of Industrial Engineering International*, 15, 271–285.

Biswas, A., Gazi, K. H., Bhaduri, P., & Mondal, S. P. (2025). Site selection for girls hostel in a university campus by MCDM based strategy. *Spectrum of Decision Making and Applications*, 2(1), 68–93.

Brans, J. P., Vincke, P., & Mareschal, B. (1986). How to select and how to rank projects: The PROMETHEE method. *European Journal of Operational Research*, 24(2), 228–238.

Casanova, L. C., di Stasis, M., Nicoletti, G., Telea, F., Habl, C., & Wismar, M. (2023). EU4Health Programme and the role of national focal points for 2023 and beyond. *Population Medicine*, 5(Supplement). doi:10.18332/popmed/164224.

Chen, L., Xu, Z., Wang, H., & Liu, S. (2018). An ordered clustering algorithm based on K-means and the PROMETHEE method. *International Journal of Machine Learning and Cybernetics*, 9, 917–926.

Del, M. S. T. T., & Tabrizi, S. K. (2020). A methodological assessment of the importance of physical values in architectural conservation using Shannon entropy method. *Journal of Cultural Heritage*, 44, 135–151.

Dincă, G., Dincă, M. S., & Andronic, M. L. (2020). The efficiency of the healthcare systems in EU countries: A DEA analysis. *Acta Oeconomica*, 70(1), 19–36.

Ecer, F., & Pamucar, D. (2022). A novel LOPCOW-DOBI multi-criteria sustainability performance assessment methodology: An application in developing country banking sector. *Omega*, 112, 102690.

EU Commission (2024). https://health.ec.europa.eu/eu-health-policy/overview_en#european-commissions-role (accessed date 10 December 2024).

Gavurova, B., Kocisova, K., & Sopko, J. (2021). Health system efficiency in OECD countries: Dynamic network DEA approach. *Health Economics Review*, 11, 1–25.

González-de-Julián, S., Vivas-Consuelo, D., & Barrachina-Martínez, I. (2024). Modelling efficiency in primary healthcare using the DEA methodology: An empirical analysis in a healthcare district. *BMC Health Services Research*, 24(1), 982.

Goswami, S. S., Behera, D. K., Afzal, A., Razak Kaladgi, A., Khan, S. A., Rajendran, P. & Asif, M. (2021). Analysis of a robot selection problem using two newly developed hybrid MCDM models of TOPSIS-ARAS and COPRAS-ARAS. *Symmetry*, 13(8), 1331.

Kargi, B., Coccia, M., & Uçkaç, B. C. (2023). Findings from the first wave of Covid-19 on the different impacts of lockdown on public health and economic growth. *International Journal of Economic Sciences*, 12(2), 21–39.

Komasi, H., Karbassi Yazdi, A., Eskandari Sani, M., & Tan, Y. (2025). Assessing the circular economy in regions of Chile by using multiple-criteria decision-making (MCDM). *Sustainability*, 17(1), 23.

Kousar, S., Ansar, A., Kausar, N., & Freen, G. (2025). Multi-criteria decision-making for smog mitigation: A comprehensive analysis of health, economic, and ecological impacts. *Spectrum of Decision Making and Applications*, 2(1), 53–67.

Liang, R. X., He, S. S., Wang, J. Q., Chen, K., & Li, L. (2019). An extended MABAC method for multi-criteria group decision-making problems based on correlative inputs of intuitionistic fuzzy information. *Computational and Applied Mathematics*, 38(3), 112.

Makan, A., & Fadili, A. (2020). Sustainability assessment of large-scale composting technologies using PROMETHEE method. *Journal of Cleaner Production*, 261, 121244.

Markovic Brankovic, J., Markovic, M., & Nikolic, D. (2018). Comparative study of hydraulic structures alternatives using PROMETHEE II complete ranking method. *Water Resources Management*, 32, 3457–3471.

Medeiros, J., & Schwierz, C. (2015). *Efficiency Estimates of Health Care Systems (No. 549).* Directorate General Economic and Financial Affairs (DG ECFIN), European Commission, Brussels, Belgium.

Miszczynska, K., & Miszczyński, P. M. (2022). Measuring the efficiency of the healthcare sector in Poland–a window-DEA evaluation. *International Journal of Productivity and Performance Management*, 71(7), 2743–2770.

Mitropoulos, P. (2021). Production and quality performance of healthcare services in EU countries during the economic crisis. *Operational Research*, 21(2), 857–873.

Nila, B., & Roy, J. (2023). A new hybrid MCDM framework for third-party logistics provider selection under sustainability perspectives. *Expert Systems with Applications*, 234, 121009.

Opricovic, S., & Tzeng, G. H. (2004). Compromise solution by MCDM methods: A comparative analysis of VIKOR and TOPSIS. *European Journal of Operational Research*, 156(2), 445–455.

Ozkaya, G., & Demirhan, A. (2023). Analysis of countries in terms of artificial intelligence technologies: PROMETHEE and GAIA method approach. *Sustainability*, 15(5), 4604.

Radulescu, C. Z., & Radulescu, M. (2024). A hybrid group multi-criteria approach based on SAW, TOPSIS, VIKOR, and COPRAS methods for complex IoT selection problems. *Electronics*, 13(4), 789.

Ranjan, R., Chatterjee, P., & Chakraborty, S. (2016). Performance evaluation of Indian states in tourism using an integrated PROMETHEE-GAIA approach. *Opsearch*, 53, 63–84.

Rechel, B., Džakula, A., Duran, A., Fattore, G., Edwards, N., Grignon, M., Smith, T. A. (2016). Hospitals in rural or remote areas: An exploratory review of policies in 8 high-income countries. *Health Policy*, 120(7), 758–769.

Sahoo, S. K., & Goswami, S. S. (2023). A comprehensive review of multiple criteria decision-making (MCDM) Methods: Advancements, applications, and future directions. *Decision Making Advances*, 1(1), 25–48.

Selamzade, F., Ersoy, Y., Ozdemir, Y., & Celik, M. Y. (2023). Health efficiency measurement of OECD countries against the COVID-19 pandemic by using DEA and MCDM methods. *Arabian Journal for Science and Engineering*, 48(11), 15695–15712.

Senvar, O., Tuzkaya, G., & Kahraman, C. (2014). Multi criteria supplier selection using fuzzy PROMETHEE method. In: *Supply Chain Management under Fuzziness: Recent Developments and Techniques* (pp. 21–34). doi:10.1007/978-3-642-53939-8_2

Singh, S., Bala, M. M., Kumar, N., & Janor, H. (2021). Application of DEA-Based Malmquist productivity index on health care system efficiency of ASEAN countries. *The International Journal of Health Planning and Management*, 36(4), 1236–1250.

Stoumpos, A. I., Kitsios, F., & Talias, M. A. (2023). Digital transformation in healthcare: Technology acceptance and its applications. *International Journal of Environmental Research and Public Health*, 20(4), 3407.

Taherdoost, H., & Madanchian, M. (2023). Multi-criteria decision making (MCDM) methods and concepts. *Encyclopedia*, 3(1), 77–87.

Tepe, S., Eti, S., Moda, H. M., Kahraman, Z. (2024). Evaluation of psychosocial risk factors encountered for energy sector employees by MAIRCA method. In: *Decision Making in Interdisciplinary Renewable Energy Projects: Navigating Energy Investments* (pp. 65–83). Springer, Cham. doi:10.1007/978-3-031-51532-3_6

Top, M., Konca, M., & Sapaz, B. (2020). Technical efficiency of healthcare systems in African countries: An application based on data envelopment analysis. *Health Policy and Technology*, 9(1), 62–68.

Torkayesh, A. E., Pamucar, D., Ecer, F., & Chatterjee, P. (2021). An integrated BWM-LBWA-CoCoSo framework for evaluation of healthcare sectors in Eastern Europe. *Socio-Economic Planning Sciences*, 78, 101052.

Tu, J., & Wu, Z. (2023). Analytic hierarchy process rank reversals: Causes and solutions. *Annals of Operations Research*, 346(2), 1785–1809.

Varabyova, Y., Blankart, C. R., Torbica, A., & Schreyögg, J. (2017). Comparing the efficiency of hospitals in Italy and Germany: Nonparametric conditional approach based on partial frontier. *Health Care Management Science*, 20, 379–394.

Willis-Shattuck, M., Bidwell, P., Thomas, S., Wyness, L., Blaauw, D., & Ditlopo, P. (2008). Motivation and retention of health workers in developing countries: A systematic review. *BMC Health Services Research*, 8, 1–8.

Yang, W., Xu, K., Lian, J., Ma, C., & Bin, L. (2018). Integrated flood vulnerability assessment approach based on TOPSIS and Shannon entropy methods. *Ecological Indicators*, 89, 269–280.

Younis, M., Ashraf, S., Abdullah, S., Shahid, T., & Kc, G. (2025). Strategic MARCOS model for optimizing renewable energy investments under Pythagorean hesitant fuzzy assessments. *Advances in Fuzzy Systems*, 2025(1), 6193403. doi:10.1155/adfs/6193403

Zavadskas, E. K., Turskis, Z., & Kildienė, S. (2014). State of art surveys of overviews on MCDM/MADM methods. *Technological and Economic Development of Economy*, 20(1), 165–179.

Žižović, M., & Albijanić, M. (2025). An implementation of the entropy method for determining weighing coefficients in a multicriteria optimization of public procurements. *Spectrum of Engineering and Management Sciences*, 3(1), 28–44.

Index

Note: **Bold** page numbers refer to tables and *italic* page numbers refer to figures.

I

J

K

L

M

N

U

V

W

X

For Product Safety Concerns and Information please contact our EU representative GPSR@taylorandfrancis.com
Taylor & Francis Verlag GmbH, Kaufingerstraße 24, 80331 München, Germany

www.ingramcontent.com/pod-product-compliance
Ingram Content Group UK Ltd.
Pitfield, Milton Keynes, MK11 3LW, UK
UKHW021513250926
475702UK00043B/279
9781032845593